Gynecological Cancers: Diagnosis and Therapeutics

Gynecological Cancers: Diagnosis and Therapeutics

Editor: Lester Price

AMERICAN
MEDICAL PUBLISHERS
www.americanmedicalpublishers.com

AMERICAN
MEDICAL PUBLISHERS
www.americanmedicalpublishers.com

Cataloging-in-Publication Data

Gynecological cancers : diagnosis and therapeutics / edited by Lester Price.
p. cm.
Includes bibliographical references and index.
ISBN 978-1-63927-678-3
1. Generative organs, Female--Cancer. 2. Generative organs, Female--Cancer--Diagnosis.
3. Generative organs, Female--Cancer--Treatment. 4. Gynecologic pathology. I. Price, Lester.
RC280.G5 G96 2023
616.994 65--dc23

American Medical Publishers,
41 Flatbush Avenue,
1st Floor, New York,
NY 11217, USA

ISBN 978-1-63927-678-3 (Hardback)

Contents

Preface

Gynecologic cancer or gynecological cancer is referred to as the cancer that begins in a woman's reproductive organs. There are five major types of cancer affecting a woman's reproductive organs, which include vaginal, ovarian, vulvar, cervical and uterine cancers. The common symptoms of gynecologic cancers are pelvic pain, abnormal vaginal bleeding, itching, burning, and sensitivity or soreness in the vulva. The tools and tests utilized to diagnose gynecologic cancer are determined by the type and location of the suspected cancer. The diagnosis also depends on other factors, such as the patient's medical history and overall health condition. Various types of diagnosis used in gynecologic cancer include transvaginal ultrasound, molecular tissue testing, endoscopy, tissue biopsies and body-fluid samples. They can be treated through a variety of methods, such as radiation therapy, surgery and chemotherapy. This book provides comprehensive insights on gynecological cancers. The readers would gain knowledge that would broaden their perspective on the diagnosis and therapeutics of these types of cancer.

This book is a result of research of several months to collate the most relevant data in the field.

When I was approached with the idea of this book and the proposal to edit it, I was overwhelmed. It gave me an opportunity to reach out to all those who share a common interest with me in this field. I had 3 main parameters for editing this text:

1. Accuracy - The data and information provided in this book should be up-to-date and valuable to the readers.

2. Structure - The data must be presented in a structured format for easy understanding and better grasping of the readers.

3. Universal Approach - This book not only targets students but also experts and innovators in the field, thus my aim was to present topics which are of use to all.

Thus, it took me a couple of months to finish the editing of this book.

I would like to make a special mention of my publisher who considered me worthy of this opportunity and also supported me throughout the editing process. I would also like to thank the editing team at the back-end who extended their help whenever required.

Editor

1

Early-Stage Ovarian Malignancy Score versus Risk of Malignancy Indices: Accuracy and Clinical Utility for Preoperative Diagnosis of Women with Adnexal Masses

Phichayut Phinyo [1], Jayanton Patumanond [2], Panprapha Saenrungmuaeng [3], Watcharin Chirdchim [4], Tanyong Pipanmekaporn [5], Apichat Tantraworasin [6], Theera Tongsong [7] and Charuwan Tantipalakorn [7,*]

1. Department of Family Medicine, Faculty of Medicine, Chiang Mai University, Chiang Mai 50200, Thailand; phichayutphinyo@gmail.com
2. Center for Clinical Epidemiology and Clinical Statistics, Faculty of Medicine, Chiang Mai University, Chiang Mai 50200, Thailand; jpatumanond@gmail.com
3. Department of Obstetrics and Gynecology, Faculty of Medicine, Mahasarakham University, Maha Sarakham 44150, Thailand; Pps2pearkabpom@gmail.com
4. Department of Obstetrics and Gynecology, Phrapokklao Hospital, Chanthaburi 22000, Thailand; watcharin.ch@cpird.in.th
5. Department of Anesthesiology, Faculty of Medicine, Chiang Mai University, Chiang Mai 50200, Thailand; tanyong24@gmail.com
6. Department of Surgery, Faculty of Medicine, Chiang Mai University, Chiang Mai 50200, Thailand; ohm_med@hotmail.com
7. Department of Obstetrics and Gynecology, Faculty of Medicine, Chiang Mai University, Chiang Mai 50200, Thailand; theera.t@cmu.ac.th

* Correspondence: nokctantipa@gmail.com

Abstract: *Background and objectives:* To compare the diagnostic accuracy and clinical utility of the Early-stage Ovarian Malignancy (EOM) score with the Risk of Malignancy Index (RMI) in the presurgical assessment of women presenting with adnexal masses. *Materials and Methods:* A secondary analysis was carried out in a retrospective cohort of women who presented with an adnexal mass and were scheduled for surgery at Phrapokklao Hospital between September 2013 and December 2017. The clinical characteristics, ultrasonographic features of the masses, and preoperative CA-125 levels were recorded. The EOM and the RMI score were calculated and compared in terms of accuracy and clinical utility. Decision curve analysis (DCA), which examined the net benefit (NB) of applying the EOM and the RMI in practice at a range of threshold probabilities, was presented. *Results:* In this study, data from 270 patients were analyzed. Fifty-four (20.0%) women in the sample had early-stage ovarian cancer. All four RMI versions demonstrated a lower sensitivity for the detection of patients with early-stage ovarian cancer compared to an EOM score $\geq$ 15. An EOM $\geq$ 15 resulted in a higher proportion of net true positive or NB than all versions of the RMIs from a threshold probability of 5% to 30%. *Conclusions:* It also showed a higher capability to reduce the number of inappropriate referrals than the RMIs at a threshold probability between 5% and 30%. The EOM score showed higher diagnostic sensitivity and has the potential to be clinically more useful than the RMIs to triage women who present with adnexal masses for referral to oncologic gynecologists. Further external validation is required to support our findings.

Keywords: ovarian cancer; adnexal mass; clinical utility; decision curve analysis; net benefit

1. Introduction

An accurate preoperative diagnosis of women who present with adnexal masses is essential for general gynecologists to arrive at the appropriate management decisions [1]. Generally, all women with ovarian tumors should be referred for subjective assessment by experienced sonographers, which is currently accepted as the most accurate and effective decision-making tool for women with ovarian tumors [2]. However, expert examiners are not widely available, especially in resource-limited settings. Thus, the clinical burden of a preoperative diagnosis of adnexal masses usually falls in the hand of general gynecologists. Women with a high probability of malignant ovarian tumors should then be referred to gynecologic oncologists for specialized oncological managements, as it is evident that this approach leads to a more favorable survival outcome for the patients [3,4]. In contrast, women with benign ovarian tumors should not be referred to avoid excessive stress for patients, creation of long waiting times, unnecessary healthcare costs, and, at the worst, overly radical surgical interventions [5]. Expectant and conservative surgical management by general gynecologists may be more appropriate in this domain of patients to reduce morbidity and preserve fertility [6].

Over the last three decades, several diagnostic algorithms and multimodal tests have been developed and recommended for use in practice to assist the differentiation of ovarian tumors. These include the International Ovarian Tumor Analysis (IOTA) systems (e.g., IOTA Simple Rules and IOTA logistic regression model (LR2)), the Risk of Ovarian Malignancy Algorithm (ROMA), and the Risk of Malignancy Index (RMI) [7,8]. Each diagnostic tool uses different predictive parameters for ovarian malignancy. The IOTA systems rely mainly on specific ultrasonographic features, whereas the ROMA focuses on serum biomarkers. The classic RMI combines multiple parameters, including menopausal status, simple ultrasonographic patterns, and serum CA-125, a widely recognized ovarian malignancy marker. A recent meta-analysis in 2014 concluded that the IOTA Simple Rules and the IOTA LR2 were the diagnostic rules with the highest accuracy level [9]. Even though the IOTA Simple Rules carried high diagnostic performance, up to about 10–20% of the examinations were inconclusive and required subsequent specialist consultations [10,11]. Due to this disadvantage of the IOTA Simple Rules, the RMI is still the most widely used and the most frequently validated decision tool for presurgical differentiation of ovarian pathology because of its simplicity and conclusive results [1,9].

The main disadvantage of the RMI is that it is heavily influenced by serum CA-125 levels, which is not a sensitive marker in the case of type I epithelial tumors (i.e., low grade serous, endometrioid, mucinous, and clear cell carcinoma) and early-stage ovarian cancer (i.e., stage I-IIA and IIIA1 according to the Fédération Internationale de Gynécologie et d'Obstétrique (FIGO) staging) [12–14]. Besides, high levels of serum CA-125 are not solely specific to ovarian cancer as it can be elevated in other benign conditions, for example, endometriosis [15]. In Thailand and some other Asian countries, there is a high prevalence of endometriosis and type I epithelial tumors; therefore, the application of RMI might not be appropriate and may lead to patient misclassification [16,17]. A validation study of all four RMI versions was done in Thailand in 2013 [18]. It was found that the diagnostic accuracy and discriminative ability of the RMI were not as high as previously claimed [19–22].

In 2019, the Early-stage Ovarian Malignancy (EOM) score was developed from a study in a cohort of women with benign ovarian tumors and early-stage ovarian cancer [23]. The EOM score was calculated based on the same parameters as the RMI. It demonstrated excellent discriminative ability with an area under the receiver operating characteristic curve of 0.88 and with good calibration. More evidence is needed to confirm the diagnostic ability and clinical usefulness of the EOM score as a proper triage tool for patient referral to specialized oncology care. This study aimed to evaluate the diagnostic accuracy and the clinical utility of the recently developed EOM score against all four versions of the RMI scoring in the presurgical assessment of women presenting with adnexal masses.

2. Materials and Methods

A secondary analysis was conducted using a retrospective cohort of women that presented with an adnexal mass at Phrapokklao Hospital from September 2013 to December 2017. Phrapokklao Hospital is a university-affiliated tertiary care hospital located in Chanthaburi Province located in the eastern seaboard of Thailand. The Research in Human Ethical Committee of Chanthaburi Province (CTIREC 046) and the Institutional Ethics Committee of the Faculty of Medicine, Chiang Mai University, approved the study protocol (Research ID: 7254 No. 179/2020). Informed consent was waived as data were collected retrospectively and anonymously. Patient data were kept confidential and in compliance with the Declaration of Helsinki.

The study included all women with an adnexal mass who presented consecutively at the hospital and were scheduled for surgery during the study period. Patients were eligible regardless of the type of ovarian operation. Key data collection comprised the preoperative clinical characteristics, the ultrasonographic features of the mass, and the tumor marker (CA-125), which were recorded during routine case management. The routine ultrasonographic assessment was generally performed by non-expert sonographers (including residents in training and general gynecologists). All ultrasonographic images were reevaluated and verified by a single gynecologic oncologist (WC). Ultrasound examination had been carried out by connecting a 3.5–5 MHz transabdominal or a 5–7.5 MHz transvaginal transducer to a sonoaceX7 (Samsung, South Korea). If multiple masses were present in a single patient, aspects of the mass with the most complex ultrasonographic features or the mass with the largest maximal diameter were collected.

The histopathologic reports of the resected masses were reviewed. Only patients with the diagnoses of benign ovarian tumors and early-stage ovarian cancer were included. In this study, early-stage ovarian cancer was defined as FIGO stage I, II, and IIIA1 (microscopic) [24,25]. Data from patients with advanced-stage ovarian cancer, recurrent ovarian cancer, metastatic cancer to the ovary, patients with a history of neoadjuvant chemotherapy, and patients with incomplete data were excluded. Patients with a pathological diagnosis of borderline ovarian tumors were included in the early-stage ovarian cancer group.

In this study, we planned to evaluate the diagnostic accuracy and the clinical utility of 5 diagnostic risk models for preoperative discrimination of benign and malignant adnexal tumors: EOM, RMI-I, RMI-II, RMI-III, and RMI-IV. Table 1 illustrates the components and score rating of each risk model.

The Early-stage Ovarian Malignancy score or the EOM score was recently developed from the dataset used in the primary data analysis prior to this study [23]. The EOM score is a combination of five simple predictors: menopausal status, tumor size, the presence of a solid component, the presence of ascites, and serum CA-125. Each component of the EOM score was rated with a different scoring regime, which was based on the logit coefficients of the prediction model. The total EOM score, ranging from 0 to 51, was derived from the summation of the score from each component. In the case of the EOM score, two cutoff points were proposed to categorize patients into low, moderate, and high-risk groups. The score cutoff point at ≥15 was intended to be used by general gynecologists to make a referral decision, whereas the score cutoff point at ≥30 was for oncologic specialists to prioritize patients for surgery or further investigation.

The Risk of Malignancy Index (RMI) is the classic diagnostic tool for preoperative diagnosis of ovarian cancer, which was developed in 1990 [19]. The RMI incorporates three main components, which are menopausal status, the ultrasound score, and the serum CA-125 level. The total score is the multiplicative product of all three components. The cutoff point for suggesting a high risk of a malignant tumor was originally set at an RMI ≥200 [26]. This cutoff point was generally used as the criteria for referring patients to a specialist. Currently, there are four versions of the RMI: RMI I [19], RMI II [20], RMI III [21], and RMI IV [22]. The differences in each version of the RMI give different score ratings for each component in RMI I to RMI III. In the fourth version of the RMI, tumor size is included in the score calculation, and a different cutoff point of >450 had been proposed.

All statistical analyses were performed using Stata version 16 (StataCorp, College Station, TX, USA). Frequency and percentage were used to describe the categorical data. The mean and standard deviation or median (interquartile range) were used to describe the continuous data, as appropriate. The comparison of categorical data was made using the exact probability test. The comparison of continuous data was made using an independent *t*-test or Mann–Whitney U test according to the data distribution. Two-tailed *p*-values < 0.05 were considered as statistically significant.

Table 1. Components of the Early-stage Ovarian Malignancy (EOM) score and Risk of Malignancy Index (RMI) I–IV.

Components	EOM	RMI †			
		I	II	III	IV
Menopausal Status					
Pre-menopause	0	1	1	1	1
Post-menopause	7	3	4	3	4
Ultrasonographic Features					
None	0	0	1	1	1
Any 1 feature		1	1	1	1
Presence of multilocularity					
Presence of solid component	3				
Bilateral lesions					
Presence of ascites	13				
Presence of intra-abdominal metastases					
≥2 Features		3	4	3	4
Tumor Size (cm)					
<7					1
≥7					2
<9	0				
9–12	10				
>12	16				
Serum CA125 (IU/L)					
<30	0				
30–200	1				
>200	12				

Abbreviations: EOM, Early-stage Ovarian Malignancy score; RMI, Risk of Malignancy Index. † For the calculation of the RMIs, the total score is the multiplicative product of the summation of the menopausal score, ultrasound score, tumor size score (for RMI IV), and serum CA-125.

Diagnostic accuracy indices, sensitivity, specificity, positive predictive values, negative predictive values, and positive likelihood ratios were calculated for each risk model. The 95% confidence intervals were estimated using the Clopper Pearson's binomial exact method. The comparison of sensitivity and specificity between the EOM score and each version of the RMI was carried out using an exact McNemar's test. The area under the receiver operating characteristic curve (AuROC) was used to represent the discriminative ability of the risk models. We compared the equality of the AuROC of each RMI model against the EOM score and used Sidak's adjustment for multiple comparisons.

To evaluate the clinical utility of the risk models, we employed the concept of decision curve analysis (DCA), which was introduced in 2006 by Vickers et al. [27]. DCA focuses on the net benefit (NB) gained from the application of risk models in practice. NB indicates the proportion of the net true positives, which remain after considering the presence of false positives. In a clinical context, the benefits of true positives and the harm of false positives are generally on different scales. Weighting factors must be used to convert false positives to the same scale as the true positives [28]. In this study, we focused on the appropriate referrals of patients to oncologic specialists. Thus, the weighting factor corresponds to the odds of the chosen threshold probability (T) to refer the patients to specialists (odds = T/1 − T). For instance, a threshold probability of 10% for patient referral implies that up to nine false positives are acceptable per one true positive (odds or benefit-to-harm ratio = 1/9). In summary, the NB is calculated as follows:

$$\text{Net Befit} = \frac{(\text{Number of True positives} - (\text{Number of False positives} \times (\text{T} \div (1 - \text{T}))}{(\text{Total sample size})}$$

where T is the threshold probability.

However, in actual practice, the choice of threshold probability varies largely depending on the discretion of each physician, as the reasonable threshold involves holistic incorporation of all potential disease outcomes. It is essential to evaluate the NB over a range of reasonable threshold probabilities within the clinical context of interest, as there is no single acceptable threshold probability [29]. In this study, we estimated the NB of all the risk models (at pre-specified cutoff points) from the risk threshold probability range of 5% to 50%, which was based on a report from a recent study on the clinical utility of the International Ovarian Tumor Analysis (IOTA) risk models [5]. We focused primarily on two important threshold probabilities, 10% and 25%, as these points were generally used as cutoff points for malignancy in the IOTA logistic regression model [30].

The decision curves were plotted to visualize the trend in NB for each model across the range of threshold probabilities. The NBs of two default strategies were also included in the graph for comparison: referring all patients or referring none. The NB of any risk model should be higher than the NB of the default strategies; otherwise, the model would be considered clinically harmful in its application. As the statistical significance and confidence intervals are not important in classical decision theory [31], we did not present the confidence intervals and p-values for the decision curve analysis.

We also presented an alternative expression of NB by calculating the net proportion of true negatives, which can be interpreted as the number of inappropriate referrals avoided per 100 patients. The equation used is as follows:

$$\text{Net proportion of True negatives} = \frac{\text{NB} - \text{NB}_{\text{ReferAll}}}{\text{Odds(T)}}$$

where NB is the net benefit; and T is the threshold probability.

3. Results

During the study period, there were 640 women with an adnexal mass scheduled for surgery and who were assessed for eligibility. Of this number, 370 women were excluded (Figure 1). Two hundred and seventy patients were therefore included in the analysis. The mean age of the patients was 44.5 ± 13.0 years. Only 25.6% of the patients ($n = 69$) were of postmenopausal age. One-third of the patients ($n = 90$, 33.3%) were nulliparous. Of the 270 patients included in the analysis, 216 (80.0%) were diagnosed with benign ovarian tumors, and 54 (20.0%) with early-stage ovarian cancer. In this dataset, there were eight patients with borderline ovarian tumors. All eight patients were included in the early-stage ovarian cancer group. The histopathological classification of all ovarian tumors included in the study is presented in Table 2. The comparison of the clinical characteristics, ultrasonographic features, and tumor marker levels between patients with ovarian cancer and patients with benign ovarian tumors are shown in Table 3.

The sensitivity of the EOM score at the cutoff point of ≥15 was significantly higher than all versions of the RMI ($p < 0.001$), while the specificity was significantly lower ($p < 0.001$ for RMI I, RMI III, and RMI IV, and $p = 0.002$ for RMI II). In contrast, the EOM score at the higher cutoff point of ≥30 showed a significantly higher specificity than that of all RMI versions ($p < 0.001$). However, at this EOM cutoff, the sensitivity was significantly lower than all RMI versions ($p < 0.001$). The other diagnostic indices (positive predictive values, negative predictive values, and positive likelihood ratios) are illustrated in Table 4. With regard to the discriminative ability via the AuROC, the EOM score was significantly more superior than RMI-I (0.88 vs. 0.73, $p < 0.001$), RMI-II (0.88 vs. 0.76, $p < 0.001$), RMI-III (0.88 vs. 0.75, $p < 0.001$), and RMI-IV (0.88 vs. 0.78, $p = 0.002$) (Figure 2).

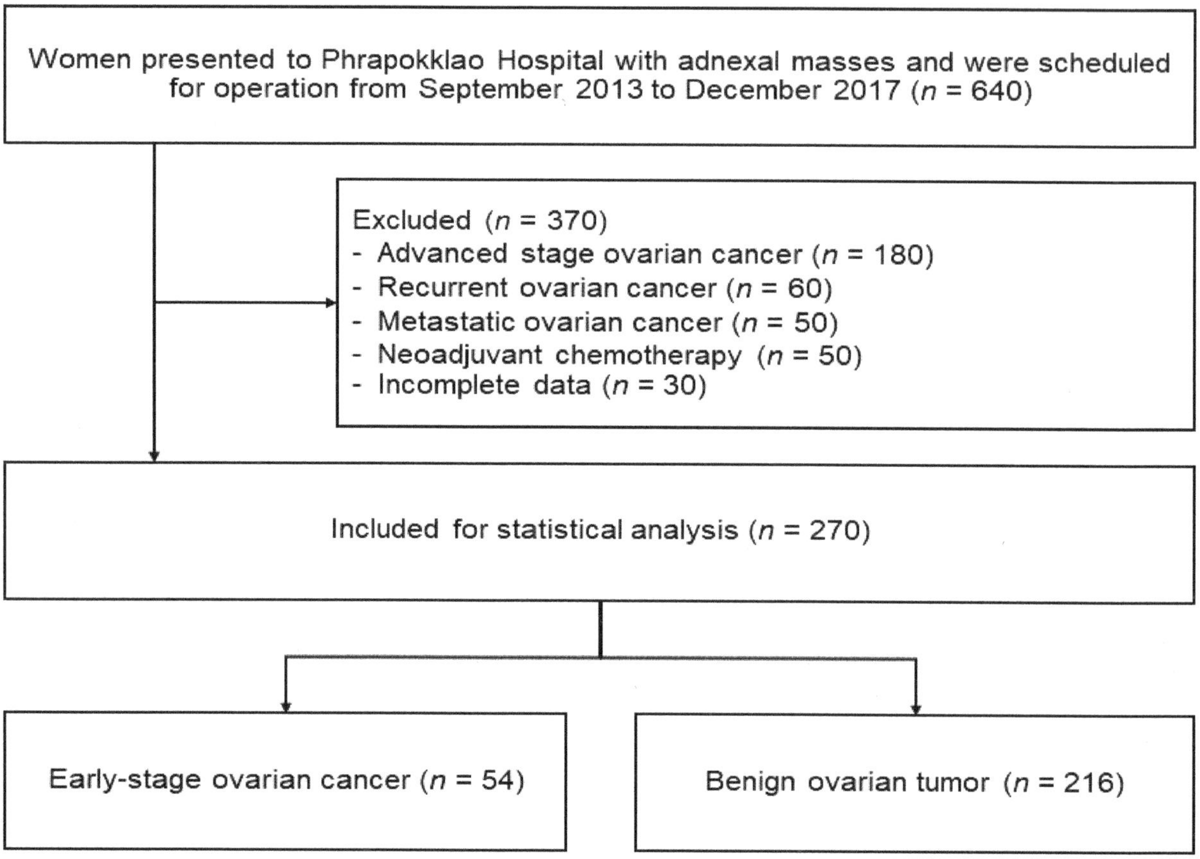

Figure 1. Study flow diagram.

Table 2. Histopathological classification of the ovarian tumors.

	n (%)
Malignant Tumors ($n = 46$)	
Endometrioid carcinoma	11 (20.4)
Serous carcinoma	10 (18.5)
Mucinous carcinoma	6 (11.1)
Adenocarcinoma	6 (11.1)
Clear cell carcinoma	5 (9.3)
Granulosa cell tumor	3 (5.6)
Other rare tumors	5 (9.3)
Borderline Tumors ($n = 8$)	
Borderline mucinous tumor	7 (12.9)
Borderline serous tumor	1 (1.8)
Borderline endometrioid tumor	0 (0)
Benign Tumors ($n = 216$)	
Endometriotic cyst	77 (35.7)
Dermoid cyst	45 (20.8)
Mucinous cystadenoma	41 (19.0)
Serous cystadenoma	26 (12.0)
Follicular cyst	11 (5.1)
Corpus luteal cyst	10 (4.6)
Others rare tumors	6 (2.8)

Regarding clinical utility, the EOM score at the cutoff point of ≥15 demonstrated a higher proportion of net true positive or NB than all versions of the RMIs at the pre-specified cutoffs from the threshold probabilities of 5% to 30% (Table 5). At the threshold probabilities of 10% and 25%, a NB of 0.158 and 0.098 by the EOM score means that there are 15.8 and 9.8 net-detected early-stage ovarian cancers per 100 patients without inappropriate referrals, respectively. At the threshold probability beyond 30%, the NB of the EOM score decreased. Using all versions of the RMI for guiding referral of patients with adnexal masses was clinically harmful at a threshold probability lower than 10%, as an approach of referral of all patients to oncologic specialists shows a higher NB. If the threshold probability for referral was between 10% and 15%, the RMIs were not considered harmful, as the NB of all the RMIs were higher than both the default strategies (refer all and refer none). However, at this risk threshold, the NB of the EOM score was higher than that of the RMIs (Figure 3a).

Table 3. Characteristics of the study patients.

Variables	Early Stage Ovarian Cancer (n = 54)		Benign Ovarian Tumor (n = 216)		p-Value
	n	(%)	n	(%)	
Clinical Characteristics					
Age (year) *	48.7	±15.4	43.5	±12.1	0.008
Nulliparity	21	(38.9)	69	(31.9)	0.337
Post-menopause	28	(51.9)	41	(19.0)	<0.001
Ultrasonographic Features					
Maximum tumor diameter (cm) *	16.4	±6.7	10.1	±5.1	<0.001
Multilocularity	38	(70.4)	145	(67.1)	0.745
Solid component	33	(61.1)	57	(26.4)	<0.001
Bilateral lesions	5	(9.3)	43	(19.9)	0.075
Ascites	11	(20.4)	2	(0.9)	<0.001
Intra-abdominal metastases	2	(3.7)	1	(0.5)	0.103
Tumor Marker					
Serum CA125 (IU/L) **	102.8	25.0, 314.0	30.8	14.8, 81.1	<0.001

Abbreviations: SD, standard deviation; IQR, interquartile range. * Mean ± SD, ** Median (IQR).

Table 4. Comparative diagnostic performance of the Early-stage Ovarian Malignancy (EOM) score and Risk of Malignancy Indices (RMI).

Scores	Cutoff	Early Stage Ovarian Cancer (n = 54)		Benign Ovarian Tumor (n = 216)		Sensitivity (%) (95% CI)	Specificity (%) (95% CI)	PPV (%) (95% CI)	NPV (%) (95% CI)	LR+ (95% CI)
		n	(row%)	n	(row%)					
EOM	≥15	51	(40.8)	74	(59.2)	94.4	65.7	40.8	97.9	2.76
	<15	3	(2.1)	142	(97.9)	(84.6–98.8)	(59.0–72.0)	(32.1–49.9)	(94.1–99.6)	(1.68–4.50)
	≥30	21	(95.5)	1	(4.6)	38.9	99.5	95.5	86.7	84.0
	<30	33	(13.3)	215	(86.7)	(25.9–53.1)	(97.4–100.0)	(77.2–99.9)	(81.8–90.7)	(12.73, 3488.41)
RMI I	≥200	31	(47.0)	35	(53.0)	57.4	83.8	47.0	88.7	3.54
	<200	23	(11.3)	181	(88.7)	(43.2–70.8)	(78.2–88.4)	(34.6–59.7)	(83.6–92.7)	(1.92–6.49)
RMI II	≥200	36	(44.4)	45	(55.6)	66.7	79.2	44.4	90.5	3.20
	<200	18	(9.5)	171	(90.5)	(52.5–78.9)	(73.1–84.4)	(33.4–55.9)	(85.4–94.3)	(1.81–5.61)
RMI III	≥200	34	(47.2)	38	(52.8)	63.0	82.4	47.2	89.9	3.58
	<200	20	(10.1)	178	(89.9)	(48.7–75.7)	(76.7–87.2)	(35.3–59.3)	(84.8–93.7)	(1.98–6.43)
RMI IV	≥450	33	(50.0)	33	(50.0)	61.1	84.7	50.0	89.7	4.00
	<450	21	(10.3)	183	(89.7)	(46.9–74.1)	(79.2–89.2)	(37.4–62.6)	(84.7–93.5)	(2.17–7.32)

Abbreviations: PPV, positive predictive value; NPV, negative predictive value; LR+, positive likelihood ratios; CI, confidence interval; EOM score, Early-stage Ovarian Malignancy score; RMI, Risk of Malignancy Index.

The EOM score also showed a higher capability to reduce inappropriate referrals than the RMIs from the threshold probabilities of 5% to 30% (Table 5) (Figure 3b). In comparison to an approach of referring all patients to oncologists, using the EOM score could reduce the number of inappropriate referrals by up to 43 per 100 patients at the risk threshold of 10% and 48 per 100 patients at the threshold probability of 20%. In contrast, at the threshold probability of 10%, only the RMI-II at the cutoff of 200 could reduce the number of inappropriate referrals by about 3 per 100 patients, whereas the other RMIs increased the number of inappropriate referrals. At a risk threshold of 25%, the EOM score reduced inappropriate referrals by between 5 and 8 (per 100 patients) more than when the RMI was used.

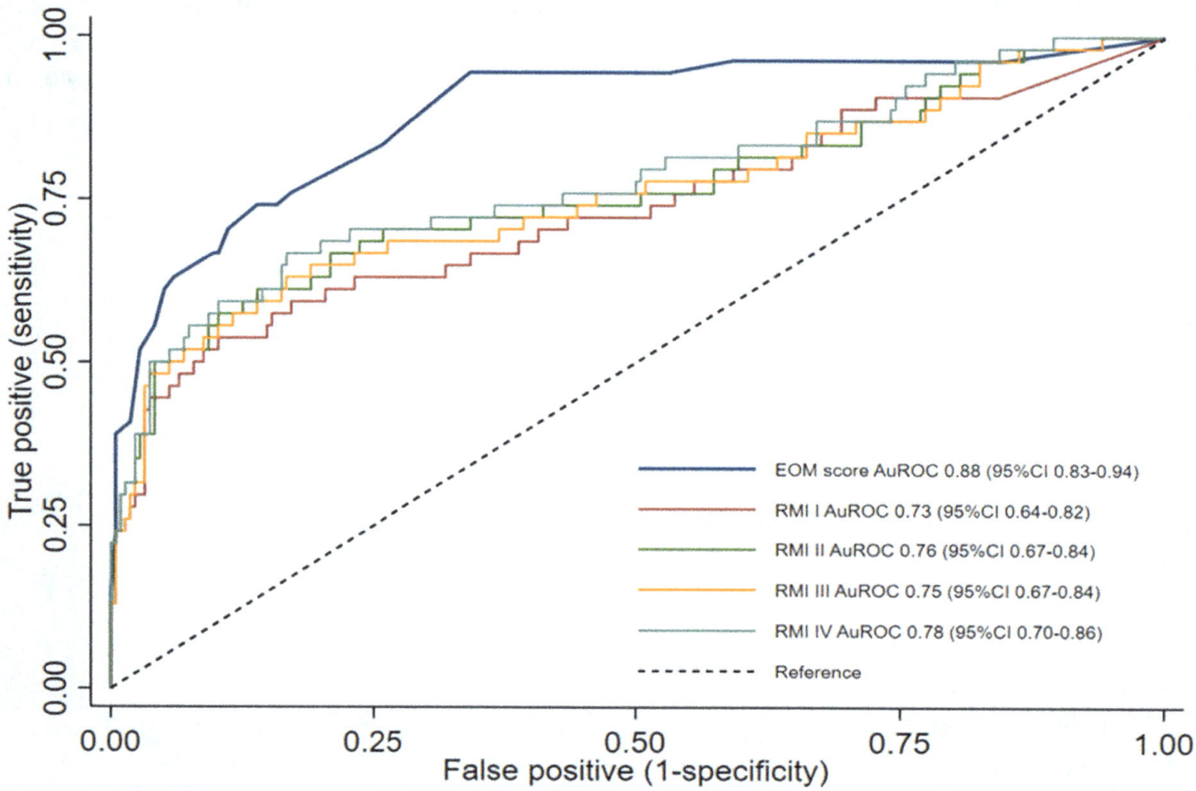

Figure 2. Comparative validation of the discriminative ability between the EOM scores and the RMIs via the receiver operating characteristic curve. Abbreviations: AuROC, area under the receiver operating characteristic curve; EOM, Early-stage Ovarian Malignancy; RMI, Risk of Malignancy Indices.

Table 5. Decision curve analysis.

Threshold Probability	Net Benefit (Proportion of Net True Positive)						Reduced Numbers of Inappropriate Referrals per 100 Patients				
	Refer all	EOM	RMI I	RMI II	RMI III	RMI IV	EOM	RMI I	RMI II	RMI III	RMI IV
5%	0.157	0.174	0.108	0.125	0.119	0.116	31.482	−94.815	−63.333	−74.815	−80.000
10%	0.111	0.158	0.100	0.115	0.110	0.109	42.593	−9.630	3.333	−0.741	−2.222
15%	0.059	0.141	0.092	0.104	0.101	0.101	46.296	18.765	25.556	23.951	23.704
20%	0	0.120	0.082	0.092	0.091	0.092	48.148	32.963	36.667	36.296	36.667
25%	−0.067	0.098	0.072	0.078	0.079	0.081	49.259	41.481	43.333	43.704	44.445
30%	−0.143	0.071	0.059	0.062	0.066	0.070	50.000	47.160	47.778	48.642	49.630
35%	−0.231	0.041	0.045	0.044	0.050	0.056	50.529	51.217	50.952	52.169	53.333
40%	−0.333	0.006	0.028	0.022	0.032	0.041	50.926	54.259	53.333	54.815	56.111
45%	−0.455	−0.035	0.009	−0.003	0.011	0.022	51.235	56.626	55.185	56.872	58.272
50%	−0.600	−0.085	−0.015	−0.033	−0.015	0	51.481	58.519	56.667	58.519	60.000

Abbreviations: EOM, Early-stage Ovarian Malignancy score; RMI, Risk of Malignancy Index.

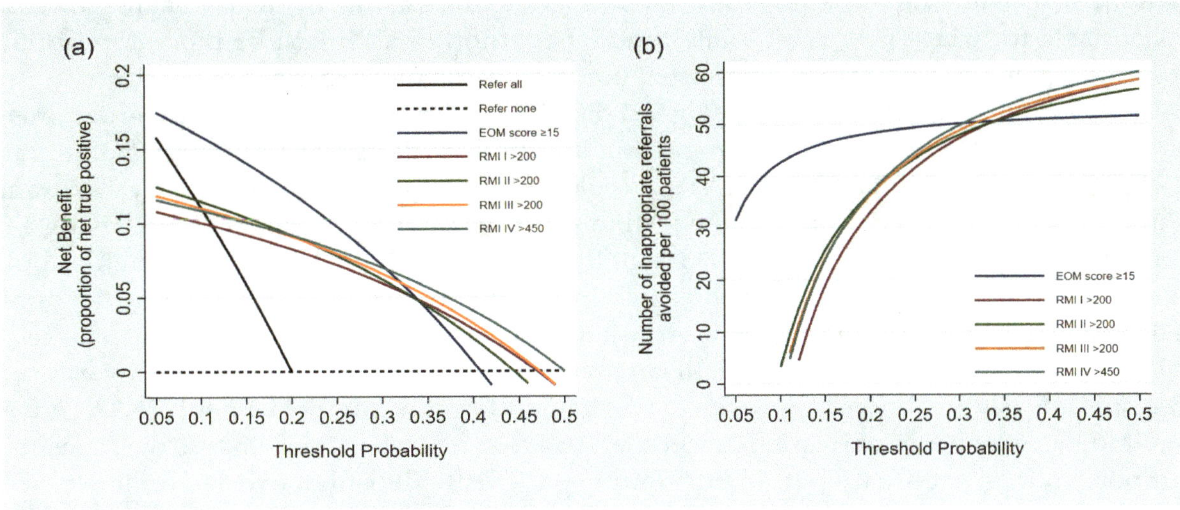

Figure 3. Comparative validation of the clinical utility between the EOM scores and Risk of Malignancy Indices via decision curves. (**a**) Decision curve plotting the net benefit against threshold probability. (**b**) Decision curve plotting a decrease in inappropriate referrals against threshold probability.

4. Discussion

In this study, all four RMI versions at their pre-specified cutoff points demonstrated a lower sensitivity for detecting patients with early-stage ovarian cancer when compared to the EOM score ≥15. Although the specificity of the EOM score at this cutoff was significantly lower than the RMI, its negative predictive value was the highest and may be more effective as a triage tool for patient referrals. An EOM score ≥15 also demonstrated clinical utility over a wide range of threshold probabilities, from as low as 5% up to 30%. The RMI had less clinical utility and was considered harmful at a low threshold probability but was beneficial at a higher threshold probability (>30%). Our findings suggest that, in some specific situations, the EOM score at the cutoff point of ≥15 should be used instead of the RMI to increase the detection of ovarian cancer cases while minimizing the number of inappropriate patient referrals.

In a recent meta-analysis, the pooled estimates of the sensitivity and specificity of the RMI I were 72.0% (95% CI: 67.0, 76.0%) and 92.0% (95% CI: 89.0, 93.0%), respectively [9]. The pooled sensitivity and specificity of the other RMI versions were comparable to the first version. The original publication of the RMI in 1990 reported the sensitivity and specificity of the RMI as 85.4% and 95.9% [19], respectively, which was significantly higher than the number reported in the meta-analysis and also from our findings. Out of all patients with malignant diseases included in the original study, around two-thirds (28/42, 66.7%) of the patients were at advanced stages of ovarian cancer or metastatic disease. As the RMI scoring is largely dependent on the serum CA-125 levels, a biomarker that is more specific to an advanced stage or type II ovarian cancer [14], the diagnostic performance of the RMI is undoubtedly disturbed in studies that include a lower proportion of these patients [18,32–35]. Our study only included patients with early-stage ovarian cancer, which probably explains the lower sensitivity of all the RMIs.

The EOM score at the cutoff point of ≥15 outperformed all four RMI versions in terms of diagnostic sensitivity in the detection of patients with early-stage ovarian cancer. The ability to discriminate between benign and early malignant conditions of the EOM score was also significantly higher than in all the RMIs. The derivation of the EOM score from a cohort of patients with benign ovarian tumors and early-stage ovarian cancer improves the ability to distinguish both conditions. Moreover, the EOM scoring system appropriately adjusts the influence of the serum CA-125 level into the model by categorizing this classic marker into three categories, assigning a weighted score to each. In our prior work, we proposed two cutoff points, at ≥15 and ≥30, for the implementation of the EOM score in practice [23]. The finding from this study adds weight to the existing evidence that the lower cutoff (≥15) is suitable for triage purposes, while the higher cutoff (≥30) might be more appropriate for diagnosis and giving guidance for the prioritization of patients for surgery.

Even though the EOM score exhibited good discrimination and calibration properties, this does not justify and establish its usefulness in making appropriate decisions for the referral of patients with a high probability of ovarian cancer to gynecologic oncologists [28]. In this study, we examined the clinical utility of the EOM score and the RMI in supporting decision-making by applying a novel decision-analytic approach, or DCA [27]. One of the most troublesome challenges to this approach lies within the definition of a reasonable threshold probability of patient referral [36], as the threshold generally depends on multiple factors, such as the judgement of the physician, patient preferences, local referral guidelines, and availability of healthcare resources [5]. As early detection of ovarian cancer would result in early treatment, appropriate staging, and survival improvements [6,37], it is more important to detect one case of ovarian cancer than to avoid referrals to oncologists (i.e., sensitivity is more important than specificity [1]). In our setting, patients with benign ovarian tumors who were misclassified and referred to specialists, or false-positive cases, usually undergo further non-invasive investigation before being scheduled for invasive surgery. In contrast, patients with ovarian cancer who otherwise would not be referred, or false-negative cases, might be subject to more unfavorable outcomes in this context, such as inadequate staging of the cancer [38,39] or suboptimal surgical management [40].

The NB of the EOM score at the cutoff point of ≥15 was higher than the approach of referring all patients, not referring any patients, and all the RMI versions from a threshold probability of 5% up to 30%. The application of the EOM score would also result in a lower number of inappropriate referrals. This was due to the higher sensitivity of the EOM score compared to the RMI. At a lower threshold probability, the detection of one ovarian cancer case weighs substantially more than one inappropriate referral. Thus, when false-positive cases are acceptable, a diagnostic rule with higher sensitivity would gain a higher NB. However, when false-positive cases are unacceptable, a prediction model with high specificity is warranted. In practice, a decision to refer patients only when the threshold probability was higher than 50% was not sufficiently reasonable, as it implies that referring false-positive cases is more harmful than not referring any patients [5]. We focused on the clinical utility of the EOM score and the RMI at two clinically relevant thresholds, 10% and 25%. We concluded that the EOM score ≥15 was clinically more useful in informing general gynecologists regarding the preoperative assessment of patients with adnexal masses than the RMI. The RMI would be useful only when the threshold probability was higher than 30%.

There were some limitations to be addressed. First, this study was a secondary analysis of a retrospective cohort study used to develop the EOM score. Thus, the accuracy and clinical utility of the EOM score might be overestimated. Further external validation studies on both aspects should be performed and are currently in process to support the findings in this study. Second, only patients with adnexal masses who were scheduled for surgery were included in this study. Patients with benign conditions who were conservatively managed were excluded, which might account for a large number of patients. However, this enables us to base all the diagnoses on the more reliable reference standard, histopathologic examinations. Third, the routine ultrasonographic evaluations were performed by non-expert sonographers, which limits the generalizability of our results to the setting where ultrasound examination was performed by an experienced sonographer. Nonetheless, by using data from a routine examination, our results could be considered as pragmatic regarding the accuracy and utility of both models. Fourth, only early-stage ovarian cancer cases were included. At this point, the transferability of our results could not be extended to patients with advanced-stage cancer or metastatic diseases. Fifth, our study included patients with FIGO stage IIIA as early-stage ovarian cancer following a previous study [25], which might not be conventional and could overestimate the discriminative ability of both the EOM score and the RMIs. However, as the overestimation occurs equally in both groups, differential bias during a comparative validation is unlikely. Finally, we did not examine the effect modification of menopausal status on the diagnostic accuracy and clinical utility as our study size in terms of menopausal women was limited and might not provide adequate statistical power. Therefore, subgroup effects might be present and should not be overlooked until further evidence is available.

5. Conclusions

In conclusion, the EOM score provides high diagnostic sensitivity, making it more suitable to use as a triage tool for referring women with an adnexal mass to specialized oncologic care than all versions of the RMI. It also demonstrates potential clinical utility by increasing the net detection of early-stage ovarian cancer cases without raising the number of inappropriate referrals. The results are promising but an external validation study would be required to confirm the diagnostic performance and clinical utility of the EOM score before being endorsed for clinical use.

Author Contributions: Conceptualization, P.P., J.P. and C.T.; methodology, P.P. and J.P.; software, P.P. and A.T.; validation, J.P., P.S., W.C., T.P., A.T., T.T., and C.T.; formal analysis, P.P.; investigation, P.P.; resources, P.S., W.C., T.T., and C.T.; data curation, P.S. and W.C.; writing—original draft preparation, P.P.; writing—review and editing, J.P., P.S., W.C., T.P., A.T., T.T., and C.T.; visualization, P.P.; supervision, J.P. and C.T.; project administration, W.C. and C.T. All authors have read and agreed to the published version of the manuscript.

References

1. Kaijser, J.; Bourne, T.; Valentin, L.; Sayasneh, A.; Van Holsbeke, C.; Vergote, I.; Testa, A.C.; Franchi, D.; Van Calster, B.; Timmerman, D. Improving strategies for diagnosing ovarian cancer: A summary of the International Ovarian Tumor Analysis (IOTA) studies. *Ultrasound Obs. Gynecol.* **2013**, *41*, 9–20. [CrossRef]
2. Valentin, L.; Hagen, B.; Tingulstad, S.; Eik-Nes, S. Comparison of 'pattern recognition' and logistic regression models for discrimination between benign and malignant pelvic masses: A prospective cross validation. *Ultrasound Obs. Gynecol.* **2001**, *18*, 357–365. [CrossRef] [PubMed]
3. Vernooij, F.; Heintz, P.; Witteveen, E.; Van Der Graaf, Y. The outcomes of ovarian cancer treatment are better when provided by gynecologic oncologists and in specialized hospitals: A systematic review. *Gynecol. Oncol.* **2007**, *105*, 801–812. [CrossRef] [PubMed]
4. Elattar, A.; Bryant, A.; Winter-Roach, B.A.; Hatem, M.; Naik, R. Optimal primary surgical treatment for advanced epithelial ovarian cancer. *Cochrane Database Syst. Rev.* **2011**, *2011*, 12. [CrossRef] [PubMed]
5. Wynants, L.; Timmerman, D.; Verbakel, J.Y.; Testa, A.; Savelli, L.; Fischerova, D.; Franchi, D.; Van Holsbeke, C.; Epstein, E.; Froyman, W.; et al. Clinical Utility of Risk Models to Refer Patients with Adnexal Masses to Specialized Oncology Care: Multicenter External Validation Using Decision Curve Analysis. *Clin. Cancer Res.* **2017**, *23*, 5082–5090. [CrossRef] [PubMed]
6. Woo, Y.L.; Kyrgiou, M.; Bryant, A.; Everett, T.; Dickinson, H.O. Centralisation of services for gynaecological cancer. *Cochrane Database Syst. Rev.* **2012**, *2012*, 5. [CrossRef]
7. American College of Obstetricians and Gynecologists. Practice Bulletin No. 174: Evaluation and Management of Adnexal Masses. *Obstet Gynecol.* **2016**, *128*, e210. [CrossRef]
8. National Collaborating Centre for Cancer (UK). *Ovarian Cancer The Recognition and Initial Management of Ovarian Cancer; National Institute for Health and Clinical Excellence: Guidance; National Collaborating Centre for Cancer (UK)*; National Collaborating Centre for Cancer (UK): Cardiff, UK, 2011; ISBN 978-0-9558265-5-9.
9. Kaijser, J.; Sayasneh, A.; Van Hoorde, K.; Ghaem-Maghami, S.; Bourne, T.; Timmerman, D.; Van Calster, B. Presurgical diagnosis of adnexal tumours using mathematical models and scoring systems: A systematic review and meta-analysis. *Hum. Reprod. Updat.* **2014**, *20*, 449–462. [CrossRef]
10. Auekitrungrueng, R.; Tinnangwattana, D.; Tantipalakorn, C.; Charoenratana, C.; Lerthiranwong, T.; Wanapirak, C.; Tongsong, T. Comparison of the diagnostic accuracy of International Ovarian Tumor Analysis simple rules and the risk of malignancy index to discriminate between benign and malignant adnexal masses. *Int. J. Gynecol. Obs.* **2019**, *146*, 364–369. [CrossRef]
11. Shetty, J.; Saradha, A.; Pandey, D.; Bhat, R.; Kumar, P.; Bharatnur, S. IOTA Simple Ultrasound Rules for Triage of Adnexal Mass: Experience from South India. *J. Obs. Gynecol. India* **2019**, *69*, 356–362. [CrossRef]

12. Hellström, I.; Raycraft, J.; Hayden-Ledbetter, M.; Ledbetter, J.A.; Schummer, M.; McIntosh, M.; Drescher, C.; Urban, N.; Hellström, K.E. The HE4 (WFDC2) protein is a biomarker for ovarian carcinoma. *Cancer Res.* **2003**, *63*, 3695–3700. [PubMed]
13. Moss, E.L.; Hollingworth, J.; Reynolds, T.M. The role of CA125 in clinical practice. *J. Clin. Pathol.* **2005**, *58*, 308–312. [CrossRef] [PubMed]
14. Chen, X.; Zhang, J.; Cheng, W.; Chang, D.Y.; Huang, J.; Wang, X.; Jia, L.; Rosen, D.G.; Zhang, W.; Yang, D.; et al. CA-125 Level as a Prognostic Indicator in Type I and Type II Epithelial Ovarian Cancer. *Int. J. Gynecol. Cancer* **2013**, *23*, 815–822. [CrossRef]
15. Buamah, P. Benign conditions associated with raised serum CA-125 concentration. *J. Surg. Oncol.* **2000**, *75*, 264–265. [CrossRef]
16. Matz, M.; Coleman, M.P.; Carreira, H.; Salmerón, D.; Chirlaque, M.D.; Allemani, C. CONCORD Working Group Worldwide comparison of ovarian cancer survival: Histological group and stage at diagnosis (CONCORD-2). *Gynecol. Oncol.* **2017**, *144*, 396–404. [CrossRef]
17. Cramer, D.W. The epidemiology of endometriosis. *Ann. N. Y. Acad. Sci.* **2002**, *955*, 11–22. [CrossRef] [PubMed]
18. Insin, P.; Prueksaritanond, N. Evaluation of Four Risk of Malignancy Indices (RMI) in the Preoperative Diagnosis of Ovarian Malignancy at Rajavithi Hospital. *Thai J. Obstet. Gynaecol.* **2013**, *201*, 163–175.
19. Jacobs, I.; Oram, D.; Fairbanks, J.; Turner, J.; Frost, C.; Grudzinskas, J.G. A risk of malignancy index incorporating CA 125, ultrasound and menopausal status for the accurate preoperative diagnosis of ovarian cancer. *BJOG* **1990**, *97*, 922–929. [CrossRef]
20. Tingulstad, S.; Hagen, B.; Skjeldestad, F.E.; Onsrud, M.; Kiserud, T.; Halvorsen, T.; Nustad, K. Evaluation of a risk of malignancy index based on serum CA125, ultrasound findings and menopausal status in the pre-operative diagnosis of pelvic masses. *BJOG* **1996**, *103*, 826–831. [CrossRef]
21. Tingulstad, S.; Hagen, B.; Skjeldestad, F.E.; Halvorsen, T.; Nustad, K.; Onsrud, M. The Risk-of-Malignancy Index to Evaluate Potential Ovarian Cancers in Local Hospitals. *Obs. Gynecol.* **1999**, *93*, 448–452. [CrossRef]
22. Yamamoto, Y.; Yamada, R.; Oguri, H.; Maeda, N.; Fukaya, T. Comparison of four malignancy risk indices in the preoperative evaluation of patients with pelvic masses. *Eur. J. Obs. Gynecol. Reprod. Biol.* **2009**, *144*, 163–167. [CrossRef] [PubMed]
23. Chirdchim, W.; Wanichsetakul, P.; Phinyo, P.; Patumanond, J.; Suwannarurk, K.; Srisomboon, J. Development and Validation of a Predictive Score for Preoperative Diagnosis of Early Stage Epithelial Ovarian Cancer. *Asian Pac. J. Cancer Prev.* **2019**, *20*, 1207–1213. [CrossRef]
24. Javadi, S.; Ganeshan, D.M.; Qayyum, A.; Iyer, R.B.; Bhosale, P.R. Ovarian Cancer, the Revised FIGO Staging System, and the Role of Imaging. *Am. J. Roentgenol.* **2016**, *206*, 1351–1360. [CrossRef] [PubMed]
25. Kleppe, M.; Van Der Aa, M.A.; Van Gorp, T.; Slangen, B.F.M.; Kruitwagen, R.F.P.M. The impact of lymph node dissection and adjuvant chemotherapy on survival: A nationwide cohort study of patients with clinical early-stage ovarian cancer. *Eur. J. Cancer* **2016**, *66*, 83–90. [CrossRef] [PubMed]
26. Håkansson, F.; Høgdall, E.V.S.; Nedergaard, L.; Lundvall, L.; Engelholm, S.A.; Pedersen, A.T.; Hartwell, D.; Høgdall, C. Danish 'Pelvic Mass' Ovarian Cancer Study Risk of malignancy index used as a diagnostic tool in a tertiary centre for patients with a pelvic mass. *Acta Obstet. Gynecol. Scand.* **2012**, *91*, 496–502.
27. Vickers, A.; Elkin, E.B. Decision Curve Analysis: A Novel Method for Evaluating Prediction Models. *Med. Decis. Mak.* **2006**, *26*, 565–574. [CrossRef]
28. Van Calster, B.; Wynants, L.; Verbeek, J.F.; Verbakel, J.Y.; Christodoulou, E.; Vickers, A.; Roobol, M.J.; Steyerberg, E.W. Reporting and Interpreting Decision Curve Analysis: A Guide for Investigators. *Eur. Urol.* **2018**, *74*, 796–804. [CrossRef]
29. Vickers, A.; Van Calster, B.; Steyerberg, E.W. Net benefit approaches to the evaluation of prediction models, molecular markers, and diagnostic tests. *BMJ* **2016**, *352*, i6. [CrossRef]
30. Testa, A.; Kaijser, J.; Wynants, L.; Fischerova, D.; Van Holsbeke, C.; Franchi, D.; Savelli, L.; Epstein, E.; Czekierdowski, A.; Guerriero, S.; et al. Strategies to diagnose ovarian cancer: New evidence from phase 3 of the multicentre international IOTA study. *Br. J. Cancer* **2014**, *111*, 680–688. [CrossRef]
31. Vickers, A.; Van Calster, B.; Steyerberg, E.W. A simple, step-by-step guide to interpreting decision curve analysis. *Diagn. Progn. Res.* **2019**, *3*, 8. [CrossRef]
32. Abdulrahman, J.G.O.; McKnight, L.; Singh, K.L. The risk of malignancy index (RMI) in women with adnexal masses in Wales. *Taiwan J. Obs. Gynecol.* **2014**, *53*, 376–381. [CrossRef] [PubMed]

33. Morgante, G.; La Marca, A.; Ditto, A.; De Leo, V. Comparison of two malignancy risk indices based on serum CA125, ultrasound score and menopausal status in the diagnosis of ovarian masses. *BJOG* **1999**, *106*, 524–527. [CrossRef] [PubMed]
34. Moolthiya, W.; Yuenyao, P. The risk of malignancy index (RMI) in diagnosis of ovarian malignancy. *APJCP* **2009**, *10*, 865–868. [PubMed]
35. Van Holsbeke, C.; Van Calster, B.; Bourne, T.; Ajossa, S.; Testa, A.C.; Guerriero, S.; Fruscio, R.; Lissoni, A.; Czekierdowski, A.; Savelli, L.; et al. External Validation of Diagnostic Models to Estimate the Risk of Malignancy in Adnexal Masses. *Clin. Cancer Res.* **2011**, *18*, 815–825. [CrossRef]
36. Fitzgerald, M.; Saville, B.R.; Lewis, R.J. Decision Curve Analysis. *JAMA* **2015**, *313*, 409–410. [CrossRef]
37. Froyman, W.; Wynants, L.; Landolfo, C.; Bourne, T.; Valentin, L.; Testa, A.C.; Sladkevicius, P.; Franchi, D.; Fischerova, D.; Savelli, L.; et al. Validation of the Performance of International Ovarian Tumor Analysis (IOTA) Methods in the Diagnosis of Early Stage Ovarian Cancer in a Non-Screening Population. *Diagnostics* **2017**, *7*, 32. [CrossRef]
38. Timmers, P.J.; Zwinderman, A.; Coens, C.; Vergote, I.; Trimbos, J. Understanding the problem of inadequately staging early ovarian cancer. *Eur. J. Cancer* **2010**, *46*, 880–884. [CrossRef]
39. Trimbos, J.B. Surgical treatment of early-stage ovarian cancer. *Best Pract. Res. Clin. Obs. Gynaecol.* **2017**, *41*, 60–70. [CrossRef]
40. Bristow, R.E.; Karlan, B.Y.; Chi, D.S. *Surgery for Ovarian Cancer: Principles and Practice*; CRC Press: Boca Raton, FL, USA, 2010.

2

Obesity Epidemic—The Underestimated Risk of Endometrial Cancer

Ludwig Kiesel [1,*], Christine Eichbaum [2], Ariane Baumeier [1] and Michael Eichbaum [3,*]

1 Department of Gynecology and Obstetrics, University of Münster Medical School, Albert-Schweitzer-Campus 1, 48149 Münster, Germany; a_baum19@uni-muenster.de
2 Department of Gynecology and Obstetrics, University of Frankfurt Medical School, Theodor-Stern-Kai 7, 60596 Frankfurt, Germany; Christine.Eichbaum@kgu.de
3 Department of Gynecology and Obstetrics, Helios Dr. Horst-Schmidt-Kliniken Wiesbaden, Ludwig-Erhard-Str. 100, 65199 Wiesbaden, Germany
* Correspondence: L.Kiesel@uni-muenster.de (L.K.); michael.eichbaum@helios-gesundheit.de (M.E.);

Simple Summary: Endometrial cancer is the most frequent gynecologic tumor in developed countries. Obesity is an established risk factor for this disease. This work provides an overview of pathophysiological interactions and pathways in obese women initiating tumorigenesis. Furthermore, the clinical impact of adiposity on the treatment of endometrial cancer is discussed as well therapeutic and preventive options.

Abstract: Endometrial cancer (EC) is the most frequently observed malignant gynecologic disease in developed countries. There is a strong association between the established risk factor obesity and the incidence of EC. Furthermore, the rate of women with a body mass index (BMI) > 30 kg/m^2 is increasing worldwide, correspondingly leading to a higher prevalence of EC. Understanding the adipose tissue as an endocrine organ, elementary pathophysiological pathways of tumorigenesis have been revealed. This includes the fundamental role of hyperglycemia, insulin resistance, and hyperestrogenemia, as well as interactions with a chronic proinflammatory microenvironment. Therapeutic options potentially include metformin or bariatric surgery. Moreover, changes in individual lifestyle such as weight reduction, physical activity, and an awareness of healthy nutrition are effective in preventing the disease.

Keywords: endometrial cancer; obesity; body mass index; hyperglycemia; proinflammatory microenvironment; metformin; surgery

---

1. Introduction

Increasing body mass index (BMI) is a phenomenon being seen not only in the classical Western world but also in developing countries [1,2]. Indeed, one-third of American women are obese, defined by a BMI > 30 kg/m^2, with about 7% presenting with severe or morbid obesity (BMI > 40 kg/m^2) [3]. There is a strong, well-established association between obesity and the development of endometrial cancer (EC) [4,5]. A meta-analysis of the American Institute for Cancer Research recently found that for every increase of five BMI units, there was a 50% increase for the risk of developing EC [6]. As a consequence, the incidence of EC is constantly increasing worldwide [7,8].

However, many women are still not aware of this very individual risk factor [3,9]. Thus, there is a strong demand to improve the common understanding of the relationship between adiposity and EC and to offer therapeutic and behavioral strategies.

This communication provides an overview of the main, known pathophysiological pathways and mechanisms connecting obesity and EC. In addition, implications for therapy and prevention are discussed.

2. Adipose-Derived Pathophysiological Mechanisms Linking EC to Adiposity

The link between obesity and EC is a highly complex system consisting of several closely intertwined pathways and mechanisms. Adiposity influences not only the metabolism but is also highly associated with hyperlipidemia, insulin resistance, hyperglycemia, and hyperinsulinemia. Fat tissue and its components have pro- and anti-inflammatory characteristics and function as a source of hormone production, thus playing a key role in endometrial proliferation. Via complex signaling pathways, receptors, and gene expression, fat tissue not only induces proliferation but also invasion and modulation of cancer cells.

2.1. Estrogen-Driven Tumorigenesis

In premenopausal women, endometrial proliferation due to cyclic estrogen expression of the ovarian tissue is essential for a healthy menstrual cycle. Naturally, estrogen levels decrease in the ovaries in postmenopausal women, and the role of peripheral and adipose tissue in estrogen synthesis gain in importance [8]. Adipose tissue expresses aromatase, an enzyme that catalyzes the endogenous conversion of androgen to estrogen [10]. Thus, with an increase in adipose tissue, estrogen levels increase (Figure 1). Similarly, the amount of sex hormone-binding globulin (SHBG), a hormone that binds and transports estrogen, decreases. Consequently, the level of bioactive estrogen in the circulating bloodstream increases further. In 1996, Potischman et al. showed that an increased risk of EC is directly associated with a high level of circulating, unopposed estrogen and a low plasma level of SHBG [11]. While both estrone and estradiol are linked to an increased risk, the highest risk was observed for unconjugated estradiol [12]. Friedenreich et al. showed in 2020 that the influence of menopause in EC emerges from estrone ($p = 0.02$), estradiol ($p = 0.006$), and, moreover, androstenedione ($p = 0.01$), but not from SHBG or testosterone [13]. The effect attributed to elevated levels of androstenedione might mainly be driven by their conversion to estrogen [14].

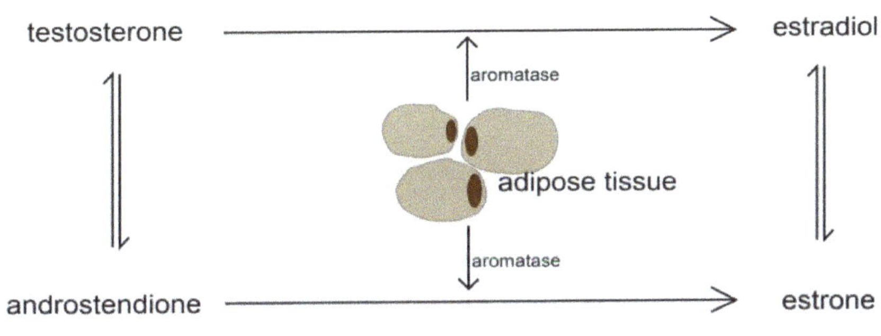

Figure 1. Adipose tissue and steroid conversions.

The oncogenic signal of estrogen is mediated through estrogen receptors α and β (ERα and ERβ), modulating transcriptional nuclear signaling [15]. In Ishikawa and KLE cell lines, ERα and Eβ promote cell invasion, migration, and proliferation, suggesting an association between receptor overexpression, invasiveness, and metastasis of EC [16]. ERs induce an overstimulation of the phosphatidylinositol 3-kinase (PI3K)/AKT/mammalian target of rapamycin (mTOR) signaling pathway in EC cell lines and thus play a role in epithelial-mesenchymal transition (EMT) [16,17]. In both types of EC, estrogen induces increased levels of phosphorylation of PI3K p85α and activates phosphorylation of mTOR and AKT [16].

Yang et al. recently discovered that estrogen-induced upregulation of prohibitin expression represents an element of endometrial tumorigenesis and the estrogen-ER signaling pathway.

By inhibiting ubiquitination, estrogen stabilizes prohibitin, while ERα mediates protein expression. High prohibitin levels are linked to a poor EC prognosis [18].

In 2011, Zhang et al. further investigated the role of fat mass and obesity-associated (FTO) gene as FTO was found to be overexpressed in endometrial tumor tissue in white, non-Hispanic [19], and Chinese women. By activating the PI3K/AKT and MPAK signal pathway, β-estradiol (E2) induced FTO evokes tumor proliferation and invasion [20]. However, E2 also interferes in EC cell invasion and migration via activation of IL-6 pathway and its target genes (Bcl-2, Mcl.1, cyclin D1 and MMP2) [21].

In addition to ERα and ERβ, estrogen also binds to G protein-coupled estrogen receptor (GPER), promoting non-nuclear-regulated apoptosis, migration, and cell growth [22].

Accordingly, the estrogen response causes tumorigenesis by damaging DNA strands, stimulating angiogenesis, and promoting cell proliferation and mutagenesis.

However, already in 1996, Potischman et al. and later Brinton et al. in 2017 reported that high estrogen levels could only partially explain the link between obesity and EC; however, BMI remained a significant hazard factor. Dossus et al. linked two other constituents in addition to steroids to elevated EC risk in postmenopausal women: insulin resistance/metabolic syndrome and inflammation [23].

2.2. *Adipose Tissue—An Endocrine Organ*

In this context, hypertrophied adipose tissue assumes the function of an endocrine organ in human metabolism. It not only secretes estrogen, but also adiponectin, visfatin, resistin, leptin, and tumor necrosis factor-α (TNFα).

High serum levels of visfatin were found to be associated with cell proliferation, differentiation, and inhibition of apoptosis in EC, especially in obese patients (BMI > 25) and correlate with tissue differentiation [24] and FIGO EC stage [25]. Likewise, Dallal et al. found high leptin serum levels as a predictive factor for EC risk [26]. Leptin binding to leptin receptors activates JAK2/STAT3, MAPK, and PI3K/Akt signaling pathways and thus modulates cell proliferation. Furthermore, leptin promotes a proinflammatory microenvironment, stimulating cytokines and T-helper 1 cells. This state of chronic inflammation modulating immune responses enhances angiogenesis and growth of cancer cells [27] (Figure 2).

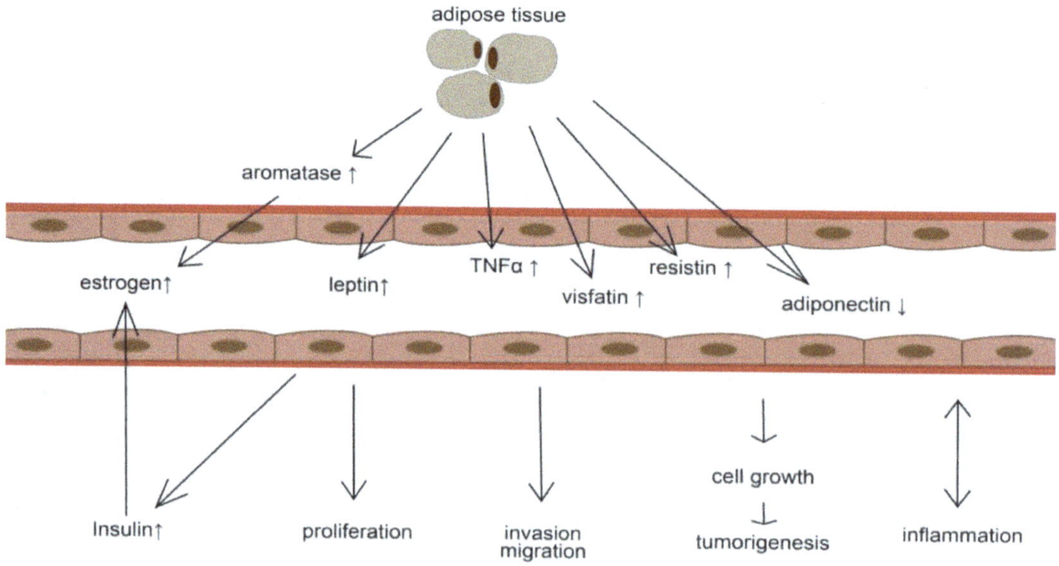

Figure 2. Simplified mechanisms of adipose tissue influence on tumorigenesis.

Likewise, adipocytes also produce adiponectin, a protein attributed to both anti-inflammatory and antiproliferative actions [28]. Serum adiponectin level was found to be decreased in women with EC and related to a poor prognosis [29]. Wang et al. were able to show an inverse correlation between adiponectin serum levels, FIGO stage, and tissue differentiation [24]. Furthermore, visfatin/adiponectin ratio and leptin/adiponectin ratio were independently associated with an increased risk for developing EC [24,30]. Although the association of hypoadiponectinemia and EC risk was shown to be independent of BMI, adiponectin secretion decreases in particular in visceral adipose tissue with increasing adiposity [31]. Weyer et al. suggested, however, that low serum levels of adiponectin were associated with hyperinsulinemia and insulin resistance independent of the degree of adiposity [32].

2.3. *The Link between Estrogen, Insulin Resistance, and Cancer*

Decrease in adiponectin and release of leptin, interleukin-6, TNFα and free fatty acids influence the response of certain body tissue to insulin [33]. Thus, adipokines, interleukins and TNFα induce insulin resistance, while adiponectin can be understood as an endogenous insulin sensitizer.

Hyperinsulinemia is considered a comorbidity of obesity and represents an estrogen-independent endometrial carcinoma risk factor [34]. Insulin and IGF-1 have been found to be associated with angiogenesis [35] and differentiation [36]. By reducing levels of IGF-binding proteins-1 and -2, insulin increases levels of IGF-1 and IGF-2 in the serum. IGF-1 inhibits cell apoptosis and promotes cell proliferation via the MAPK and PI3K/mTOR signaling pathway [37]. High levels of IGF-1 and insulin then depress SHBG synthesis again in the liver and induce steroidogenesis, increasing bioavailable estrogen levels.

Analogous to hypoadiponectemia, hyperinsulinemia was found to be a risk factor of EC independently of BMI [38,39]. Another comorbidity of adiposity is hypercholesterolemia, which recently was linked to cancer growth as the potentially missing link between obesity and cancer. As a cholesterol metabolite, 27-hydroxycholesterol (27HC) functions as an endogenous selective ER modulator (SERM). Serum concentrations of ER increase with age and with serum cholesterol levels [40].

Obesity constitutes a risk factor for EC; therefore, adipose tissue must be seen as a highly complex, multifactorial component in tumorigenesis. Adipose tissue functions as an endocrine organ; thus, obesity results in a dysregulated secretion of proinflammatory cytokines, adipocytes, dysfunction, and infiltration of immune cells, inducing damaged DNA strands, angiogenesis, cell proliferation, and mutagenesis. Weihe et al. found that this association started during childhood and adolescence, which increases cancer risk in adulthood [41]. However, certain risk factors, such as hyperinsulinemia, insulin resistance, and hypoadiponectinemia, were shown to be independent of BMI, partially explaining mechanisms of endometrial carcinogenesis in nonobese women. Cancer-inducing interactions among all involved components are still not fully understood. Nonetheless, these risk factors, seen as comorbidities, are related to adiposity, underscoring the relevance of obesity in endometrial tumorigenesis.

3. Clinical Management and Treatment

3.1. *Metformin*

The biguanide metformin is commonly used as antidiabetic drug, mainly as standard medication for patients suffering from type 2 diabetes mellitus. However, preclinical studies also confirmed an antineoplastic activity of this molecule. On the one hand, metformin influences several cellular growth and proliferation signaling pathways, in particular the PI3K/AKT/mTOR or PI3K/AKT/MDM2 pathway [42,43]. On the other hand, there is evidence that metformin inhibits EMT, for example, by increasing E-cadherin expression [44]. Recent reports also demonstrated that metformin inhibited PD-L1 in an EC cell line model and thereby can suppress cancer cell growth [45].

There is increasing evidence that these antineoplastic effects can be used to prevent and treat EC [46]. In 2017, Meireles and colleagues published a systematic review of 19 relatively heterogeneous studies showing that metformin reversed atypic endometrial hyperplasia [46,47]. In addition, another systematic review demonstrated that metformin treatment was associated with a significantly decreased mortality among postmenopausal EC patients [48]. In contrast to these reports, in a systematic review of seven studies in 2019, Chu and colleagues could not confirm a risk reduction for EC by metformin [49].

Nevertheless, the same authors proved that relapse in EC patients was significantly reduced and overall survival significantly prolonged (HR = 0.47, 95% CI 0.33–0.67, $p < 0.05$).

Whether metformin can be directly used as an antineoplastic agent for the treatment of EC is currently still the topic of controversial debate [46,50–55].

3.2. *Obesity and Its Consequences for Surgical Treatment*

Total laparoscopic hysterectomy with bilateral salpingoophorectomy is a routine surgical procedure with curative intent in patients with early-stage EC [56]. One advantage of minimally invasive surgery in obese patients is that major perioperative morbidity associated with wound breakdown of larger mid-line incision scars can be avoided [57]. Furthermore, significantly less blood loss is attributed to laparoscopic interventions than to open surgery and patients can be mobilized faster during the postoperative period. Thus, the risk of thrombosis can be reduced and reconvalescence can be improved [58]. Gambacorti-Passerini and colleagues confirmed these findings in an observational study on 83 patients, pointing out that laparoscopic surgery can be safely offered to obese patients with EC [59].

However, the Trendelenburg position is mandatory for laparoscopic hysterectomy. A recently published systematic review and meta-analysis of 51 observational studies on 10,800 patients found a conversion rate of 7% for morbidly obese patients undergoing laparoscopic surgery, whereas in 31% of these cases, the reason for conversion was an intolerance of Trendelenburg position [60]. In that study, the authors also found that robotic surgery was better able to avoid conversions.

Nevertheless, there is consensus that adiposity is associated with a highly increased rate of perioperative complications and morbidity following laparotomy, including greater blood loss, wound infections, secondary wound breakdown, thrombosis, and hospital stay [61]. Finally, in cases of extreme morbid obesity, any surgical access might be impossible, either because anesthesiological surveillance of the patient is insufficient or because there is no surgical route to the surgically relevant structures in the pelvis mainly due to the intra-abdominal adiposity.

3.3. *Possible Complications of Chemotherapy and Radiotherapy Due to Obesity*

There is some evidence that obese patients show differences in pharmacokinetics and metabolic dysregulation compared to non-obese patients [62]. However, there is very little evidence that these differences lead to increased toxicity among obese patients [63]. Moreover, the main risk factor for obese patients under chemotherapy can be seen in the fact that the treatment might be underdosed. Fearing potential—but not really proven—toxicities, physicians still tend to cap the maximum dosage of standard chemotherapy regimens at 2.0 m^2 body surface area (BSA) instead of applying the full standard dosage. In 2012, a special ASCO guideline focused on this issue, after stating that in 2012 up to 40% of all obese cancer patients were treated with suboptimally dosed chemotherapy regimens [64]. In line with these data, in 2009 Schwartz et al. reported on a retrospective study on 59 obese patients with a BSA > 2.0 m^2 receiving adjuvant chemotherapy with carboplatin and paclitaxel for endometrial or ovarian cancer [65]. A total of 50 patients were treated with standard paclitaxel dosages according to the actual body weight, whereas in nine patients, the paclitaxel dosages were capped at a BSA of 2.0 m^2. Interestingly, the authors did not find any significant differences between both groups in rates of toxicity or dose modification. Thus, they concluded that any empiric dose reduction is unnecessary and may lead to suboptimal cancer treatment.

Radiotherapy is also a cornerstone of standard treatment of primary endometrial cancer. In parallel to the chemotherapy-related effects discussed above, there is also a lack of evidence regarding the effects of obesity on potential radiotherapy complications. In 2017, Smits and colleagues reported the result of a retrospective cohort study on 159 women diagnosed with endometrial cancer who received radiotherapy as part of their general primary treatment including external beam radiotherapy as well as vaginal brachytherapy [66]. In the analyzed cohort, 63 women had a BMI < 30 kg/m^2 and 47 women were obese. As main result of this study, BMI was not associated with the incidence of acute and late radiation toxicities in the different radiotherapy groups and there were no differences in individual complication between the BMI groups.

4. Weight Reduction and Its Value as Prevention Measure

4.1. Lifestyle

There is increasing evidence that intentional weight loss significantly reduces incidence and mortality of EC in obese patients. The Women's Health Initiative Study (WHI), for example, demonstrated that an intentional weight loss of >5% was associated with a significantly reduced EC risk [46,67,68]. This was also confirmed in a systematic review and meta-analysis by Zhang et al. in 2019. The authors reported that intentional weight loss and maintaining a stable, healthy weight were associated with a significantly lower risk of EC (RR range 0.61–0.96) [69].

The question of weight loss is relevant as Haggerty and colleagues pointed out in 2017. They conducted a survey among patients with stage I EC and found that 59% of the patients reported great interest in using weight loss as a preventive method against recurrence [3].

Intentional weight loss can, on the one hand, be achieved by maintaining a healthy and effective diet to reasonably reduce weight. On the other hand, increasing physical activity, for example, by exercise is also a potential method of losing weight. There is consensus that physical activity is beneficial for reducing individual cancer risk [70–72]. In particular, the risk for developing EC can be positively affected [73,74].

4.2. Bariatric Surgery

Bariatric surgery interventions can lead to substantial weight loss. In 2007, Sjostrom and colleagues reported the results of the Swedish Obese Subjects (SOS) study [75]. In this trial, 1420 obese women who underwent bariatric surgery were observed and compared to a control group that received "conventional", conservative obesity treatment such as diet, increase in physical activity, etc. In this trial, bariatric surgery led to a significantly reduced incidence of EC (HR = 0.56, $p = 0.014$) after a median follow-up period of 18.2 years [46,76]. These findings were recently confirmed and underscored by data from a systematic review published by Winder et al. [77]. The authors analyzed the results of five prospective trials comparing women who underwent bariatric surgery with a control group with respect to their risk of developing EC. As a key result of this study, a significant risk reduction for EC was found for the bariatric surgery group (OR = 0.317, 95% CI = 0.161–0.627).

The pathophysiological mechanism underlying the effects of bariatric surgery is still not fully understood. One possible pathway of action might be the decrease in glucose levels as well as beneficial influences from insulin levels and associated cytokines. In addition, bariatric surgery was reported to decrease serum levels of proinflammatory cytokines [78].

4.3. Implications of Weight Loss after Diagnosis of Endometrial Cancer

In contrast to the presented evidence for the beneficial effects of weight reduction in order to prevent the origination of endometrial cancer, there is little information on the effects of weight loss after diagnosis of the disease. In 2012 in a retrospective study El-Safadi and co-authors analyzed 705 patients with endometrial cancer under follow-up. The records of all patients were reviewed for body weight after the diagnosis of EC and during follow-up [79]. Finally, the recurrence-free interval was determined. Interestingly, in this study a moderate weight gain of ≤ 1 kg/m^2 was associated with the best prognosis among these patients. In contrast, patients who showed a weight loss, had a worse prognosis. However, the authors did not differentiate between intentional and non-intentional weight-loss. In addition, the statistical power of this retrospective analysis was low. Nevertheless, currently there is no strong evidence given that once an endometrial cancer has been originated weight reduction would lead to definite improvement of outcome.

5. Conclusions

Endometrial cancer (EC) is the most frequently observed malignant gynecologic disease in developed countries.

Obesity presents one risk factor in tumorigenesis of EC as adipose tissue can been understood as an endocrine organ resulting in a disbalanced levels of estrogen, pro- and anti-inflammatory cytokines and adipocytes. This imbalance leads to a dysregulation of insulin resistance and hyperglycemia, to an infiltration of immune cells, inducing damaged DNA strands, angiogenesis, increased cell proliferation rates and mutagenesis. The interactions of all these components in tumorigenesis are still not fully understood. Understanding these risk factors as comorbidities related to adiposity, they emphasize the relevance of obesity in endometrial tumorigenesis.

There is broad evidence that the antidiabetic agent metformin has antineoplastic properties and can be used in the prevention and treatment of endometrial cancer.

Obesity has a major impact on surgery for EC and is also of relevance for chemotherapy and radiotherapy.

Intentional weight loss as well as bariatric surgery are effective to reduce the risk for the origination of endometrial cancer.

Author Contributions: L.K.—conceptualization, L.K., M.E., A.B., C.E.—writing, original draft preparation, L.K., M.E., A.B., C.E.—review and editing. All authors have read and agreed to the published version of the manuscript.

References

1. GBD 2015 Obesity Collaborators; Afshin, A.; Forouzanfar, M.H.; Reitsma, M.B.; Sur, P.; Estep, K.; Lee, A.; Marczak, L.; Mokdad, A.H.; Moradi-Lakeh, M.; et al. Health effects of overweight and obesity in 195 countries over 25 years. *N. Engl. J. Med.* **2017**, *377*, 13–27.
2. Friedenreich, C.M.; Ryder-Burbidge, C.; McNeil, J. Physical activity, obesity and sedentary behavior in cancer etiology: Epidemiologic evidence and biologic mechanisms. *Mol. Oncol.* **2020**. [CrossRef] [PubMed]
3. Haggerty, A.F.; Sarwer, D.B.; Schmitz, K.H.; Ko, E.M.; Allison, K.C.; Chu, C.S. Obesity and Endometrial Cancer: A Lack of Knowledge but Opportunity for Intervention. *Nutr. Cancer* **2017**, *69*, 990–995. [CrossRef] [PubMed]
4. Reeves, G.K.; Pirie, K.; Beral, V.; Green, J.; Spencer, E.; Bull, D. Cancer incidence and mortality in relation to body mass index in the Million Women Study: Cohort study. *BMJ* **2007**, *335*, 1134. [CrossRef] [PubMed]
5. Onstad, M.A.; Schmandt, R.E.; Lu, K.H. Addressing the Role of Obesity in Endometrial Cancer Risk, Prevention, and Treatment. *J. Clin. Oncol.* **2016**, *34*, 4225–4230. [CrossRef]
6. World Cancer Research Fund/American Institute for Cancer Research: Continuous Update Project Report. Food: Nutrition, Physical Activity, and the Prevention of Endometrial Cancer. 2013. Available online: http://www.dietandcancerreport.org (accessed on 1 November 2020).
7. Bray, F.; Ferlay, J.; Soerjomataram, I.; Siegel, R.L.; Torre, L.A.; Jemal, A. Global cancer statistics 2018: GLOBOCAN estimates of incidence and mortality worldwide for 36 cancers in 185 countries. *CA Cancer J. Clin.* **2018**, *68*, 394–424. [CrossRef]
8. Moore, K.; Brewer, M.A. Endometrial Cancer: Is This a New Disease? *Am. Soc. Clin. Oncol. Educ. Book* **2017**, *37*, 435–442. [CrossRef]
9. Connor, E.V.; Raker, C.A.; Clark, M.A.; Stuckey, A.R. Obesity risk awareness in women with endometrial cancer. *Arch. Gynecol. Obstet.* **2017**, *295*, 965–969. [CrossRef]
10. Simpson, E.R.; Mahendroo, M.S.; Means, G.D.; Kilgore, M.W.; Hinshelwood, M.M.; Graham-Lorence, S.; Amarneh, B.; Ito, Y.; Fisher, C.R.; Michael, M.D.; et al. Aromatase Cytochrome P450, The Enzyme Responsible for Estrogen. Biosynthesis. *Endocr. Rev.* **1994**, *15*, 342–355.
11. Potischman, N.; Hoover, R.N.; Brinton, L.A.; Siiteri, P.; Dorgan, J.F.; Swanson, C.A.; Berman, M.L.; Mortel, R.; Twiggs, L.B.; Barrett, R.J.; et al. Case—Control Study of Endogenous Steroid Hormones and Endometrial Cancer. *J. Natl. Cancer Inst.* **1996**, *88*, 1127–1135. [CrossRef]

12. Brinton, L.A.; Trabert, B.; Anderson, G.L.; Falk, R.T.; Felix, A.S.; Fuhrman, B.J.; Gass, M.L.; Kuller, L.H.; Pfeiffer, R.M.; Rohan, T.E.; et al. Serum Estrogens and Estrogen Metabolites and Endometrial Cancer Risk among Postmenopausal Women. *Cancer Epidemiol. Biomark. Prev.* **2016**, *25*, 1081–1089. [CrossRef] [PubMed]
13. Friedenreich, C.M.; Derksen, J.; Speidel, T.; Brenner, D.R.; Heer, E.; Courneya, K.S.; Cook, L.S. Case—control study of endogenous sex steroid hormones and risk of endometrial cancer. *Cancer Causes Control* **2020**, *31*, 161–171. [CrossRef] [PubMed]
14. Lukanova, A.; Lundin, E.; Micheli, A.; Arslan, A.; Ferrari, P.; Rinaldi, S.; Krogh, V.; Lenner, P.; Shore, R.E.; Biessy, C.; et al. Circulating levels of sex steroid hormones and risk of endometrial cancer in postmenopausal women. *Int. J. Cancer* **2004**, *108*, 425–432. [CrossRef] [PubMed]
15. Rodriguez, A.C.; Blanchard, Z.; Maurer, K.A.; Gertz, J. Estrogen Signaling in Endometrial Cancer: A Key Oncogenic Pathway with Several Open Questions. *Horm. Cancer* **2019**, *10*, 51–63. [CrossRef] [PubMed]
16. Hou, X.; Zhao, M.; Wang, T.; Zhang, G. Upregulation of estrogen receptor mediates migration, invasion and proliferation of endometrial carcinoma cells by regulating the PI3K/AKT/mTOR pathway. *Oncol. Rep.* **2014**, *31*, 1175–1182. [CrossRef] [PubMed]
17. Guo, R.X.; Wei, L.H.; Tu, Z.; Sun, P.M.; Wang, J.L.; Zhao, D.; Li, X.P.; Tang, J.M. 17 beta-estradiol activates PI3K/Akt signaling pathway by estrogen receptor (ER)-dependent and ER-independent mechanisms in endometrial cancer cells. *J. Steroid Biochem. Mol. Biol.* **2006**, *99*, 9–18. [CrossRef] [PubMed]
18. Yang, B.; Chen, R.; Liang, X.; Shi, J.; Wu, X.; Zhang, Z.; Chen, X. Estrogen Enhances Endometrial Cancer Cells Proliferation by Upregulation of Prohibitin. *J. Cancer* **2019**, *10*, 1616–1621. [CrossRef]
19. Lurie, G.; Gaudet, M.M.; Spurdle, A.B.; Carney, M.E.; Wilkens, L.R.; Yang, H.P.; Weiss, N.S.; Webb, P.M.; Thompson, P.J.; Terada, K.; et al. The obesity-associated polymorphisms FTO rs9939609 and MC4R rs17782313 and endometrial cancer risk in non-Hispanic white women. *PLoS ONE* **2011**, *6*, e16756. [CrossRef]
20. Zhang, Z.; Zhou, D.; Lai, Y.; Liu, Y.; Tao, X.; Wang, Q.; Zhao, G.; Gu, H.; Liao, H.; Zhu, Y.; et al. Estrogen induces endometrial cancer cell proliferation and invasion by regulating the fat mass and obesity-associated gene via PI3K/AKT and MAPK signaling pathways. *Cancer Lett.* **2012**, *319*, 89–97. [CrossRef]
21. Che, Q.; Xiao, X.; Xu, J.; Liu, M.; Lu, Y.; Liu, S.; Dong, X. 17β-Estradiol promotes endometrial cancer proliferation and invasion through IL-6 pathway. *Endocr. Connect.* **2019**, *8*, 961–968. [CrossRef]
22. Prossnitz, E.R.; Barton, M. The G-protein-coupled estrogen receptor GPER in health and disease. *Nat. Rev. Endocr.* **2011**, *7*, 715–726. [CrossRef] [PubMed]
23. Dossus, L.; Lukanova, A.; Rinaldi, S.; Allen, N.; Cust, A.E.; Becker, S.; Tjonneland, A.; Hansen, L.; Overvad, K.; Chabbert-Buffet, N.; et al. Hormonal, metabolic, and inflammatory profiles and endometrial cancer risk within the EPIC cohort–a factor analysis. *Am. J. Epidemiol.* **2013**, *177*, 787–799. [CrossRef] [PubMed]
24. Wang, Z.; Gao, S.; Sun, C.; Li, J.; Gao, W.; Yu, L. Clinical significance of serum adiponectin and visfatin levels in endometrial cancer. *Int. J. Gynaecol. Obstet.* **2019**, *145*, 34–39. [CrossRef] [PubMed]
25. Tian, W.; Zhu, Y.; Wang, Y.; Teng, F.; Zhang, H.; Liu, G.; Ma, X.; Sun, D.; Rohan, T.; Xue, F. Visfatin, a potential biomarker and prognostic factor for endometrial cancer. *Gynecol. Oncol.* **2013**, *129*, 505–512. [CrossRef] [PubMed]
26. Dallal, C.M.; Brinton, L.A.; Bauer, D.C.; Buist, D.S.; Cauley, J.A.; Hue, T.F.; Lacroix, A.; Tice, J.A.; Chia, V.M.; Falk, R.; et al. Obesity-related hormones and endometrial cancer among postmenopausal women: A nested case—control study within the B~FIT cohort. *Endocr.-Relat. Cancer* **2013**, *20*, 151–160. [CrossRef] [PubMed]
27. Atoum, M.F.; Alzoughool, F.; Al-Hourani, H. Linkage Between Obesity Leptin and Breast Cancer. *Breast Cancer Basic Clin. Res.* **2020**, *14*. [CrossRef]
28. Tumminia, A.; Vinciguerra, F.; Parisi, M.; Graziano, M.; Sciacca, L.; Baratta, R.; Frittitta, L. Adipose Tissue, Obesity and Adiponectin: Role in Endocrine Cancer Risk. *Int. J. Mol. Sci.* **2019**, *20*, 2863. [CrossRef]
29. Soliman, P.T.; Wu, D.; Tortolero-Luna, G.; Schmeler, K.M.; Slomovitz, B.M.; Bray, M.S.; Gershenson, D.M.; Lu, K.H. Association between adiponectin, insulin resistance, and endometrial cancer. *Cancer* **2006**, *106*, 2376–2381. [CrossRef]
30. Ashizawa, N.; Yahata, T.; Quan, J.; Adachi, S.; Yoshihara, K.; Tanaka, K. Serum leptin-adiponectin ratio and endometrial cancer risk in postmenopausal female subjects. *Gynecol. Oncol.* **2010**, *119*, 65–69. [CrossRef]
31. Reneau, J.; Goldblatt, M.; Gould, J.; Kindel, T.; Kastenmeier, A.; Higgins, R.; Rengel, L.R.; Schoyer, K.; James, R.; Obi, B.; et al. Effect of adiposity on tissue-specific adiponectin secretion. *PLoS ONE* **2018**, *13*, e0198889. [CrossRef]

32. Weyer, C.; Funahashi, T.; Tanaka, S.; Hotta, K.; Matsuzawa, Y.; Pratley, R.E.; Tataranni, P.A. Hypoadiponectinemia in obesity and type 2 diabetes: Close association with insulin resistance and hyperinsulinemia. *J. Clin. Endocrinol. Metab.* **2001**, *86*, 1930–1935. [CrossRef] [PubMed]
33. Wajchenberg, B.L. Subcutaneous and visceral adipose tissue: Their relation to the metabolic syndrome. *Endocr. Rev.* **2000**, *21*, 697–738. [CrossRef] [PubMed]
34. Gunter, M.J.; Hoover, D.R.; Yu, H.; Wassertheil-Smoller, S.; Manson, J.E.; Li, J.; Harris, T.G.; Rohan, T.E.; Xue, X.; Ho, G.Y.; et al. A prospective evaluation of insulin and insulin-like growth factor-I as risk factors for endometrial cancer. *Cancer Epidemiol. Biomark. Prev.* **2008**, *17*, 921–929. [CrossRef]
35. Kluge, A.; Zimmermann, R.; Münkel, B.; Mohri, M.; Sack, S.; Schaper, J.; Schaper, W. Insulin-like growth factor I is involved in inflammation linked angiogenic processes after microembolisation in porcine heart. *Cardiovasc. Res.* **1995**, *29*, 407–415. [CrossRef]
36. Khandwala, H.M.; McCutcheon, I.E.; Flyvbjerg, A.; Friend, K.E. The effects of insulin-like growth factors on tumorigenesis and neoplastic growth. *Endocr. Rev.* **2000**, *21*, 215–244. [CrossRef]
37. Vrachnis, N.; Iavazzo, C.; Iliodromiti, Z.; Sifakis, S.; Alexandrou, A.; Siristatidis, C.; Grigoriadis, C.; Botsis, D.; Creatsas, G. Diabetes mellitus and gynecologic cancer: Molecular mechanisms, epidemiological, clinical and prognostic perspectives. *Arch. Gynecol. Obstet.* **2016**, *293*, 239–246. [CrossRef]
38. Nead, K.T.; Sharp, S.J.; Thompson, D.J.; Painter, J.N.; Savage, D.B.; Semple, R.K.; Barker, A.; Australian National Endometrial Cancer Study Group (ANECS); Perry, J.R.; Attia, J.; et al. Evidence of a Causal Association Between Insulinemia and Endometrial Cancer: A Mendelian Randomization Analysis. *J. Nat. Cancer Inst.* **2015**, *107*, djv178. [CrossRef] [PubMed]
39. Troisi, R.; Potischman, N.; Hoover, R.N.; Siiteri, P.; Brinton, L.A. Insulin and Endometrial Cancer. *Am. J. Epidemiol.* **1997**, *146*, 476–482. [CrossRef]
40. Asghari, A.; Umetani, M. Obesity and Cancer: 27-Hydroxycholesterol, the Missing Link. *Int. J. Mol. Sci.* **2020**, *21*, E4822. [CrossRef]
41. Weihe, P.; Spielmann, J.; Kielstein, H.; Henning-Klusmann, J.; Weihrauch-Blüher, S. Childhood Obesity and Cancer Risk in Adulthood. *Curr. Obes. Rep.* **2020**. Advance online publication. [CrossRef]
42. Zhao, Y.; Sun, H.; Feng, M.; Zhao, J.; Zhao, X.; Wan, Q.; Cai, D. Metformin is associated with reduced cell proliferation in human endometrial cancer by inbibiting PI3K/AKT/mTOR signaling. *Gynecol. Endocrinol.* **2018**, *34*, 428–432. [CrossRef] [PubMed]
43. Qiang, P.; Shao, Y.; Sun, Y.P.; Zhang, J.; Chen, L.J. Metformin inhibits proliferation and migration of endometrial cancer cells through regulating PI3K/AKT/MDM2 pathway. *Eur. Rev. Med. Pharmacol. Sci.* **2019**, *23*, 1778–1785. [PubMed]
44. Liu, Z.; Qi, S.; Zhao, X.; Li, M.; Ding, S.; Lu, J.; Zhang, H. Metformin inhibits 17β-estradiol-induced epithelial-to-mesenchymal transition via βKlotho-related ERK1/2 signaling and AMPKα signaling in endometrial adenocarcinoma cells. *Oncotargets* **2016**, *19*, 21315–21331. [CrossRef]
45. Xue, J.; Li, L.; Li, N.; Li, F.; Qin, X.; Li, T.; Liu, M. Metformin suppresses cancer cell growth i n endometrial carcinoma by inhibiting PD-L1. *Eur. J. Pharmacol.* **2019**, *15*, 859. [CrossRef]
46. Byrne, F.L.; Martin, A.R.; Kosasih, M.; Caruana, B.T.; Farrell, R. The Role of Hyperglycemia in Endometrial Cancer Pathogenesis. *Cancers* **2020**, *8*, 1191. [CrossRef]
47. Meireles, C.G.; Pereira, S.A.; Valadares, L.P.; Rego, D.F.; Simeoni, L.A.; Guerra, E.N.S.; Lofrano-Porto, A. Effects of metformin on endometrial cancer: Systematic review and meta-analysis. *Gynecol. Oncol.* **2017**, *147*, 167–180. [CrossRef]
48. Perez-Lopez, F.R.; Pasupuleti, V.; Gianuzzi, X.; Palma-Ardiles, G.; Hernandez-Fernandez, W.; Adrian, V.H. Systematic review and meta-analysis of the effect of metformin treatment on overall mortality rates in women with endometrial cancer and type 2 diabetes mellitus. *Maturitas* **2017**, *101*, 6–11. [CrossRef]
49. Chu, D.; Wu, J.; Wang, K.; Zhao, M.; Wang, C.; Li, L.; Guo, R. Effect of metformin use on the risk and prognosis of endometrial cancer: A systematic review and meta-analysis. *BMC Cancer* **2018**, *18*, 438. [CrossRef]
50. Nevadunsky, N.S.; Van Arsdale, A.; Strickler, H.D.; Moadel, A.; Kaur, G.; Frimer, M.; Conroy, E.; Goldberg, G.L.; Einstein, M.H. Metformin use and endometrial cancer survival. *Gynecol. Oncol.* **2014**, *132*, 236–240. [CrossRef]
51. Ko, E.M.; Walter, P.; Jackson, A.; Clark, L.; Franasiak, J.; Bolac, C.; Havrilesky, L.J.; Secord, A.A.; Moore, D.T.; Gehrig, P.A.; et al. Metformin is associated with improved survival in endometrial cancer. *Gynecol. Oncol.* **2014**, *132*, 438–442. [CrossRef]

52. Al Hilli, M.M.; Bakkum-Gamez, J.N.; Mariani, A.; Cliby, W.A.; Mc Gree, M.E.; Weaver, A.L.; Dowdy, S.C.; Podratz, K.C. The effect of diabetes and metformin on clinical outcomes is negligible in risk-adjusted endometrial cancer cohorts. *Gynecol. Oncol.* **2016**, *140*, 270–276. [CrossRef] [PubMed]
53. Lemanska, A.; Zaborowski, M.; Spaczynski, M.; Nowak-Markwitz, E. Do endometrial cancer patients benefit from metformin intake? *Ginekol. Pol.* **2015**, *86*, 419–423. [CrossRef] [PubMed]
54. Seebacher, V.; Bergmeister, B.; Grimm, C.; Koelbl, H.; Reinthaller, A.; Polterauer, S. The prognostic role of metformin in patients with endometrial cancer: A retrospective study. *Eur. J. Obstet. Gynecol. Reprod. Biol.* **2016**, *203*, 291–296. [CrossRef] [PubMed]
55. Arima, R.; Hautakoski, A.; Marttila, M.; Arffman, M.; Sund, R.; Ilanne-Parikka, P.; Kangaskokko, J.; Hinkula, M.; Puistola, U.; Läärä, E. Cause-specific mortality in endometrioid endometrial cancer patients with type 2 diabetes using metformin or other types of antidiabetic medication. *Gynecol. Oncol.* **2017**, *147*, 678–683. [CrossRef]
56. Janda, M.; Gebski, V.; Davies, L.C.; Forder, P.; Brand, A.; Hogg, R.; Jobling, T.W.; Land, R.; Manolitsas, T.; Nascimento, M.; et al. Effect of Total Laparoscopic Hysterectomy vs. Total Abdominal Hysterectomy on Disease-Free Survival Among Women with Stage I Endometrial Cancer: A Randomized Clinical Trial. *JAMA* **2017**, *317*, 1224–1233. [CrossRef]
57. Mahdi, H.; Jernigan, A.M.; Aljebori, Q.; Lockhart, D.; Moslemi-Kebria, M. The impact of obesity on the 30-day morbidity and mortality after surgery for endometrial cancer. *J. Minim. Invasive Gynecol.* **2015**, *22*, 94–102. [CrossRef]
58. Al Sawah, E.; Salemi, J.L.; Hoffman, M.; Imudia, A.N.; Mikhail, E. Association between Obesity, Surgical Route, and Perioperative Outcomes in Patients with Uterine Cancer. *Minim. Invasive Surg.* **2018**, *19*, 5130856. [CrossRef]
59. Gambacorti-Passerini, Z.M.; López-De la Manzanara Cano, C.; Pérez Parra, C.; Cespedes Casas, M.C.; Sánchez Hipólito, L.; Martín Francisco, C.; Muñoz-Rodríguez, J.R. Obesity in Patients with Endometrial Cancer: May It Affect the Surgical Outcomes of Laparoscopic Approach? *Obes. Surg.* **2019**, *29*, 3285–3290. [CrossRef]
60. Cusimano, M.C.; Simpson, A.N.; Dossa, F.; Liani, V.; Kaur, Y.; Acuna, S.A.; Robertson, D.; Satkunaratnam, A.; Bernardini, M.Q.; Ferguson, S.E.; et al. Laparoscopic and robotic hysterectomy in endometrial cancer patients with obesity: A systematic review and meta-analysis of conversions and complications. *Arch. Gynecol. Obstet.* **2017**, *295*, 965–969.
61. Orekoya, O.; Samson, M.E.; Trivedi, T.; Vyas, S.; Steck, S.E. The impact of obesity on surgical outcome in endometrial cancer patients: A systematic review. *J. Gynecol. Surg.* **2016**, *32*, 149–157. [CrossRef]
62. Horowitz, N.S.; Wright, A.A. Impact of obesity on chemotherapy management and outcomes in women with gynecologic malignancies. *Gynecol. Oncol.* **2015**, *138*, 201–206. [CrossRef]
63. Ottaiano, A.; De Divitiis, C.; Capozzi, M.; Avallone, A.; Pisano, C.; Pignata, S.; Tafuto, S. Obesity and Cancer: Biological Links and Treatment Implications. *Curr. Cancer Drug Targ.* **2018**, *18*, 231–238. [CrossRef]
64. Griggs, J.J.; Mangu, P.B.; Anderson, H.; Balaban, E.P.; Dignam, J.J.; Hryniuk, W.M.; Morrison, V.A.; Pini, T.M.; Runowicz, C.D.; Rosner, G.L.; et al. American Society of Clinical Oncology. Appropriate chemotherapy dosing for obese adult patients with cancer: American Society of Clinical Oncology clinical practice guideline. *J. Clin. Oncol.* **2012**, *30*, 1553–1561. [CrossRef]
65. Schwartz, J.; Toste, B.; Dizon, D.S. Chemotherapy toxicity in gynecologic cancer patients with a body surface area (BSA)>2 m2. *Gynecol. Oncol.* **2009**, *114*, 53–56. [CrossRef] [PubMed]
66. Smits, A.; McGrane, J.; Lopes, A.; Kent, E.; Bekkers, R.; Massuger, L.; Simpson, N.; Galaal, K. Radiation-related toxicities and outcomes in endometrial cancer: Are obese women at a disadvantage? *Int. J. Clin. Oncol.* **2017**, *22*, 945–953. [CrossRef] [PubMed]
67. Luo, J.; Chlebowski, R.T.; Hendryx, M.; Rohan, T.; Wactawski-Wende, J.; Thomson, C.A.; Felix, A.S.; Chen, C.; Barrington, W.; Coday, M.; et al. Intentional weight loss and endometrial cancer risk. *J. Clin. Oncol.* **2017**, *35*, 1189–1193. [CrossRef] [PubMed]
68. Luo, J.; Hendryx, M.; Manson, J.E.; Figueiredo, J.C.; LeBlanc, E.S.; Barrington, W.; Rohan, T.E.; Howard, B.V.; Reding, K.; Ho, G.Y.; et al. Intentional weight loss and obesity-related cancer risk. *JNCI Cancer Spectr.* **2019**, *3*, pkz054. [CrossRef]

69. Zhang, X.; Rhoades, J.; Caan, B.J.; Cohn, D.E.; Salani, R.; Noria, S.; Suarez, A.A.; Paskett, E.D.; Felix, A.S. Intentional weight loss, weight cycling, and endometrial cancer risk: A systematic review and meta-analysis. *Int. J. Gynecol. Cancer* **2019**, *29*, 1361–1371. [CrossRef]
70. Moore, S.C.; Lee, I.; Weiderpass, E.; Campbell, P.T.; Sampson, J.N.; Kitahara, C.M.; Keadle, S.K.; Arem, H.; Berrington de Gonzalez, A.; Hartge, P.; et al. Association of leisure-time physical activity with risk of 26 types of cancer in 1.44 million adults. *Complement Ther. Med.* **2019**, *44*, 9–13. [CrossRef]
71. Lugo, D.; Pulido, A.L.; Mihos, C.G.; Issa, O.; Cusnir, M.; Horvath, S.A.; Lin, J.; Santana, O. The effects of physical activity on cancer prevention, treatment and prognosis: A review of the literature. *JAMA Intern. Med.* **2016**, *176*, 816–825. [CrossRef]
72. Kerr, J.; Anderson, C.; Lippman, S.M. Physical activity, sedentary behaviour, diet, and cancer: An update and emerging new evidence. *Lancet Oncol.* **2017**, *18*, e457–e471. [CrossRef]
73. Koutoukidis, D.A.; Knobf, M.T.; Lanceley, A. Obesity, diet, physical activity, and health-related quality of life in endometrial cancer survivors. *Nutr. Rev.* **2015**, *73*, 399–408. [CrossRef] [PubMed]
74. Demark-Wahnefried, W.; Morey, M.C.; Sloane, R.; Snyder, D.C.; Miller, P.E.; Hartman, T.J.; Cohenet, H.J. Reach out to enhance wellness home-based diet-exercise intervention promotes reproducible and sustainable long-term improvements in health behaviors, body weight, and physical functioning in older, overweight/obese cancer survivors. *J. Clin. Oncol.* **2012**, *30*, 2354–2361. [CrossRef] [PubMed]
75. Sjostrom, L.; Narbro, K.; Sjostrom, C.D.; Karason, K.; Larsson, B.; Wedel, H.; Lystig, T.; Sullivan, M.; Bouchard, C.; Carlsson, B.; et al. Effects of bariatric surgery on mortality in Swedish obese subjects. *N. Engl. J. Med.* **2007**, *357*, 741–752. [CrossRef] [PubMed]
76. Anveden, Å.; Taube, M.; Peltonen, M.; Jacobson, P.; Andersson-Assarsson, J.C.; Sjöholm, K.; Svensson, P.-A.; Carlsson, L.M.S. Long-term incidence of female-specific cancer after bariatric surgery or usual care in the Swedish Obese Subjects Study. *Gynecol. Oncol.* **2017**, *145*, 224–229. [CrossRef] [PubMed]
77. Winder, A.A.; Kularatna, M.; MacCormick, A.D. Does bariatric surgery affect the incidence of endometrial cancer development? A systematic review. *Obes. Surg.* **2018**, *28*, 1433–1440. [CrossRef]
78. Izquierdo, A.G.; Carreira, M.C.; Rodriguez-Carnero, G.; Fernandez-Quintela, A.; Sueiro, A.M.; Martinez-Olmos, M.A.; Guzman, G.; De Luis, D.; Pinhel, M.A.S.; Nicoletti, C.F.; et al. Weight loss normalizes enhanced expression of the oncogene survivin in visceral adipose tissue and blood leukocytes from individuals with obesity. *Int. J. Obes.* **2020**. Online ahead of print. [CrossRef]
79. El-Safadi, S.; Sauerbier, A.; Hackethal, A.; Münstedt, K. Body weight changes after the diagnosis of endometrial cancer and their influences on disease-related prognosis. *Arch. Gynecol. Obstet.* **2012**, *285*, 1725–1729. [CrossRef]

3

Genetic Susceptibility to Endometrial Cancer: Risk Factors and Clinical Management

Thilo Dörk [1,*], Peter Hillemanns [1], Clemens Tempfer [2], Julius Breu [3] and Markus C. Fleisch [3]

1 Department of Gynecology and Obstetrics, Comprehensive Cancer Center, Hannover Medical School, 30625 Hannover, Germany; hillemanns.peter@mh-hannover.de
2 Department of Gynaecology, Marien-Hospital, Ruhr University of Bochum, 44625 Herne, Germany; Clemens.Tempfer@elisabethgruppe.de
3 Department of Gynecology and Obstetrics, University of Witten/Herdecke, 42283 Wuppertal, Germany; Julius.Breu@helios-gesundheit.de (J.B.); Markus.Fleisch@helios-gesundheit.de (M.C.F.)
* Correspondence: doerk.thilo@mh-hannover.de

Abstract: Endometrial cancer (EC) is the most common cancer affecting the female reproductive organs in higher-income states. Apart from reproductive factors and excess weight, genetic predisposition is increasingly recognized as a major factor in endometrial cancer risk. Endometrial cancer is genetically heterogeneous: while a subgroup of patients belongs to cancer predisposition syndromes (most notably the Lynch Syndrome) with high to intermediate lifetime risks, there are also several common genomic polymorphisms contributing to the spectrum of germline predispositions. Germline variants and somatic events may act in concert to modulate the molecular evolution of the tumor, where mismatch-repair deficiency is common in endometrioid endometrial tumors whereas homologous recombinational repair deficiency has been described for non-endometrioid endometrial tumors. In this review, we will survey the currently known genomic predispositions for endometrial cancer and discuss their relevance for clinical management in terms of counseling, screening and novel treatments.

Keywords: endometrium; carcinoma; genetics; Lynch syndrome; Cowden syndrome; targeted therapy

1. Risk Factors, Biology and Genetics

1.1. Epidemiology

Endometrial cancer (EC) develops in the inner layer of the uterus from the glandular epithelial sheet that covers the luminal surface and secretes substances essential for normal menstruation and embryonic development. Endometrial cancer is the most common cancer affecting the female reproductive organs in higher-income states [1–3]. Women in the US have a 2.6% lifetime risk of developing endometrial cancer, with some racial disparity documented [4]. It is commonly encountered in postmenopausal patients, although some 25% of cases occur prior to menopause, with some 5% in patients younger than 40 years old [1,5]. Most women diagnosed with endometrial cancer (EC) have well-differentiated cancers with endometrioid histology associated with early-stage disease and favorable outcomes, however there are clinically aggressive histologic subtypes of the disease, such as the serous histotype [2]. Five year overall survival ranges from 74% to 91% in patients without metastatic disease [3].

Endometrial cancer is the most strongly hormone- and excess weight-related cancer [1,6,7]. Both factors are correlated through the elevated estrogen levels associated with greater body weight in older women, since after menopause, androgens are converted to estrogens through the enzyme aromatase, found in adipose cells. Other risk factors, including reproductive factors such as parity, may also reflect the influence of sex steroid hormones. The endometrium is a dynamic tissue that undergoes frequent remodeling in response to oscillating levels of estrogen and progesterone, implying a recurrent need for clonal expansion and repopulation from progenitor cells [8,9].

However, risk factors in patients with uterine serous carcinoma seem to differ from those in women with endometrioid carcinoma, suggesting that there may be at least two different pathways of endometrial carcinogenesis. While a strong association was observed for high body mass index (BMI) in the endometrioid carcinoma cases, serous carcinomas were not strongly associated with BMI [10]. Parity, oral contraceptive use, cigarette smoking, age at menarche and diabetes were associated with both histological groups to similar extents [10,11].

1.2. Biology

The genomic landscapes accompanying clonal proliferation and malignant transformation of endometrial cells have been studied through next-generation sequencing in endometrial cancer as well as in normal endometrial epithelium [12–16]. Clonal expansion and a basal mutational burden can already be observed in single glands of normal endometrium, which accumulate somatic variants by age at an estimated rate of 29 variants per gland per year [16]. The basal mutational rate is about five times higher in endometrial cancer cells, which additionally can adopt a mutator phenotype with highly increased levels of specific mutational signatures indicating defective repair of mismatches, oxidative damage or breaks in their genomic DNA [12–14,16]. Large-scale molecular analysis of endometrial tumors grouped endometrial cancers into four molecular classifications: POLE-ultramutated, microsatellite instability-hypermutated, copy-number low (also called endometrioid-like) and copy-number high (also called serous-like) [12]. There is marked correlation between molecular and histological data: endometrioid histology is mostly represented in the first three clusters, which are distinguished by different degrees of microsatellite instability, DNA methylation and copy-number alterations, whereas the copy-number-high cluster covers most of the serous histology and tends to be a high grade and stage, with a high rate of recurrence and poor disease related outcome [12]. A comparison of frequently mutated genes revealed that activating variants in a group of known cancer driver genes, such as *PIK3CA*, *PIK3R1*, *ERBB2* or *KRAS*, can already be found in separate glands of normal epithelium and may occur as early as in the first two decades of life [16]. On the other hand, cancer driver genes known to be commonly mutated in endometrial cancer such as *TP53*, *PTEN* or *CTNNB1* were rarely mutated in the normal endometrium. This suggests a model in which single endometrial glands may first acquire driver mutations in genes that aid in tissue homeostasis but have limited capacity of malignant transformation. Endometrial cancer may then develop from these cells after additional mutational or epigenetic events impairing additional tumor suppressor or caretaker genes [16,17]. In this model, both stages would be driven by age-dependent accumulation of somatic variants and the neoplastic evolution started in early lifetime can take several decades, but the development would be accelerated if there is inherited variation in any of the cancer driver genes or in genes impacting on mutational repair, resulting in a genetic predisposition. Pathological examinations indicate that the first very subtle tissue alterations in a genetically predisposed woman can be seen in endometrial glands where cells ultimately lose the expression of the affected mismatch repair gene [18].

1.3. Genetic Predisposition

1.3.1. Spectrum of Hereditary Factors

A family history of endometrial cancer is associated with a two-to-threefold increased risk of endometrial cancer [19,20]. Although some of the associations between family history and endometrial cancer risk may be attributable to shared environmental or lifestyle risk factors, twin studies have estimated heritability between 27% and 52% [20–23]. Furthermore, colorectal, breast and stomach cancers co-occur with endometrial cancer at significantly higher frequencies in patient compared to control families [20]. A genetic predisposition for both colorectal and endometrial cancer was first observed in women with Lynch Syndrome, a hereditary cancer syndrome that accounts for 2–3% of all endometrial cancer cases [24,25]. However, family history is still associated with a risk of endometrial cancer after excluding Lynch Syndrome patients, indicating that additional genetic risk factors exist for familial endometrial cancer [20]. More recent work has uncovered further endometrial cancer susceptibility candidate genes [26] as well as several genomic loci harboring common low-risk variants [27] (Figure 1, Table 1); the current status of this ongoing research will be briefly reviewed below, followed by a survey and discussion of the clinical implications.

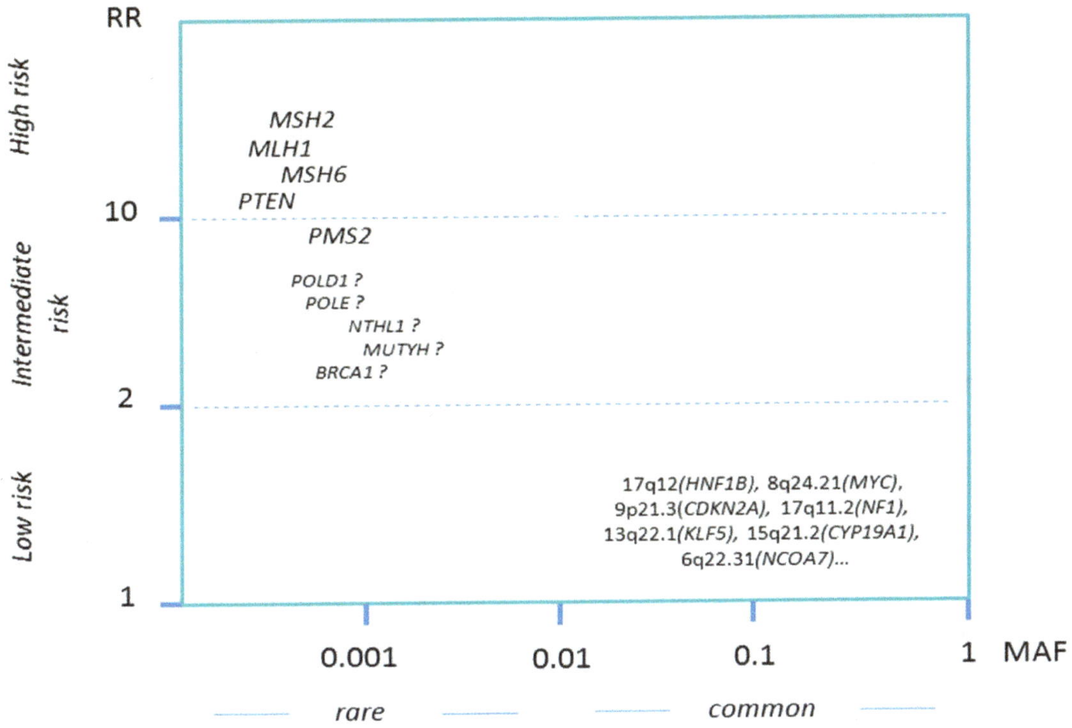

Figure 1. Schematic illustration of hereditary risk factors with risk estimates plotted against frequency. RR, relative risk; MAF, minor allele frequency. Risk estimates refer to classical pathogenic variants and may vary depending on the nature of the specific gene variant. Candidate intermediate risk factors are indicated with question mark (see Section 1.3 for further discussion). Low-risk genome-wide case-control association studies (GWAS) loci are indicated by their chromosomal region with plausibly predicted nearby genes given in brackets. MAF values refer to the abundance of loss-of-function variants estimated from the gnomAD database (https://gnomad.broadinstitute.org/). As a note of caution, these MAFs may substantially differ between distinct populations, some missense variants are not covered and only a subgroup of variants in *POLD1* and *POLE* may cause cancer (see Section 1.3.4). Figure not drawn to scale.

1.3.2. Lynch Syndrome

Lynch Syndrome (LS) represents one of the most common hereditary cancer syndromes [24], occurring at an incidence of 1/100–1/180 [28]. Due to its involvement of colorectal carcinomas, it is also known as Hereditary Non-Polyposis Colorectal Cancer (HNPCC). However, already the first LS pedigrees described had shown a high incidence of cancers within the uterus [29,30], and it is now well established that endometrial cancer is a frequent part of the cancer spectrum in LS [20,31,32]. Endometrial tumors from LS patients are often poorly differentiated, tend to have tumor-infiltrating lymphocytes and tend to involve the low uterine segment [4]. By contrast with patients who have sporadic endometrioid low-grade tumors, LS patients do not tend to have a particularly high body mass index [33].

Table 1. Established and candidate endometrial cancer risk genes.

Gene	Location	Frequency *	Associated Syndrome		Lifetime Risk EC	Other Cancers
			Biallelic	Monoallelic		
Established						
MLH1	3p22.2	1/1500	CMMRD	Lynch Syndrome	~40–45%	Colon, Ovary, Stomach, Pancreas, Brain **, HS **
MSH2	2p21-16	1/10,000	CMMRD	Lynch Syndrome	~50%	Colon, Ovary, Skin, Brain **, HS **
MSH6	2p16.3	1/2500	CMMRD	Lynch Syndrome	~40–45%	Colon, Ovary, Stomach, Pancreas, Breast?, Brain **, HS **
PMS2	7p22.1	1/600	CMMRD	Lynch Syndrome	~15–20%	Colon, Ovary, Breast?, Brain **, HS **
PTEN	10q23.31	1/10,000	unknown	Cowden Syndrome	~25%	Breast, Thyroid, Kidney, Colon, Skin
Candidates						
POLD1	19q13.33	not defined *	unknown	Lynch Syndrome-like	likely increased	Colon
POLE	12q24.33	not defined *	(FILS or IMAGEI Syndrome)	Lynch Syndrome-like	likely increased	Colon
NTHL1	16p13.3	1/250	NTHL1 multicancer syndrome	–	likely increased for homozygotes	Colon, Breast
MUTYH	1p34.1	1/200	MUTYH-associated polyposis	MUTYH-associated polyposis	possibly increased for homozygotes	Colon
BRCA1	17q21.31	1/600	Fanconi Anemia S	Hereditary Breast and Ovarian Cancer	possibly increased for serous EC	Breast, Ovary, Skin, Pancreas

Established and candidate endometrial cancer risk genes. Summarized for each gene are chromosomal location, carrier frequency estimates for loss-of-function variants in the general population, clinical syndromes associated with biallelic or monoallelic variants, estimated lifetime risk for endometrial cancer and common cancer sites apart from the endometrium. Lifetime risks for established genes refer to heterozygote risks. * carrier frequency for loss-of-function variants does not cover non-truncating variants. Note that *POLD1* and *POLE* truncating variants are associated with FILS or IMAGEI syndromes while cancer-associated variants are missense variants. ** Brain tumors and hematological cancers are common in patients with biallelic mismatch repair (MMR) gene variants. ES, endometrial cancer; HS, hematopoietic system; CMMRD, "Constitutional MisMatch Repair Deficiency"; FILS, "Facial dysmorphism, Immunodeficiency, Livedo, and Short stature"; IMAGEI, "Intrauterine growth retardation, Metaphyseal dysplasia, Adrenal hypoplasia congenita, GEnital anomalies, and Immunodeficiency".

LS is caused by germline pathogenic variants affecting one of four genes encoding the DNA mismatch repair (MMR) system components: *MLH1*, *MSH2*, *MSH6* and *PMS2*. These genes encode proteins that are required for the repair of mismatches in the base-pairing of genomic DNA, thereby ensuring the integrity of genomic information [34]. MMR deficiency results in a hypermutability with 100–1000 fold increased mutational rates [35]. Due to slippage in the replication process, runs of repetitive nucleotides are prone to base-pairing errors, resulting in the diagnostic observation of "microsatellite instability" in MMR-deficient tumors. As MMR proteins also signal through the ATM/ATR pathway, MMR-deficient cells fail to undergo damage-induced cell cycle arrest and apoptosis [28,36–38].

Individuals with LS are usually heterozygous for a pathogenic MMR gene variant, and somatic inactivation of the second allele ("second hit") is required to develop a carcinoma from the respective cell type. This commonly occurs via a loss of heterozygosity, e.g., through deletion of the second allele. Another mode of somatic inactivation is gene promoter methylation, which is the main cause of sporadic tumors with MMR deficiency, particularly for *MLH1* [39,40]. In a small proportion of patients, the hypermethylation can be induced by constitutional deletions of the neighboring gene *EPCAM* (adjacent to *MSH2*); these germline deletions thus represent additional hereditary factors [41,42]. Constitutional hypermethylation has also been reported for *MHL1*, with some cases occurring de novo in non-transmissible Lynch Syndrome, but in other cases the underlying epimutations can be inherited [41,43,44]. In addition, few reports exist about deletions or inversions affecting both *MLH1* and *LRRFIP2* (upstream of *MLH1*) that either create expressed, but non-functional, gene fusions or inactivation of both genes [45–47].

Rare cases with biallelic hereditary variants in MMR genes and a constitutional MMR deficiency (CMMRD) have also been described, including few endometrial cancer patients [48–50]. The syndrome is also known as Turcot Syndrome. In such patients, where the "second hit" is already inherited, hematological or brain tumors in addition to LS-associated carcinomas already manifest at childhood and endometrial cancer can occur in young females, suggesting intensified gynecological surveillance starting at age 20 [49].

Data from the Prospective Lynch Syndrome Database (PLSD) indicate that the average lifetime risks of LS-associated endometrial cancers in heterozygotes are high. Risks to age 75 years for heterozygous *MLH1* variant carriers were 37% (30–47%), for *MSH2* variant carriers 49% (40–61%), for *MSH6* variant carriers 41% (29–62%) and for *PMS2* variant carriers 13% (5–50%) [32]. These risk estimates are in a similar range as for colorectal cancer and are 3–4 times higher than for ovarian cancer [24,32]. *PMS2* variants seem to confer a somewhat lower endometrial cancer risk than variants in the other three genes [32,51]. Perhaps consistent with a more moderate penetrance, it has turned out that *PMS2* variants may be more common in colon cancer patients with a less pronounced family history that would not fulfill the Amsterdam criteria for LS syndrome [52]. It remains to be seen whether this holds true for endometrial cancer.

MMR deficiency in endometrial cancer may be best assessed using immunohistochemical (IHC) staining for the four major DNA mismatch repair proteins (MLH1, MSH2, MSH6 and PMS2), which appears to outperform the classical microsatellite instability testing [53]. Loss or abnormality of nuclear staining for any of the proteins would indicate MMR deficiency. This is a common observation also in sporadic endometrial tumors of the endometrioid type [54], and genetic testing at the germline level will then be required to distinguish between LS and sporadic origin. As will be discussed later, this will make an important difference in the medical counseling and surveillance of these patients.

1.3.3. Cowden Syndrome

Cowden Syndrome (CS), named after the first described patient Rachel Cowden, is an autosomal dominant syndrome that has been associated with a germline mutation in *PTEN* [55–57] (for review see [58]). This gene encodes a phosphatase involved in cell signaling pathways affecting cell proliferation and survival. CS is a hamartoma and cancer syndrome that affects about 1 in 200,000 individuals and predisposes to an increased lifetime risk for cancers of the breast, thyroid, kidney, endometrium, colon and for melanoma [59]. Endometrial cancer occurs in 21–28% of CS patients [60–62] and can develop at a very early age [63,64]. Immunohistochemistry shows loss of PTEN staining in endometrial cancers of CS patients, however, somatic mutation of *PTEN* and therefore loss of PTEN expression are also common observations in sporadic endometrial cancer [65,66]. Germline pathogenic *PTEN* variants are very rare in endometrial cancer patients outside of CS families [67].

CS is genetically heterogeneous, however, and at less stringent criteria only some 25% of CS patients harbored germline *PTEN* loss-of-function variants [68]. About 10% of Cowden and Cowden-like syndrome individuals without a detected *PTEN* variant have been found to carry germline gain-of-function variants in *AKT1* or *PIK3CA* that are predicted to act in the same PI3K/AKT signaling pathway, which is inhibited by PTEN [68]. The relative proportion of endometrial cancers in this group of CS patients remains to be established.

1.3.4. Further Candidate Genes

POLE and *POLD1*

Germline variants within the exonuclease domains of the DNA replication and proof-reading polymerases POLD1 and POLE have been identified as dominantly inherited predispositions in colorectal cancer and have also been implicated in susceptibility to endometrial cancer [69–73]. At the presently low numbers, the relative risks for endometrial cancer have not yet been quantified but pedigrees were consistent with a hereditary predisposition. Biallelic *POLE* variants have also been found to cause a growth retardation and immunodeficiency syndrome [74,75]; however, the loss-of-function variants causing this syndrome seem to be distinct from the missense variants in the catalytic domain that confer the non-syndromic susceptibility to cancer [74].

MUTYH

The *MUTYH* gene encodes a protein of the base excision repair system, which repairs oxidative DNA damage. MUTYH-associated polyposis is an autosomal recessively inherited predisposition to adenomatous polyposis and colorectal cancer. While biallelic variants have been associated with a 75% lifetime risk of colon cancer, monoallelic variants may confer an only 7% lifetime risk of colon cancer [76]. Some results have been presented that heterozygotes for *MUTYH* variants may also carry an about two-fold increased risk for endometrial cancer [77,78]. However, the evidence is limited so far and larger replication studies are warranted. A splice variant of *MUTYH*, c.934-2A>G, occurs at a carrier frequency of up to 3% in East Asian populations but has not firmly been linked to disease.

NTHL1

The *NTLH1* gene encodes another protein of the base excision repair system in which mutations were reported as an autosomal recessively inherited predisposition to adenomatous polyposis and colorectal cancer [79]. Homozygosity for a germline nonsense variant in *NTLH1* was identified in multiple polyposis-affected patients from three unrelated families, all including women who developed an endometrial malignancy [79]. A subsequent study of another 17 families with biallelic *NTLH1* variants indicated a high incidence of polyposis coli and breast carcinomas but also identified endometrial cancer patients in 4 of the 17 families [80]. According to these findings, constitutional *NTHL1* deficiency underlies a high-risk hereditary multitumor syndrome that appears to predispose homozygotes to colon cancer, breast cancer and endometrial cancer. It is unknown whether *NTHL1* monoallelic variants also confer some increase in cancer risk, as has been suggested for *MUTYH* heterozygotes, but from the available evidence the heterozygote risk, if any, is likely to be small.

BRCA1

A multinational cohort study of the Breast Cancer Linkage Consortium involving 11,847 *BRCA1* variant carriers reported a significant two-to-three-fold increase in the risk of endometrial cancer [81]. However, the interpretation of these results is complicated by the fact that *BRCA1* variant carriers may take tamoxifen, which is known to increase endometrial cancer risk (for a more extensive review see [26]). Subsequent studies identified a larger risk for those women taking tamoxifen compared to those without, and conflicting results have been obtained whether there is any tamoxifen-independent residual risk of endometrial cancer for carriers of a pathogenic *BRCA1* or *BRCA2* variant [82,83]. Evidence has been presented that *BRCA1* variant carriers after risk-reducing salpingo-oophorectomy may have an increased risk of the more aggressive but rarer serous/serous-like endometrial cancers, though no significant risk of the endometrioid subtype cancer [84], and that these *BRCA1*-associated endometrial cancers are associated with an unfavorable outcome [85]. However, more research is required to corroborate these observations.

1.3.5. Low-Penetrance Susceptibility Loci

A growing body of evidence has linked single-nucleotide variants with polymorphic frequencies at various genomic regions to an altered risk of endometrial carcinoma. This has mainly been accomplished through genome-wide case-control association studies (GWAS) conducted by the Endometrial Cancer Association Consortium [27]. A first genome-wide significant endometrial cancer susceptibility region was identified in the 5′-portion of the gene *HNF1B* [86]. Subsequent GWAS with higher coverage and larger sample size yielded additional 15 genomic risk loci so far [27,87–89], including some known pan-cancer gene loci such as *MYC*, *CDKN2A* or *NF1*. Interestingly, a comparison with GWAS results from other clinical entities revealed an overlap of six loci with traits associated with steroid hormone levels [27]. Furthermore, credible causal endometrial cancer risk variants were enriched at epigenetic marks that were activated by estrogen stimulation in endometrial cancer cells, supporting the causal role of estrogen in this cancer (see O'Mara et al., 2019 [27]). One initially genome-wide significant hit was the genomic locus for *AKT1*, a gene also implicated in Cowden Syndrome (see Section 1.3.3). Subsequent functional studies showed that the most likely causal variant in this region, the risk allele of rs2494737, generates a binding site for the transcription factor YY1 that would stimulate *AKT1* expression [90]. However, with increasing sample size the *AKT1* locus has fallen below the genome-wide significance threshold, and further studies will be needed to finally prove its relevance.

Although each of the 16 identified genome-wide significant variants has only a small effect on risk, they are common polymorphisms with a cumulative contribution to the familial relative risk of the disease. It has been estimated that common genetic variants of the type that can be tagged by standard GWAS arrays potentially account for approximately 28% of the familial relative risk of endometrial cancer, and that the 16 risk variants identified to date account for approximately one quarter of this figure, suggesting that many more genetic risk variants remain to be found [27,89]. Meta-analyses are presently being performed to identify additional variants relevant for endometrial cancer and a related disease. For instance, a cross-cancer GWAS for endometrial and colon cancer identified a risk variant in *SH2B3* [91], and a cross-disease GWAS for endometriosis and endometrial cancer identified a risk region within the *PTPRD* gene [92]. It is likely that more such meta-analyses will uncover additional loci.

With increasing number of low-penetrance variants for endometrial cancer, it may be possible to construct polygenic risk scores that should be helpful in future genetic risk prediction and counseling [93]. Equally importantly, every newly identified region adds to our knowledge about the etiology of the disease and can point to possible pharmacological targets. In addition, single nucleotide polymorphism genotypes have already proven very helpful in corroborating epidemiological and clinical observations by detecting potentially causal relationships between physiological traits and endometrial cancer through Mendelian randomization analyses [27,94–97].

2. Clinical Implications and Management

2.1. *Screening for Hereditary Syndromes among Patients with Endometrial Cancer*

In order to identify recently published relevant clinical studies in the field we performed a PubMed search using a strategy as presented in Figure 2 and checked cross references.

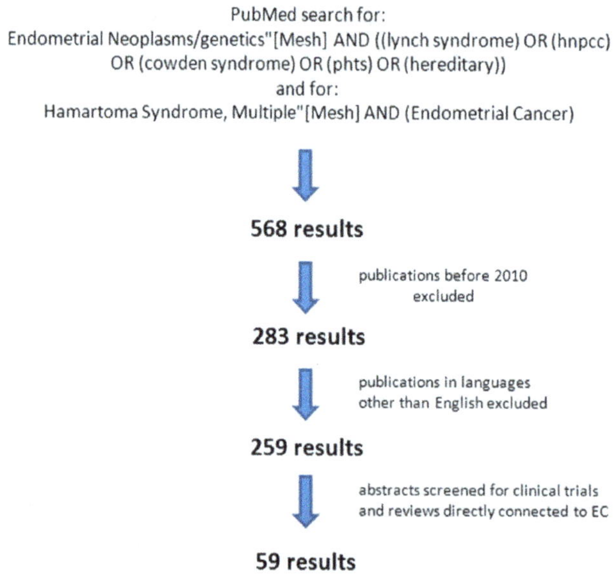

Figure 2. PubMed search strategy.

Patients with hereditary forms of endometrial cancer are mostly diagnosed at a younger mean age (48 years) compared to patients in an unscreened population (68 years). About 10% of all patients are diagnosed prior to age 50. Moreover, in female Lynch Syndrome mutation carriers, endometrial cancer often precedes other cancers and therefore can be considered a "sentinel" cancer allowing identification of patients with mutations in MMR genes [98].

Investigations of screening strategies mainly focused on the most frequent hereditary syndrome, represented by the LS. Due to their low prevalence, Cowden and other hereditary tumor syndromes with EC risk are just rarely diagnosed in an unscreened EC population. A targeted genomic search for specific non-LS mutations appears to be only useful, if individual or family history suggests so. With the Amsterdam criteria and the Bethesda guidelines, two criteria sets mainly based on patients history have been established to identify LS individuals and screen individuals at risk for further genetic testing [99].

Several cohort studies have investigated the best screening strategy and target group for LS associated EC [39,100–105] (Table 2, see Figure 2 for PubMed search strategy). Despite the lower mean age of patients with hereditary forms of EC, a considerable number of LS-associated cancers (62% and 64% in the two biggest cohorts) were diagnosed after the age of 50, and about 37% of cases did not fulfill clinical criteria (Amsterdam/revised Bethesda) especially in cases age 50 and older. These numbers demonstrate that a screening strategy based on individual or family history or early disease manifestation (prior to age 50) alone has a low sensitivity. Therefore, some authors advocate a universal somatic screening strategy for LS independent of these factors below an age threshold (<60 years or <70 years), which still needs to be defined [39,100,101,104].

Table 2. Cohort studies investigating screening strategies for hereditary syndromes among endometrial cancer (EC) patients.

Study	Number	Design	Patients	Strategy	Results
Backes et al., 2009 [94]	$n = 140$	Prospective	Unselected EC patients	IHC MMR proteins → invitation for genetic counseling when suggestive for LS.	30 patients (21%) with loss of one or more MMR proteins, 15/30 invited to genetic counseling, 2/15 accepted both negative for LS.
Buchanan et al., 2014 [35]	$n = 702$	Prospective (multicentric)	Unselected EC patients	IHC MMR proteins + DNA *MLH1* methylation status for all tumors exhibiting MLH1/PMS2 loss → genetic testing in IHC MRD patients.	170 (24%) of 702 patients showed MMR loss. 158/170 available for genetic testing. 22/158 truncating gene variants. Overall carrier frequency 3%. Testing MMR loss by IHC in women <60 years at diagnosis was optimal regarding sensitivity and cost-effectiveness.
Egoavil et al., 2013 [88]	$n = 173$	Prospective (monocentric)	Unselected EC patients	MMR-IHC and MSI testing MMR mutation testing in positive cases. If MMR gene mutation was detected or *MLH1* methylation in the blood test was positive, patients were classified as LS positive.	61/173 patients had abnormal IHC or MSI results. 8/61 patients tested positive for LS (prevalence 4.6% (8/173)).
Ferguson et al., 2014 [89]	$n = 117$	Prospective (monocentric)	Unselected EC patients	Family history assessment, IHC screening for MMR, MSI testing, tumor morphology followed by germline testing for MMR gene mutations.	34/117 had MMR deficiency in IHC. 27/117 had MSI, 7/27 LS (5.9%). IHC < 60 had sensitivity of 100%, specificity of 86.1%, with PPV of 58.3% and NPV of 100%, family history and tumor morphology had poorest performance with a specificity of 42.1%.

Table 2. *Cont.*

Study	Number	Design	Patients	Strategy	Results
Gausachs et al., 2012 [96]	n.a.	n.a.	n = 122 CRC patients with MMRD, 57 LS, 48 MSS cancers and positive family history for CRC, 73 sporadic CRC.	*BRAF* mutation and *MLH1* promoter hypermethylation were assessed and a decision model was developed to estimate incremental costs of alternative case finding methods for detecting *MLH1* mutation carriers.	Sensitivity of the absence of *BRAF* mutations for depiction of LS patients was 96% (23/24) and specificity was 28% (13/47). Specificity of *MLH1* promoter hypermethylation for depiction of sporadic tumors was 66% (31/47) and sensitivity of 96% (23/24). The cost per additional mutation detected by hypermethylation analysis lower when compared with *BRAF* and germinal *MLH1* mutation study.
Hampel et al., 2006 [90]; Hampel et al., 2007 [91]	n = 562	Prospective (multicentric)	Unselected EC patients	MSI testing, if positive germline mutations in MMR genes were tested.	119/562 were MSI positive, 11 germline mutations in at least one MMR gene, one patient not MSI positive but germline mutation in *MSH6*, one patient's MSI test failed. 8/13 patients w/o criteria for HNPCC syndrome, 8/13 diagnosed >50 years.
Leenen et al., 2012 [92]	n = 179	Prospective (multicentric)	Unselected EC patients	MSI/IHC for MMR proteins. *MLH1* promoter hypermethylation if MSI high and MLH1 absent. Tumors classified as: (1) likely to be caused by LS, (MSI high and MMR protein deficiency) (2) sporadic MSI-H (MSI high, MLH1 absent, and *MLH1* promoter hyper-methylated), or (3) MSS.	Eleven EC patients found likely to have LS (6%) Germline analyses revealed 7 MMR mutations. Ten patients likely to have LS (92%) were >50 years. 31 sporadic MSI-H tumors with *MLH1* promoter hypermethylation (17%; 95% CI 13–24%) identified.
Moline et al., 2013 [95]	n = 245	Prospective	EC patients <50 years or suspicious personal history or histo-pathologic features. EC <69 years or at any age with suspicious features	MSI and IHC, later IHC for two proteins, and *MLH1* promoter methylation analysis when indicated. Genetic counselor contacted patients to offer counseling appointments.	245 EC screened. 62 (25%) abnormal results, 42 patients referred for genetic counseling. 34/42 patients underwent genetic counseling, 28 pursued genetic testing, 11 LS. Age and pathology overlooked 27 eligible cases, 3 cases of LS were only found by clinician request.

Cohort studies investigating screening strategies for hereditary syndromes among EC patients (IHC, Immunohistochemistry; MMR, Mismatch repair; LS, Lynch-Syndrome; MMRD, Mismatch Repair Deficiency; MSI, microsatellite instability; MSS, microsatellite stability; n.a., not applicable; NPV, negative predictive value; PPV, positive predictive value; CRC, colorectal cancer; EC, endometrial cancer).

Immunohistochemical staining for MMR proteins (MLH1, MSH2, MSH6 and PMS2) in tumor specimen can serve as a screening test and is highly concordant with or even outperforms microsatellite instability testing in endometrial cancer [53]. If IHC screening reveals a loss of expression of one or more MMR proteins and if gene methylation can be excluded (*MLH1* promoter), tumor sequencing may uncover the underlying pathogenic variants and germ line testing will reveal whether there is a hereditary predisposition in LS patients [39,100–102,104–110]. MMR protein loss or high microsatellite instability is present in 23–35% of unselected endometrial cancers.

The identification of a pathogenic germline mutation in an endometrial cancer patient (index patient) allows the predictive genetic testing of unaffected family members (individuals at risk). This helps to identify LS among endometrial cancer patients and to counsel and to subject them to intensified cancer screening programs. Importantly, if individual or family history is suspicious and loss of MMR proteins is demonstrated by IHC of tumor tissue, LS must be suspected even if germline analysis cannot confirm the mutation. According to the largest published series, the mutation detection rate (positive predictive value, PPV) of an immunohistochemistry staining of MMR proteins in order to identify LS associated endometrial cancers is 46% if all unselected endometrial cancer cases below age 60 are analyzed, IHC is eventful and methylation as a cause of MLH1/PMS2 loss can be excluded. The authors conclude that this screening strategy provides the highest PPV regarding the identification of mutation carriers with the lowest number of diagnostic tests and therefore appears to be the most effective strategy analyzed in this series [39]. This relatively low PPV for Lynch syndrome is probably due to unrecognized MMR gene somatic mutations, so the underlying tumor biology could still be driven by mismatch repair deficiency.

In a prospective cohort study different screening strategies for LS including IHC, family history and tumor morphology were investigated and compared regarding test performance criteria. IHC in women aged <60 years had the best performance characteristics, with a sensitivity of 100%, a specificity of 86.1%, a positive predictive value of 58.3% and a negative predictive value of 100%. Family history and tumor morphology both had the lowest sensitivity at 71.4%. Overall tumor morphology had the poorest performance, with a specificity of 42.1% [101].

Hence, IHC for MMR proteins has proven to be most sensitive and may be favored over MSI (microsatellite instability) testing, which still can serve as a backup strategy. Patients with MMR-deficient tumors could then undergo targeted next-generation-sequencing and methylation testing of their tumor tissue and/or, if family history or age criteria are suspicious, targeted next-generation sequencing of MMR genes in their germline (blood) samples. Possible paths to LS diagnosis are illustrated in Figure 3.

2.2. Gynecologic Surveillance in Families with Hereditary EC

Recommendations for gynecologic surveillance strategies in LS families differ between guidelines and countries. Overall, there is no evidence to support a systematic screening for endometrial cancer as no study has demonstrated a true survival benefit. In an unscreened population, endometrial cancers are mostly detected at early stages as most postmenopausal patients present with uterine bleedings and seek medical advice early. Gynecologic examination and finally hysteroscopy, dilation and curettage will lead to the diagnosis. At early stages, standard therapy consisting of total hysterectomy plus bilateral salpingo-oophorectomy (BSO) and pelvic washings will result in a remarkable 5-year survival rate between 75% and 83%. Considering the overall good prognosis of EC due to usually early detection, it appears difficult to demonstrate a true survival benefit of a general systematic screening strategy even in a high risk group.

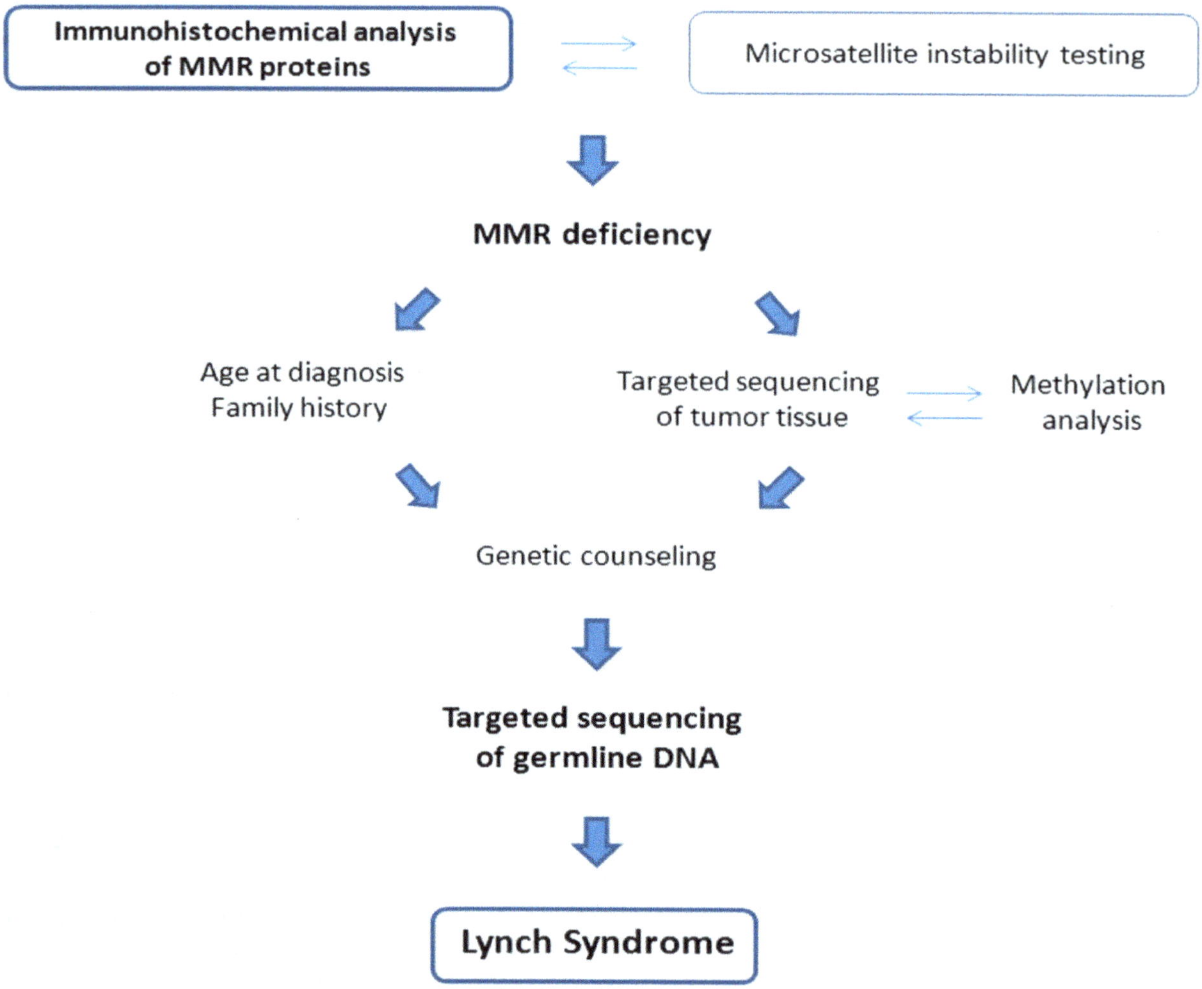

Figure 3. Paths to a Lynch Syndrome diagnosis, starting from the detection of MMR (mismatch repair) deficiency through IHC (immunohistochemical) or MSI (microsatellite instability) analysis. Patients with clinical criteria of Lynch Syndrome may be tested directly for germline predispositions (left arm). Targeted sequencing of MMR genes in tumor tissue, perhaps complemented by methylation analyses, may also reveal pathogenic variants that would qualify to be tested in the germline and may ultimately lead to a LS diagnosis (right arm).

However, as LS patients on average are diagnosed twenty years earlier than patients with sporadic endometrial cancer, they are not rarely pre- or peri-menopausal and irregular bleedings as a cardinal symptom of endometrial cancer harder to identify in this group. Therefore EC might potentially be detected later and at later stages. This provides the rationale for a systematic screening especially in the population of pre- and perimenopausal LS mutation carriers. A number of cohort studies investigated which screening strategy is the most effective (Table 3, see Figure 2 for PubMed search strategy). Transvaginal ultrasound alone seemed not to be sufficient for early detection of endometrial cancers in LS patients especially in pre- and peri-menopausal patients [111–113]. In another study on 175 LS patients (759 patient years) investigating transvaginal sonography (TVS) in combination with endometrial biopsy (EB), 4 of 14 endometrial cancers were detected by TVS and 8 by EB alone [114], which in addition also detected 14 premalignant hyperplasias in the cohort.

Table 3. Studies on different gynecologic surveillance strategies in families with hereditary EC.

Study	Number	Design	Patients	Intervention	Results
Dove-Edwin et al., 2002 [100]	$n = 269$	Prospective (multicentric)	Unselected women from HNPCC or HNPCC-like families.	Annual or biannual TVU.	During surveillance two EC, none detected by screening.
Helder-Woolderink et al., 2013 [106]	$n = 75$	Prospective (monocentric)	Women >30 years with LS or first-degree relatives with LS.	Period 1 TVU and CA 125; Period 2 TVU, CA 125 and EB to detect EC or precancerous lesions.	Six pre-malignancies and one EC detected. 0/6 would have been missed without EB, annual TVU seems to detect pre-malignancies in women with LS or first-degree relatives with LS.
Lécuru et al., 2008 [104]	$n = 62$	Prospective (monocentric)	Unselected women with LS/meeting Amsterdam II Criteria.	Women with least one hysteroscopy and EB during standard screening.	Three possibly malignant lesions detected, none of them missed w/o hysteroscopy due to abnormal uterine bleeding.
Manchanda et al., 2012 [105]	$n = 41$	Prospective observational	Unselected women with LS.	Annual OHES vs. annual TVS.	OHES detected 4/4 EC/AEH, TVS 2/4; OHES has similar specificity, higher PLR and lower NLR.
Renkonen-Sinisalo et al., 2007 [103]	$n = 175$	Prospective Cohort Study	Unselected women with LS.	TVU and EB.	14/175 patients diagnosed with EC. 11/14 diagnosed by surveillance. 4/11 diagnosed by TVUS only. EB detected 14 cases of potentially premalignant hyperplasia. Cases detected by surveillance at more favorable disease stage. 0/14 detected patients but 6/83 symptomatic LS patients died of EC (n.s., $p = 0.4$).
Rijcken et al., 2003 [101]	$n = 41$	Prospective	Women with LS.	Annual TVU and serum level CA 125.	17/179 TVUs suggested biopsy. 3/17 AEH. One EC as an interval carcinoma, no OC.
Ryan et al., 2017 [107]	$n = 162$	Retrospective	Unselected women with LS diagnosed with EC.	Comparison of mutated MMR genes and type of mutation.	Patients with *MSH6* variants and those with truncating *MLH1* variants diagnosed with EC at later age (median difference 6.6 years; 95% CI 2.7–10.4; $p = 0.002$ for truncating *MLH1* variants).

Cohort studies on different gynecologic surveillance strategies in families with hereditary EC. (HNPCC, hereditary non-polyposis coli; TVU, transvaginal ultrasound; TVS, transvaginal sonography; CA, cancer-antigen; EB, endometrial biopsy; OHES, Outpatient hysteroscopy and endometrial sampling; EC, endometrial cancer; AEH, atypical endometrial hyperplasia; PLR/NLR, positive/negative likelihood ratio; OC, ovarian cancer).

The results of three prospective endometrial cancer screening studies are inconsistent. However, these studies had a low number of cases and short follow-up. In 58 LS patients, 2 endometrial cancers were detected combining TVS and EB [115]. A second study on 41 LS patients screened by annual TVS, outpatient hysteroscopy and EB half of all endometrial cancers were not detected by TVS, concluding that EB enhanced sensitivity of screening significantly [116]. These results are contrasted by the results of the third study on 75 LS patients (300 women years) in which all 6 premalignant lesions and endometrial cancers were detected by ultrasound [117].

Taking the published data on screening together, the evidence for a general endometrial cancer screening in LS or CS patients remains weak. However, there is evidence that annual EB is superior to TVS for identification of endometrial cancer and other premalignant endometrial lesions. Although a group of European experts recommends a screening for all mutation carriers using TVS and EB starting from age 35 to 40 [49], the best age of onset of cancer surveillance remains unclear. A retrospective cohort study utilizing the Genetic Register Lynch Syndrome Database from the Manchester Centre for Genomic Medicine identified 568 female LS carriers and investigated whether mutated gene and type of mutation influence age at onset of LS associated cancers [118]. In this cohort 162 endometrial cancers (38%) were diagnosed. Of all cases, 38% were attributable to *MSH6*, 30% to *MSH2* and 27% to *MLH1* mutations. Women with *MSH6* mutations with endometrial cancer were older compared to women carrying other mutations. The mean ages of endometrial cancer onset were 49 (range 17–71), 47 (range 32–72) and 53 (range 42–66) for women with *MLH1*, *MSH2* and *MSH6* mutations, respectively. There were no endometrial cancer patients with *PMS2* mutations in this series. In the Prospective Lynch Syndrome Database (PLSD), as discussed above, the risk for endometrial cancer at age 75 in *PMS2* variant carriers was estimated at only 13% [32]. This would suggest a potential role for a stratified rather than uniform surveillance strategy depending on the underlying genomic alteration.

2.3. Prophylactic Surgery

BSO should be considered when child-bearing is completed ideally at around age 40 [119]. A retrospective analysis revealed a significant decrease in endometrial cancer incidence after prophylactic hysterectomy in LS patients. However, prospective data showing long-term quality of life and investigations on potential negative effects are still missing [120]. In view of the high lifetime risk to develop endometrial cancer, also the psychological benefit after completion of family planning and prophylactic hysterectomy needs to be considered. When offered, many LS patients opt for a prophylactic operation. German colon cancer guidelines recommend offering prophylactic hysterectomy if laparotomy or laparoscopy is scheduled for other reasons to avoid re-laparotomy/laparoscopy when endometrial cancer is diagnosed later in life.

Basis for the recommendation of prophylactic BSO is the fact that there are no effective screening strategies for ovarian cancer available as demonstrated in numerous studies on patients with hereditary breast and ovarian cancer. The only effective measure to improve survival is prophylactic BSO. In LS, the risk for ovarian cancer is increased with a lifetime incidence of about 12% but to a lesser extent than in carriers of a pathogenic *BRCA1* or *BRCA2* variant. However, negative effects of premenopausal BSO and therefore endocrine deprivation on quality of life, sexual function, bone density and cardiovascular morbidity also need consideration. Moreover, OC risk for pathologic *MSH6* variants carriers appears to be low and is not even measurable in *PMS2* variant carriers [28]. According to the prospective Lynch syndrome database the prognosis of LS associated OC with an approximate 10 year survival of over 80%, which is significantly better than survival in pathologic *BRCA1* or *BRCA2* variant carriers [28]. Accordingly, a general recommendation regarding prophylactic BSO in particular for premenopausal LS patients cannot be given. However, all patients need counseling regarding the pros and cons in order to make an informed choice for or against prophylactic BSO.

In a series of 39 prophylactic hysterectomy specimens in LS patients with a mean age of 45 years and without clinical or imaging signs of endometrial cancer, Bartosch and coworkers [121] found three invasive endometrial cancers and four atypical hyperplasias, which are considered to be precancerous lesions. This finding of incidental endometrial cancers and atypical hyperplasias was also confirmed in case series of other investigators, demonstrating that prophylactic surgery is effective and can prevent advances stage disease in asymptomatic patients [122].

2.4. MSI and Defective Mismatch Repair as Therapeutic Target in Mutation Carriers with EC

There are clinical trials ongoing for metastatic EC investigating the effect of targeted or immunotherapy drugs. POLE mutated ECs and ECs with MSI similar to triple negative breast cancers express multiple neoantigens. These interact with activated T-lymphocytes and thereby trigger a potentially strong antitumor immune response in the tissue. Accordingly, recent studies found LS EC to be highly immunogenic [123,124].

Tumor cells expressing Programmed cell death 1 ligand 1 (PD-L1, also known as CD274) bind the T-cell receptor PD-1, which suppresses the immune response and helps tumor cells to survive. The PD-L1/PD-1 interaction is targeted by check point inhibitors like pembrolizumab. The FDA has recently granted an accelerated approval to pembrolizumab for the treatment of cancers with defective MMR-repair (including EC) based on the positive results of a phase two basket study including various cancer types (Keynote-028) [125]. At the 2019 ESMO conference, the results of a phase Ib/II Study (Keynote-146) investigating the combination of pembrolizumab and lenvatinib (oral multikinase inhibitor targeting VEGF-1–3, FGFR 1–4, PDGFRα, RET and KIT) in 124 patients with progressive metastatic EC after $\leq$2 courses of chemotherapy were presented. The objective response rate was 38% in the overall cohort, and remarkable 63.6% for patients with MSI or defective MMR [126].

Preclinical studies have further suggested that Poly-ADP-Ribose-Polymerase (PARP) inhibitors, perhaps in combination with PI3-kinase inhibitors, could be useful in endometrial cancer treatment as most endometrial tumors are PTEN-deficient [127,128]. Twelve clinical trials including PARP inhibitors are presently ongoing [129]. Such medication may also prove effective in high-grade non-endometrioid endometrial cancers that have been shown to be deficient in homologous recombinational DNA repair [130].

3. Conclusions

Endometrial cancer is a genetically heterogeneous disease with a prominent contribution of mismatch repair gene mutations that cause Lynch Syndrome. Immunohistochemical staining of MMR proteins is an effective screening strategy to identify those patients and to provide genetic counseling and cancer surveillance to their blood relatives. Prophylactic hysterectomy and bilateral salpingo-oophorectomy are effective preventive surgeries but need to be considered on an individual basis. With the identification of frequently targeted cancer driver genes, stratified treatments are emerging and might prove useful in the future. A few endometrial cancer susceptibility genes beyond Lynch Syndrome have been identified more recently, but their pathogenic variants are collectively rare. More common polymorphisms contribute to endometrial cancer risk in an additive fashion and have already provided insight into novel disease-associated molecular pathways. Larger case-control studies are needed to fully explore the genomic landscape of endometrial cancer predisposition.

References

1. Olson, S.H.; Jewell, E.; Rastogi, R.M. Endometrial Cancer. In *Women and Health*, 2nd ed.; Academic Press: Cambridge, MA, USA; Elsevier: Amsterdam, The Netherlands, 2013; pp. 1147–1158. ISBN 978-0-12-384978-6. [CrossRef]
2. Amant, F.; Moerman, P.; Neven, P.; Timmerman, D.; van Limbergen, E.; Vergote, I. Endometrial cancer. *Lancet* **2005**, *366*, 491–505. [CrossRef]

3. Morice, P.; Leary, A.; Creutzberg, C.; Abu-Rustum, N.; Darai, E. Endometrial cancer. *Lancet* **2016**, *387*, 1094–1108. [CrossRef]
4. Shai, A.; Segev, Y.; Narod, S. Genetics of endometrial cancer. *Fam. Cancer* **2014**, *13*, 499–505. [CrossRef]
5. Benedet, J.L.; Miller, D.M. Gynaecologic Cancer. In *UICC International Union against Cancer Manual of Clinical Oncology*, 7th ed.; Pollack, R.E., Ed.; Wiley: New York, NY, USA, 1999; pp. 537–562.
6. Calle, E.E.; Rodriguez, C.; Walker-Thurmond, K.; Thun, M.J. Overweight, obesity, and mortality from cancer in a prospectively studied cohort of US adults. *N. Engl. J. Med.* **2003**, *348*, 1625–1638. [CrossRef]
7. Reeves, G.K.; Pirie, K.; Beral, V.; Green, J.; Spencer, E.; Bull, D.; Million Women Study Collaboration. Cancer incidence and mortality in relation to body mass index in the million women study: Cohort study. *BMJ* **2007**, *335*, 1134. [CrossRef]
8. Kaitu'u-Lino, T.J.; Ye, L.; Gargett, C.E. Reepithelialization of the uterine surface arises from endometrial glands: Evidence from a functional mouse model of breakdown and repair. *Endocrinology* **2010**, *151*, 3386–3395. [CrossRef]
9. Gargett, C.E.; Schwab, K.E.; Deane, J.A. Endometrial stem/progenitor cells: The first 10 years. *Hum. Reprod. Update* **2016**, *22*, 137–163. [CrossRef]
10. Sherman, M.E.; Sturgeon, S.; Brinton, L.A.; Potischman, N.; Kurman, R.J.; Berman, M.L.; Mortel, R.; Twiggs, L.B.; Barrett, R.J.; Wilbanks, G.D. Risk factors and hormone levels in patients with serous and endometrioid uterine carcinomas. *Mod. Pathol.* **1997**, *10*, 963–968.
11. Setiawan, V.W.; Yang, H.P.; Pike, M.C.; McCann, S.E.; Yu, H.; Xiang, Y.B.; Wolk, A.; Wentzensen, N.; Weiss, N.S.; Webb, P.M.; et al. Type I and II endometrial cancers: Have they different risk factors? *J. Clin. Oncol.* **2013**, *31*, 2607–2618. [CrossRef]
12. Cancer Genome Atlas Research Network; Kandoth, C.; Schultz, N.; Cherniack, A.D.; Akbani, R.; Liu, Y.; Shen, H.; Robertson, A.G.; Pashtan, I.; Shen, R.; et al. Integrated genomic characterization of endometrial carcinoma. *Nature* **2013**, *497*, 67–73. [CrossRef]
13. Suda, K.; Nakaoka, H.; Yoshihara, K.; Ishiguro, T.; Tamura, R.; Mori, Y.; Yamawaki, K.; Adachi, S.; Takahashi, T.; Kase, H.; et al. Clonal Expansion and Diversification of Cancer-Associated Mutations in Endometriosis and Normal Endometrium. *Cell Rep.* **2018**, *24*, 1777–1789. [CrossRef]
14. Alexandrov, L.B.; Kim, J.; Haradhvala, N.J.; Huang, M.N.; Tian Ng, A.W.; Wu, Y.; Boot, A.; Covington, K.R.; Gordenin, D.A.; Bergstrom, E.N.; et al. The repertoire of mutational signatures in human cancer. *Nature* **2020**, *578*, 94–101. [CrossRef] [PubMed]
15. Dou, Y.; Kawaler, E.A.; Cui Zhou, D.; Gritsenko, M.A.; Huang, C.; Blumenberg, L.; Karpova, A.; Petyuk, V.A.; Savage, S.R.; Satpathy, S.; et al. Clinical Proteomic Tumor Analysis Consortium. Proteogenomic Characterization of Endometrial Carcinoma. *Cell* **2020**, *180*, 729–748.e26. [CrossRef] [PubMed]
16. Moore, L.; Leongamornlert, D.; Coorens, T.; Sanders, M.A.; Ellis, P.; Dentro, S.C.; Dawson, K.J.; Butler, T.; Rahbari, R.; Mitchell, T.J.; et al. The mutational landscape of normal human endometrial epithelium. *Nature* **2020**, *580*, 640–646. [CrossRef] [PubMed]
17. Bae-Jump, V.L.; Levine, D.A. A catalogue of cancer-driving mutations in healthy tissue. *Nature* **2020**, *580*, 595–596. [CrossRef]
18. McKenzie, R.; Scott, R.J.; Otton, G.; Scurry, J. Early changes of endometrial neoplasia revealed by loss of mismatch repair gene protein expression in a patient diagnosed with Lynch syndrome. *Pathology* **2016**, *48*, 78–80. [CrossRef]
19. Win, A.K.; Reece, J.C.; Ryan, S. Family history and risk of endometrial cancer: A systematic review and meta-analysis. *Obstet. Gynecol.* **2015**, *125*, 89–98. [CrossRef]
20. Johnatty, S.E.; Tan, Y.Y.; Buchanan, D.D.; Bowman, M.; Walters, R.J.; Obermair, A.; Quinn, M.A.; Blomfield, P.B.; Brand, A.; Leung, Y.; et al. Family history of cancer predicts endometrial cancer risk independently of Lynch Syndrome: Implications for genetic counselling. *Gynecol. Oncol.* **2017**, *147*, 381–387. [CrossRef]
21. Lichtenstein, P.; Holm, N.V.; Verkasalo, P.K.; Iliadou, A.; Kaprio, J.; Koskenvuo, M.; Pukkala, E.; Skytthe, A.; Hemminki, K. Environmental and heritable factors in the causation of cancer–analyses of cohorts of twins from Sweden, Denmark, and Finland. *N. Engl. J. Med.* **2000**, *343*, 78–85. [CrossRef]
22. Lu, Y.; Ek, W.E.; Whiteman, D.; Vaughan, T.L.; Spurdle, A.B.; Easton, D.F.; Pharoah, P.D.; Thompson, D.J.; Dunning, A.M.; Hayward, N.K.; et al. Most common 'sporadic' cancers have a significant germline genetic component. *Hum. Mol. Genet.* **2014**, *23*, 6112–6118. [CrossRef]

23. Mucci, L.A.; Hjelmborg, J.B.; Harris, J.R.; Czene, K.; Havelick, D.J.; Scheike, T.; Graff, R.E.; Holst, K.; Möller, S.; Unger, R.H.; et al. Familial risk and heritability of cancer among twins in Nordic countries. *J. Am. Med. Assoc.* **2016**, *315*, 68–76. [CrossRef] [PubMed]
24. Lynch, H.T.; Lynch, P.M.; Lanspa, S.J.; Snyder, C.L.; Lynch, J.F.; Boland, C.R. Review of the Lynch syndrome: History, molecular genetics, screening, differential diagnosis, and medicolegal ramifications. *Clin. Genet.* **2009**, *76*, 1–18. [CrossRef] [PubMed]
25. Resnick, K.E.; Hampel, H.; Fishel, R.; Cohn, D.E. Current and emerging trends in Lynch syndrome identification in women with endometrial cancer. *Gynecol. Oncol.* **2009**, *114*, 128–134. [CrossRef] [PubMed]
26. Spurdle, A.B.; Bowman, M.A.; Shamsani, J.; Kirk, J. Endometrial cancer gene panels: Clinical diagnostic vs research germline DNA testing. *Mod. Pathol.* **2017**, *30*, 1048–1068. [CrossRef] [PubMed]
27. O'Mara, T.A.; Glubb, D.M.; Kho, P.F.; Thompson, D.J.; Spurdle, A.B. Genome-Wide Association Studies of Endometrial Cancer: Latest Developments and Future Directions. *Cancer Epidemiol. Biomark. Prev.* **2019**, *28*, 1095–1102. [CrossRef]
28. Cerretelli, G.; Ager, A.; Arends, M.J.; Frayling, I.M. Molecular pathology of Lynch syndrome. *J. Pathol.* **2020**, *250*, 518–531. [CrossRef]
29. Warthin, A.S. Heredity with reference to carcinoma. *Arch. Intern. Med.* **1913**, *12*, 546–555. [CrossRef]
30. Lynch, H.T.; Shaw, M.W.; Magnuson, C.W.; Larsen, A.L.; Krush, A.J. Hereditary factors in cancer: Study of two large Midwestern kindreds. *Arch. Intern. Med.* **1966**, *117*, 206–212. [CrossRef]
31. Møller, P.; Seppälä, T.T.; Bernstein, I.; Holinski-Feder, E.; Sala, P.; Gareth Evans, D.; Lindblom, A.; Macrae, F.; Blanco, I.; Sijmons, R.H.; et al. Cancer risk and survival in path_MMR carriers by gene and gender up to 75 years of age: A report from the prospective Lynch syndrome database. *Gut* **2018**, *67*, 1306–1316. [CrossRef]
32. Dominguez-Valentin, M.; Sampson, J.R.; Seppälä, T.T.; Ten Broeke, S.W.; Plazzer, J.P.; Nakken, S.; Engel, C.; Aretz, S.; Jenkins, M.A.; Sunde, L.; et al. Cancer risks by gene, age, and gender in 6350 carriers of pathogenic mismatch repair variants: Findings from the prospective Lynch syndrome database. *Genet. Med.* **2020**, *22*, 15–25. [CrossRef]
33. Joehlin-Price, A.S.; Perrino, C.M.; Stephens, J.; Backes, F.J.; Goodfellow, P.J.; Cohn, D.E.; Suarez, A.A. Mismatch repair protein expression in 1049 endometrial carcinomas, associations with body mass index, and other clinicopathologic variables. *Gynecol. Oncol.* **2014**, *133*, 43–47. [CrossRef] [PubMed]
34. Modrich, P.; Lahue, R. Mismatch repair in replication fidelity, genetic recombination, and cancer biology. *Annu. Rev. Biochem.* **1996**, *65*, 101–133. [CrossRef] [PubMed]
35. Preston, B.D.; Albertson, T.M.; Herr, A.J. DNA replication fidelity and cancer. *Semin. Cancer Biol.* **2010**, *20*, 281–293. [CrossRef] [PubMed]
36. Brown, K.D.; Rathi, A.; Kamath, R.; Beardsley, D.I.; Zhan, Q.; Mannino, J.L.; Baskaran, R. The mismatch repair system is required for S-phase checkpoint activation. *Nat. Genet.* **2003**, *33*, 80–84. [CrossRef]
37. Stojic, L.; Brun, R.; Jiricny, J. Mismatch repair and DNA damage signalling. *DNA Repair* **2004**, *3*, 1091–1101. [CrossRef]
38. Yoshioka, K.; Yoshioka, Y.; Hsieh, P. ATR kinase activation mediated by MutSalpha and MutLalpha in response to cytotoxic O6-methylguanine adducts. *Mol. Cell* **2006**, *22*, 501–510. [CrossRef]
39. Buchanan, D.D.; Tan, Y.Y.; Walsh, M.D.; Clendenning, M.; Metcalf, A.M.; Ferguson, K.; Arnold, S.T.; Thompson, B.A.; Lose, F.A.; Parsons, M.T.; et al. Tumor mismatch repair immunohistochemistry and DNA MLH1 methylation testing of patients with endometrial cancer diagnosed at age younger than 60 years optimizes triage for population-level germline mismatch repair gene mutation testing. *J. Clin. Oncol.* **2014**, *32*, 90–100. [CrossRef]
40. Pasanen, A.; Loukovaara, M.; Bützow, R. Clinicopathological significance of deficient DNA mismatch repair and MLH1 promoter methylation in endometrioid endometrial carcinoma. *Mod. Pathol.* **2020**, *33*, 1443–1452. [CrossRef]
41. Niessen, R.C.; Hofstra, R.M.; Westers, H.; Ligtenberg, M.J.; Kooi, K.; Jager, P.O.; de Groote, M.L.; Dijkhuizen, T.; Olderode-Berends, M.J.; Hollema, H.; et al. Germline hypermethylation of MLH1 and EPCAM deletions are a frequent cause of Lynch syndrome. *Genes Chromos. Cancer* **2009**, *48*, 737–744. [CrossRef]
42. Kempers, M.J.; Kuiper, R.P.; Ockeloen, C.W.; Chappuis, P.O.; Hutter, P.; Rahner, N.; Schackert, H.K.; Steinke, V.; Holinski-Feder, E.; Morak, M.; et al. Risk of colorectal and endometrial cancers in EPCAM deletion-positive Lynch syndrome: A cohort study. *Lancet Oncol.* **2011**, *12*, 49–55. [CrossRef]

43. Crépin, M.; Dieu, M.C.; Lejeune, S.; Escande, F.; Boidin, D.; Porchet, N.; Morin, G.; Manouvrier, S.; Mathieu, M.; Buisine, M.P. Evidence of constitutional MLH1 epimutation associated to transgenerational inheritance of cancer susceptibility. *Hum. Mutat.* **2012**, *33*, 180–188. [CrossRef]
44. Morak, M.; Ibisler, A.; Keller, G.; Jessen, E.; Laner, A.; Gonzales-Fassrainer, D.; Locher, M.; Massdorf, T.; Nissen, A.M.; Benet-Pagès, A.; et al. Comprehensive analysis of the MLH1 promoter region in 480 patients with colorectal cancer and 1150 controls reveals new variants including one with a heritable constitutional MLH1 epimutation. *J. Med. Genet.* **2018**, *55*, 240–248. [CrossRef]
45. Pinheiro, M.; Pinto, C.; Peixoto, A.; Veiga, I.; Mesquita, B.; Henrique, R.; Baptista, M.; Fragoso, M.; Sousa, O.; Pereira, H.; et al. A novel exonic rearrangement affecting MLH1 and the contiguous LRRFIP2 is a founder mutation in Portuguese Lynch syndrome families. *Genet. Med.* **2011**, *13*, 895–902. [CrossRef]
46. Morak, M.; Koehler, U.; Schackert, H.K.; Steinke, V.; Royer-Pokora, B.; Schulmann, K.; Kloor, M.; Höchter, W.; Weingart, J.; Keiling, C.; et al. Biallelic MLH1 SNP cDNA expression or constitutional promoter methylation can hide genomic rearrangements causing Lynch syndrome. *J. Med. Genet.* **2011**, *48*, 513–519. [CrossRef] [PubMed]
47. Meyer, C.; Brieger, A.; Plotz, G.; Weber, N.; Passmann, S.; Dingermann, T.; Zeuzem, S.; Trojan, J.; Marschalek, R. An interstitial deletion at 3p21.3 results in the genetic fusion of MLH1 and ITGA9 in a Lynch syndrome family. *Clin. Cancer Res.* **2009**, *15*, 762–769. [CrossRef]
48. Sjursen, W.; Bjørnevoll, I.; Engebretsen, L.F.; Fjelland, K.; Halvorsen, T.; Myrvold, H.E. A homozygote splice site PMS2 mutation as cause of Turcot syndrome gives rise to two different abnormal transcripts. *Fam. Cancer* **2009**, *8*, 179–186. [CrossRef]
49. Vasen, H.F.; Ghorbanoghli, Z.; Bourdeaut, F.; Cabaret, O.; Caron, O.; Duval, A.; Entz-Werle, N.; Goldberg, Y.; Ilencikova, D.; Kratz, C.P.; et al. Guidelines for surveillance of individuals with constitutional mismatch repair-deficiency proposed by the European Consortium "Care for CMMR-D" (C4CMMR-D). *J. Med. Genet.* **2014**, *51*, 283–293. [CrossRef]
50. Lavoine, N.; Colas, C.; Muleris, M.; Bodo, S.; Duval, A.; Entz-Werle, N.; Coulet, F.; Cabaret, O.; Andreiuolo, F.; Charpy, C.; et al. Constitutional mismatch repair deficiency syndrome: Clinical description in a French cohort. *J. Med. Genet.* **2015**, *52*, 770–778. [CrossRef]
51. ten Broeke, S.W.; Brohet, R.M.; Tops, C.M.; van der Klift, H.M.; Velthuizen, M.E.; Bernstein, I.; Capellá Munar, G.; Gomez Garcia, E.; Hoogerbrugge, N.; Letteboer, T.G.; et al. Lynch syndrome caused by germline PMS2 mutations: Delineating the cancer risk. *J. Clin. Oncol.* **2015**, *33*, 319–325. [CrossRef]
52. Blount, J.; Prakash, A. The changing landscape of Lynch syndrome due to PMS2 mutations. *Clin. Genet.* **2018**, *94*, 61–69. [CrossRef]
53. Crosbie, E.J.; Ryan, N.; Arends, M.J.; Bosse, T.; Burn, J.; Cornes, J.M.; Crawford, R.; Eccles, D.; Frayling, I.M.; Ghaem-Maghami, S.; et al. The Manchester International Consensus Group recommendations for the management of gynecological cancers in Lynch syndrome. *Genet. Med.* **2019**, *21*, 2390–2400. [CrossRef]
54. Modica, I.; Soslow, R.A.; Black, D.; Tornos, C.; Kauff, N.; Shia, J. Utility of immunohistochemistry in predicting microsatellite instability in endometrial carcinoma. *Am. J. Surg. Pathol.* **2007**, *31*, 744–751. [CrossRef]
55. Lloyd, K.M., 2nd; Dennis, M. Cowden's disease. A possible new symptom complex with multiple system involvement. *Ann. Intern. Med.* **1963**, *58*, 136–142. [CrossRef]
56. Nelen, M.R.; Padberg, G.W.; Peeters, E.A.; Lin, A.Y.; van den Helm, B.; Frants, R.R.; Coulon, V.; Goldstein, A.M.; van Reen, M.M.; Easton, D.F.; et al. Localization of the gene for Cowden disease to chromosome 10q22-23. *Nat. Genet.* **1996**, *13*, 114–116. [CrossRef]
57. Liaw, D.; Marsh, D.J.; Li, J.; Dahia, P.L.; Wang, S.I.; Zheng, Z.; Bose, S.; Call, K.M.; Tsou, H.C.; Peacocke, M.; et al. Germline mutations of the PTEN gene in Cowden disease, an inherited breast and thyroid cancer syndrome. *Nat. Genet.* **1997**, *16*, 64–67. [CrossRef]
58. Pilarski, R. PTEN Hamartoma Tumor Syndrome: A Clinical Overview. *Cancers* **2019**, *11*, 844. [CrossRef]
59. Mester, J.; Eng, C. Cowden syndrome: Recognizing and managing a not so-rare hereditary cancer syndrome. *J. Surg. Oncol.* **2015**, *111*, 125–130. [CrossRef]
60. Tan, M.H.; Mester, J.L.; Ngeow, J.; Rybicki, L.A.; Orloff, M.S.; Eng, C. Lifetime cancer risks in individuals with germline PTEN mutations. *Clin. Cancer Res.* **2012**, *18*, 400–407. [CrossRef] [PubMed]
61. Bubien, V.; Bonnet, F.; Brouste, V.; Hoppe, S.; Barouk-Simonet, E.; David, A.; Edery, P.; Bottani, A.; Layet, V.; Caron, O.; et al. French Cowden Disease Network. High cumulative risks of cancer in patients with PTEN hamartoma tumour syndrome. *J. Med. Genet.* **2013**, *50*, 255–263. [CrossRef]

62. Nieuwenhuis, M.H.; Kets, C.M.; Murphy-Ryan, M.; Yntema, H.G.; Evans, D.G.; Colas, C.; Møller, P.; Hes, F.J.; Hodgson, S.V.; Olderode-Berends, M.J.; et al. Cancer risk and genotype-phenotype correlations in PTEN hamartoma tumor syndrome. *Fam. Cancer* **2013**, *13*, 57–63. [CrossRef]
63. Elnaggar, A.C.; Spunt, S.L.; Smith, W.; Depas, M.; Santoso, J.T. Endometrial cancer in a 15-year-old girl: A complication of Cowden syndrome. *Gynecol. Oncol. Case Rep.* **2012**, *3*, 18–19. [CrossRef] [PubMed]
64. Baker, W.D.; Soisson, A.P.; Dodson, M.K. Endometrial cancer in a 14-year old girl with Cowden syndrome: A case report. *J. Obstet. Gynaecol. Res.* **2013**, *39*, 876–878. [CrossRef]
65. Mutter, G.L.; Lin, M.C.; Fitzgerald, J.T.; Kum, J.B.; Baak, J.P.; Lees, J.A.; Weng, L.P.; Eng, C. Altered PTEN expression as a diagnostic marker for the earliest endometrial precancers. *J. Natl. Cancer Inst.* **2000**, *92*, 924–930. [CrossRef]
66. Djordjevic, B.; Barkoh, B.A.; Luthra, R.; Broaddus, R.R. Relationship between PTEN, DNA mismatch repair, and tumor histotype in endometrial carcinoma: Retained positive expression of PTEN preferentially identifies sporadic non-endometrioid carcinomas. *Mod. Pathol.* **2013**, *26*, 1401–1412. [CrossRef]
67. Black, D.; Bogomolniy, F.; Robson, M.E.; Offit, K.; Barakat, R.R.; Boyd, J. Evaluation of germline PTEN mutations in endometrial cancer patients. *Gynecol. Oncol.* **2005**, *96*, 21–24. [CrossRef]
68. Orloff, M.S.; He, X.; Peterson, C.; Chen, F.; Chen, J.L.; Mester, J.L.; Eng, C. Germline PIK3CA and AKT1 Mutations in Cowden and Cowden-like Syndromes. *Am. J. Hum. Genet.* **2013**, *92*, 76–80. [CrossRef]
69. Palles, C.; Cazier, J.B.; Howarth, K.M.; Domingo, E.; Jones, A.M.; Broderick, P.; Kemp, Z.; Spain, S.L.; Guarino, E.; Salguero, I.; et al. Germline mutations affecting the proofreading domains of POLE and POLD1 predispose to colorectal adenomas and carcinomas. *Nat. Genet.* **2013**, *45*, 136–144. [CrossRef]
70. Elsayed, F.A.; Kets, C.M.; Ruano, D.; van den Akker, B.; Mensenkamp, A.R.; Schrumpf, M.; Nielsen, M.; Wijnen, J.T.; Tops, C.M.; Ligtenberg, M.J.; et al. Germline variants in POLE are associated with early onset mismatch repair deficient colorectal cancer. *Eur. J. Hum. Genet.* **2014**, *23*, 1080–1084. [CrossRef]
71. Rohlin, A.; Zagoras, T.; Nilsson, S.; Lundstam, U.; Wahlström, J.; Hultén, L.; Martinsson, T.; Karlsson, G.B.; Nordling, M. A mutation in POLE predisposing to a multi-tumour phenotype. *Int. J. Oncol.* **2014**, *45*, 77–81. [CrossRef]
72. Bellido, F.; Pineda, M.; Aiza, G.; Valdés-Mas, R.; Navarro, M.; Puente, D.A.; Pons, T.; González, S.; Iglesias, S.; Darder, E.; et al. POLE and POLD1 mutations in 529 kindreds with familial colorectal cancer and/or polyposis: Review of reported cases and recommendations for genetic testing and surveillance. *Genet. Med.* **2016**, *18*, 325–332. [CrossRef]
73. Siraj, A.K.; Parvathareddy, S.K.; Bu, R.; Iqbal, K.; Siraj, S.; Masoodi, T.; Concepcion, R.M.; Ghazwani, L.O.; AlBadawi, I.; Al-Dayel, F.; et al. Germline POLE and POLD1 proofreading domain mutations in endometrial carcinoma from Middle Eastern region. *Cancer Cell Int.* **2019**, *19*, 334. [CrossRef]
74. Logan, C.V.; Murray, J.E.; Parry, D.A.; Robertson, A.; Bellelli, R.; Tarnauskaitė, Ž; Challis, R.; Cleal, L.; Borel, V.; Fluteau, A.; et al. DNA Polymerase Epsilon Deficiency Causes IMAGe Syndrome with Variable Immunodeficiency. *Am. J. Hum. Genet.* **2018**, *103*, 1038–1044. [CrossRef] [PubMed]
75. Pachlopnik Schmid, J.; Lemoine, R.; Nehme, N.; Cormier-Daire, V.; Revy, P.; Debeurme, F.; Debré, M.; Nitschke, P.; Bole-Feysot, C.; Legeai-Mallet, L.; et al. Polymerase ε1 mutation in a human syndrome with facial dysmorphism, immunodeficiency, livedo, and short stature ("FILS syndrome"). *J. Exp. Med.* **2012**, *209*, 2323–2330. [CrossRef]
76. Win, A.K.; Dowty, J.G.; Cleary, S.P.; Kim, H.; Buchanan, D.D.; Young, J.P.; Clendenning, M.; Rosty, C.; MacInnis, R.J.; Giles, G.G.; et al. Risk of colorectal cancer for carriers of mutations in MUTYH, with and without a family history of cancer. *Gastroenterology* **2014**, *146*, 1208–1211.e5. [CrossRef] [PubMed]
77. Vogt, S.; Jones, N.; Christian, D.; Engel, C.; Nielsen, M.; Kaufmann, A.; Steinke, V.; Vasen, H.F.; Propping, P.; Sampson, J.R.; et al. Expanded extracolonic tumor spectrum in MUTYH-associated polyposis. *Gastroenterology* **2009**, *137*, 1976–1985.e10. [CrossRef] [PubMed]
78. Win, A.K.; Reece, J.C.; Dowty, J.G.; Buchanan, D.D.; Clendenning, M.; Rosty, C.; Southey, M.C.; Young, J.P.; Cleary, S.P.; Kim, H.; et al. Risk of extracolonic cancers for people with biallelic and monoallelic mutations in MUTYH. *Int. J. Cancer* **2016**, *139*, 1557–1563. [CrossRef] [PubMed]
79. Weren, R.D.; Ligtenberg, M.J.; Kets, C.M.; de Voer, R.M.; Verwiel, E.T.; Spruijt, L.; van Zelst-Stams, W.A.; Jongmans, M.C.; Gilissen, C.; Hehir-Kwa, J.Y.; et al. A germline homozygous mutation in the base-excision repair gene NTHL1 causes adenomatous polyposis and colorectal cancer. *Nat. Genet.* **2015**, *47*, 668–671. [CrossRef]

80. Grolleman, J.E.; de Voer, R.M.; Elsayed, F.A.; Nielsen, M.; Weren, R.; Palles, C.; Ligtenberg, M.; Vos, J.R.; Ten Broeke, S.W.; de Miranda, N.; et al. Mutational Signature Analysis Reveals NTHL1 Deficiency to Cause a Multi-tumor Phenotype. *Cancer Cell* **2019**, *35*, 256–266. [CrossRef] [PubMed]
81. Thompson, D.; Easton, D.F.; Breast Cancer Linkage Consortium. Cancer Incidence in BRCA1 mutation carriers. *J. Natl. Cancer Inst.* **2002**, *94*, 1358–1365. [CrossRef]
82. Beiner, M.E.; Finch, A.; Rosen, B.; Lubinski, J.; Møller, P.; Ghadirian, P.; Lynch, H.T.; Friedman, E.; Sun, P.; Narod, S.A.; et al. The risk of endometrial cancer in women with BRCA1 and BRCA2 mutations. A prospective study. *Gynecol. Oncol.* **2007**, *104*, 7–10. [CrossRef]
83. Segev, Y.; Iqbal, J.; Lubinski, J.; Gronwald, J.; Lynch, H.T.; Møller, P.; Ghadirian, P.; Rosen, B.; Tung, N.; Kim-Sing, C.; et al. The incidence of endometrial cancer in women with BRCA1 and BRCA2 mutations: An international prospective cohort study. *Gynecol. Oncol.* **2013**, *130*, 127–131. [CrossRef] [PubMed]
84. Shu, C.A.; Pike, M.C.; Jotwani, A.R.; Friebel, T.M.; Soslow, R.A.; Levine, D.A.; Nathanson, K.L.; Konner, J.A.; Arnold, A.G.; Bogomolniy, F.; et al. Uterine cancer after risk-reducing salpingo-oophorectomy without hysterectomy in women with BRCA mutations. *JAMA Oncol.* **2016**, *2*, 1434–1440. [CrossRef] [PubMed]
85. de Jonge, M.M.; Ritterhouse, L.L.; de Kroon, C.D.; Vreeswijk, M.; Segal, J.P.; Puranik, R.; Hollema, H.; Rookus, M.A.; van Asperen, C.J.; van Leeuwen, F.E.; et al. Germline BRCA-Associated Endometrial Carcinoma Is a Distinct Clinicopathologic Entity. *Clin. Cancer Res.* **2019**, *25*, 7517–7526. [CrossRef]
86. Spurdle, A.B.; Thompson, D.J.; Ahmed, S.; Ferguson, K.; Healey, C.S.; O'Mara, T.; Walker, L.C.; Montgomery, S.B.; Dermitzakis, E.T.; Australian National Endometrial Cancer Study Group; et al. Genome-wide association study identifies a common variant associated with risk of endometrial cancer. *Nat. Genet.* **2011**, *43*, 451–454. [CrossRef]
87. Chen, M.M.; O'Mara, T.A.; Thompson, D.J.; Painter, J.N.; Australian National Endometrial Cancer Study Group (ANECS); Attia, J.; Black, A.; Brinton, L.; Chanock, S.; Chen, C.; et al. GWAS meta-analysis of 16 852 women identifies new susceptibility locus for endometrial cancer. *Hum. Mol. Genet.* **2016**, *25*, 2612–2620. [CrossRef]
88. Cheng, T.H.; Thompson, D.J.; O'Mara, T.A.; Painter, J.N.; Glubb, D.M.; Flach, S.; Lewis, A.; French, J.D.; Freeman-Mills, L.; Church, D.; et al. Five endometrial cancer risk loci identified through genome-wide association analysis. *Nat. Genet.* **2016**, *48*, 667–674. [CrossRef]
89. O'Mara, T.A.; Glubb, D.M.; Amant, F.; Annibali, D.; Ashton, K.; Attia, J.; Auer, P.L.; Beckmann, M.W.; Black, A.; Bolla, M.K.; et al. Identification of nine new susceptibility loci for endometrial cancer. *Nat. Comm.* **2018**, *9*, 3166. [CrossRef]
90. Painter, J.N.; Kaufmann, S.; O'Mara, T.A.; Hillman, K.M.; Sivakumaran, H.; Darabi, H.; Cheng, T.; Pearson, J.; Kazakoff, S.; Waddell, N.; et al. A Common Variant at the 14q32 Endometrial Cancer Risk Locus Activates AKT1 through YY1 Binding. *Am. J. Hum. Genet.* **2016**, *98*, 1159–1169. [CrossRef]
91. Cheng, T.H.; Thompson, D.; Painter, J.; O'Mara, T.; Gorman, M.; Martin, L.; Palles, C.; Jones, A.; Buchanan, D.D.; Win, A.K.; et al. Meta-analysis of genome-wide association studies identifies common susceptibility polymorphisms for colorectal and endometrial cancer near SH2B3 and TSHZ1. *Sci. Rep.* **2015**, *5*, 17369. [CrossRef]
92. Painter, J.N.; O'Mara, T.A.; Morris, A.P.; Cheng, T.; Gorman, M.; Martin, L.; Hodson, S.; Jones, A.; Martin, N.G.; Gordon, S.; et al. Genetic overlap between endometriosis and endometrial cancer: Evidence from cross-disease genetic correlation and GWAS meta-analyses. *Cancer Med.* **2018**, *7*, 1978–1987. [CrossRef]
93. O'Mara, T.A.; Crosbie, E.J. Polygenic risk score opportunities for early detection and prevention strategies in endometrial cancer. *Br. J. Cancer* **2020**, in press. [CrossRef]
94. Nead, K.T.; Sharp, S.J.; Thompson, D.J.; Painter, J.N.; Savage, D.B.; Semple, R.K.; Barker, A.; Australian National Endometrial Cancer Study Group (ANECS); Perry, J.R.; Attia, J.; et al. Evidence of a causal association between insulinemia and endometrial cancer: A mendelian randomization analysis. *J. Natl. Cancer Inst.* **2015**, *107*. [CrossRef] [PubMed]
95. Painter, J.N.; O'Mara, T.A.; Marquart, L.; Webb, P.M.; Attia, J.; Medland, S.E.; Cheng, T.; Dennis, J.; Holliday, E.G.; McEvoy, M.; et al. Genetic risk score Mendelian randomization shows that obesity measured as body mass index, but not waist:hip ratio, is causal for endometrial cancer. *Cancer Epidemiol. Biomark. Prev.* **2016**, *25*, 1503–1510. [CrossRef] [PubMed]

96. Thompson, D.J.; O'Mara, T.A.; Glubb, D.M.; Painter, J.N.; Cheng, T.; Folkerd, E.; Doody, D.; Dennis, J.; Webb, P.M.; Australian National Endometrial Cancer Study Group (ANECS); et al. CYP19A1 fine-mapping and Mendelian randomization: Estradiol is causal for endometrial cancer. *Endocr. Relat. Cancer* **2016**, *23*, 77–91. [CrossRef] [PubMed]
97. Kho, P.-F.; Amant, F.; Annibali, D.; Ashton, K.; Attia, J.; Auer, P.L.; Beckmann, M.W.; Black, A.; Brinton, L.; Buchanan, D.D.; et al. Mendelian randomization analyses suggest a role for cholesterol in the development of endometrial cancer. *Int. J. Cancer* **2020**, in press. [CrossRef]
98. Lu, K.H.; Dinh, M.; Kohlmann, W.; Watson, P.; Green, J.; Syngal, S.; Bandipalliam, P.; Chen, L.M.; Allen, B.; Conrad, P.; et al. Gynecologic cancer as a "sentinel cancer" for women with hereditary nonpolyposis colorectal cancer syndrome. *Obstet Gynecol.* **2005**, *105*, 569–574. [CrossRef]
99. Lipton, L.R.; Johnson, V.; Cummings, C.; Fisher, S.; Risby, P.; Eftekhar Sadat, A.T.; Cranston, T.; Izatt, L.; Sasieni, P.; Hodgson, S.V.; et al. Refining the Amsterdam Criteria and Bethesda Guidelines: Testing algorithms for the prediction of mismatch repair mutation status in the familial cancer clinic. *J. Clin. Oncol.* **2004**, *22*, 4934–4943, with published correction in *J. Clin. Oncol.* **2005**, *23*, 3652. [CrossRef]
100. Egoavil, C.; Alenda, C.; Castillejo, A.; Paya, A.; Peiro, G.; Sánchez-Heras, A.B.; Castillejo, M.I.; Rojas, E.; Barberá, V.M.; Cigüenza, S.; et al. Prevalence of Lynch syndrome among patients with newly diagnosed endometrial cancers. *PLoS ONE* **2013**, *8*, e79737. [CrossRef]
101. Ferguson, S.E.; Aronson, M.; Pollett, A.; Eiriksson, L.R.; Oza, A.M.; Gallinger, S.; Lerner-Ellis, J.; Alvandi, Z.; Bernardini, M.Q.; MacKay, H.J.; et al. Performance characteristics of screening strategies for Lynch syndrome in unselected women with newly diagnosed endometrial cancer who have undergone universal germline mutation testing. *Cancer* **2014**, *120*, 3932–3939. [CrossRef]
102. Hampel, H.; Frankel, W.; Panescu, J.; Lockman, J.; Sotamaa, K.; Fix, D.; Comeras, I.; La Jeunesse, J.; Nakagawa, H.; Westman, J.A.; et al. Screening for Lynch syndrome (hereditary nonpolyposis colorectal cancer) among endometrial cancer patients. *Cancer Res.* **2006**, *66*, 7810–7817. [CrossRef]
103. Hampel, H.; Panescu, J.; Lockman, J.; Sotamaa, K.; Fix, D.; Comeras, I.; LaJeunesse, J.; Nakagawa, H.; Westman, J.A.; Prior, T.W.; et al. Comment on: Screening for Lynch Syndrome (Hereditary Nonpolyposis Colorectal Cancer) among Endometrial Cancer Patients. *Cancer Res.* **2007**, *67*, 9603. [CrossRef] [PubMed]
104. Leenen, C.H.; van Lier, M.G.; van Doorn, H.C.; van Leerdam, M.E.; Kooi, S.G.; de Waard, J.; Hoedemaeker, R.F.; van den Ouweland, A.M.; Hulspas, S.M.; Dubbink, H.J.; et al. Prospective evaluation of molecular screening for Lynch syndrome in patients with endometrial cancer ≤ 70 years. *Gynecol. Oncol.* **2012**, *125*, 414–420. [CrossRef] [PubMed]
105. Snowsill, T.; Huxley, N.; Hoyle, M.; Jones-Hughes, T.; Coelho, H.; Cooper, C.; Frayling, I.; Hyde, C. A systematic review and economic evaluation of diagnostic strategies for Lynch syndrome. *Health Technol. Assess.* **2014**, *18*, 1–406. [CrossRef]
106. Backes, F.J.; Leon, M.E.; Ivanov, I.; Suarez, A.; Frankel, W.L.; Hampel, H.; Fowler, J.M.; Copeland, L.J.; O'Malley, D.M.; Cohn, D.E. Prospective evaluation of DNA mismatch repair protein expression in primary endometrial cancer. *Gynecol. Oncol.* **2009**, *114*, 486–490. [CrossRef]
107. Moline, J.; Mahdi, H.; Yang, B.; Biscotti, C.; Roma, A.A.; Heald, B.; Rose, P.G.; Michener, C.; Eng, C. Implementation of tumor testing for lynch syndrome in endometrial cancers at a large academic medical center. *Gynecol. Oncol.* **2013**, *130*, 121–126. [CrossRef]
108. Gausachs, M.; Mur, P.; Corral, J.; Pineda, M.; González, S.; Benito, L.; Menéndez, M.; Espinàs, J.A.; Brunet, J.; Iniesta, M.D.; et al. MLH1 promoter hypermethylation in the analytical algorithm of Lynch syndrome: A cost-effectiveness study. *Eur. J. Hum. Genet.* **2012**, *20*, 762–768. [CrossRef] [PubMed]
109. Deng, G.; Bell, I.; Crawley, S.; Gum, J.; Terdiman, J.P.; Allen, B.A.; Truta, B.; Sleisenger, M.H.; Kim, Y.S. BRAF mutation is frequently present in sporadic colorectal cancer with methylated hMLH1, but not in hereditary nonpolyposis colorectal cancer. *Clin. Cancer Res.* **2004**, *10 Pt 1*, 191–195. [CrossRef] [PubMed]
110. Kawaguchi, M.; Yanokura, M.; Banno, K.; Kobayashi, Y.; Kuwabara, Y.; Kobayashi, M.; Nomura, H.; Hirasawa, A.; Susumu, N.; Aoki, D. Analysis of a correlation between the BRAF V600E mutation and abnormal DNA mismatch repair in patients with sporadic endometrial cancer. *Int. J. Oncol.* **2009**, *34*, 1541–1547. [CrossRef] [PubMed]
111. Dove-Edwin, I.; Boks, D.; Goff, S.; Kenter, G.G.; Carpenter, R.; Vasen, H.F.; Thomas, H.J. The outcome of endometrial carcinoma surveillance by ultrasound scan in women at risk of hereditary nonpolyposis colorectal carcinoma and familial colorectal carcinoma. *Cancer* **2002**, *94*, 1708–1712. [CrossRef]

112. Rijcken, F.E.; Mourits, M.J.; Kleibeuker, J.H.; Hollema, H.; van der Zee, A.G. Gynecologic screening in hereditary nonpolyposis colorectal cancer. *Gynecol. Oncol.* **2003**, *91*, 74–80. [CrossRef]
113. Auranen, A.; Joutsiniemi, T. A systematic review of gynecological cancer surveillance in women belonging to hereditary nonpolyposis colorectal cancer (Lynch syndrome) families. *Acta Obstet. Gynecol. Scand.* **2011**, *90*, 437–444. [CrossRef]
114. Renkonen-Sinisalo, L.; Bützow, R.; Leminen, A.; Lehtovirta, P.; Mecklin, J.P.; Järvinen, H.J. Surveillance for endometrial cancer in hereditary nonpolyposis colorectal cancer syndrome. *Int. J. Cancer* **2006**, *120*, 821–824. [CrossRef] [PubMed]
115. Lécuru, F.; Le Frère Belda, M.A.; Bats, A.S.; Tulpin, L.; Metzger, U.; Olschwang, S.; Laurent-Puig, P. Performance of office hysteroscopy and endometrial biopsy for detecting endometrial disease in women at risk of human non-polyposis colon cancer: A prospective study. *Int. J. Gynecol. Cancer* **2008**, *18*, 1326–1331. [CrossRef] [PubMed]
116. Manchanda, R.; Saridogan, E.; Abdelraheim, A.; Johnson, M.; Rosenthal, A.N.; Benjamin, E.; Brunell, C.; Side, L.; Gessler, S.; Jacobs, I.; et al. Annual outpatient hysteroscopy and endometrial sampling (OHES) in HNPCC/Lynch syndrome (LS). *Arch. Gynecol. Obstet.* **2012**, *286*, 1555–1562. [CrossRef]
117. Helder-Woolderink, J.M.; De Bock, G.H.; Sijmons, R.H.; Hollema, H.; Mourits, M.J. The additional value of endometrial sampling in the early detection of endometrial cancer in women with Lynch syndrome. *Gynecol. Oncol.* **2013**, *131*, 304–308. [CrossRef] [PubMed]
118. Ryan, N.; Morris, J.; Green, K.; Lalloo, F.; Woodward, E.R.; Hill, J.; Crosbie, E.J.; Evans, D.G. Association of Mismatch Repair Mutation With Age at Cancer Onset in Lynch Syndrome: Implications for Stratified Surveillance Strategies. *JAMA Oncol.* **2017**, *3*, 1702–1706. [CrossRef]
119. Vasen, H.F.; Blanco, I.; Aktan-Collan, K.; Gopie, J.P.; Alonso, A.; Aretz, S.; Bernstein, I.; Bertario, L.; Burn, J.; Capella, G.; et al. Revised guidelines for the clinical management of Lynch syndrome (HNPCC): Recommendations by a group of European experts. *Gut* **2013**, *62*, 812–823. [CrossRef]
120. Schmeler, K.M.; Lynch, H.T.; Chen, L.M.; Munsell, M.F.; Soliman, P.T.; Clark, M.B.; Daniels, M.S.; White, K.G.; Boyd-Rogers, S.G.; Conrad, P.G.; et al. Prophylactic surgery to reduce the risk of gynecologic cancers in the Lynch syndrome. *N. Engl. J. Med.* **2006**, *354*, 261–269. [CrossRef]
121. Bartosch, C.; Pires-Luís, A.S.; Meireles, C.; Baptista, M.; Gouveia, A.; Pinto, C.; Shannon, K.M.; Jerónimo, C.; Teixeira, M.R.; Lopes, J.M.; et al. Pathologic Findings in Prophylactic and Nonprophylactic Hysterectomy Specimens of Patients With Lynch Syndrome. *Am. J. Surg. Pathol.* **2016**, *40*, 1177–1191. [CrossRef]
122. Shaw, P.A.; Clarke, B.A. Prophylactic gynecologic specimens from hereditary cancer carriers. *Surg. Pathol. Clin.* **2016**, *9*, 307–328. [CrossRef]
123. Ramchander, N.C.; Ryan, N.; Walker, T.; Harries, L.; Bolton, J.; Bosse, T.; Evans, D.G.; Crosbie, E.J. Distinct Immunological Landscapes Characterize Inherited and Sporadic Mismatch Repair Deficient Endometrial Cancer. *Front. Immunol.* **2020**, *10*, 3023. [CrossRef] [PubMed]
124. Bohaumilitzky, L.; von Knebel Doeberitz, M.; Kloor, M.; Ahadova, A. Implications of Hereditary Origin on the Immune Phenotype of Mismatch Repair-Deficient Cancers: Systematic Literature Review. *J. Clin. Med.* **2020**, *9*, 1741. [CrossRef]
125. Ott, P.A.; Bang, Y.J.; Berton-Rigaud, D.; Elez, E.; Pishvaian, M.J.; Rugo, H.S.; Puzanov, I.; Mehnert, J.M.; Aung, K.L.; Lopez, J.; et al. Safety and Antitumor Activity of Pembrolizumab in Advanced Programmed Death Ligand 1-Positive Endometrial Cancer: Results From the KEYNOTE-028 Study. *J. Clin. Oncol.* **2017**, *35*, 2535–2541. [CrossRef]
126. Makker, V.; Rasco, D.; Vogelzang, N.J.; Brose, M.S.; Cohn, A.L.; Mier, J.; Di Simone, C.; Hyman, D.M.; Stepan, D.E.; Dutcus, C.E.; et al. Lenvatinib plus pembrolizumab in patients with advanced endometrial cancer: An interim analysis of a multicentre, open-label, single-arm, phase 2 trial. *Lancet Oncol.* **2019**, *20*, 711–718. [CrossRef]
127. Dedes, K.J.; Wetterskog, D.; Mendes-Pereira, A.M.; Natrajan, R.; Lambros, M.B.; Geyer, F.C.; Vatcheva, R.; Savage, K.; Mackay, A.; Lord, C.J.; et al. PTEN deficiency in endometrioid endometrial adenocarcinomas predicts sensitivity to PARP inhibitors. *Sci. Transl. Med.* **2010**, *2*, 53ra75. [CrossRef] [PubMed]
128. Bian, X.; Gao, J.; Luo, F.; Rui, C.; Zheng, T.; Wang, D.; Wang, Y.; Roberts, T.M.; Liu, P.; Zhao, J.J.; et al. PTEN deficiency sensitizes endometrioid endometrial cancer to compound PARP-PI3K inhibition but not PARP inhibition as monotherapy. *Oncogene* **2018**, *37*, 341–351. [CrossRef]

4

Long-Term Evaluation of Women Referred to a Breast Cancer Family History Clinic (Manchester UK 1987–2020)

Anthony Howell [1,2,3,*], Ashu Gandhi [1,2,3], Sacha Howell [1,2,3], Mary Wilson [1], Anthony Maxwell [1,4,*], Susan Astley [1,2,4], Michelle Harvie [1], Mary Pegington [1,3], Lester Barr [1], Andrew Baildam [1,5], Elaine Harkness [1,4], Penelope Hopwood [1,6], Julie Wisely [1,7], Andrea Wilding [1], Rosemary Greenhalgh [1], Jenny Affen [1], Andrew Maurice [1], Sally Cole [1], Julia Wiseman [1], Fiona Lalloo [1,8], David P. French [9] and D. Gareth Evans [1,2,4,8,10,11]

1 Nightingale Breast Screening Centre & Prevent Breast Cancer Unit Wythenshawe Hospital, Manchester University NHS Foundation Trust, Manchester M23 9LT, UK; ashu.gandhi@mft.nhs.uk (A.G.); sacha.howell@manchester.ac.uk (S.H.); mary.wilson@mft.nhs.uk (M.W.); Sue.astley@manchester.ac.uk (S.A.); michelle.harvie@manchester.ac.uk (M.H.); Mary.pegington@manchester.ac.uk (M.P.); lester.barr@mft.nhs.uk (L.B.); aetab2@btinternet.com (A.B.); elaine.harkness@manchester.ac.uk (E.H.); penny.hopwood@icr.ac.uk (P.H.); julie.wisely@mft.nhs.uk (J.W.); Andrea.Wilding@MFT.NHS.UK (A.W.); rosemary.greenhalgh@mft.nhs.uk (R.G.); jenny.affen@mft.nhs.uk (J.A.); Andrew.maurice@nhs.net (A.M.); Sally.cole@mft.nhs.uk (S.C.); julia.wiseman@mft.nhs.uk (J.W.); fiona.lalloo@mft.nhs.uk (F.L.); Gareth.Evans@mft.nhs.uk (D.G.E.)

2 Manchester Breast Centre, The Christie Hospital, Manchester M23 9LT, UK

3 Division of Cancer Sciences, Medicine and Health, University of Manchester, Manchester Academic Health Science Centre, Manchester M23 9LT, UK

4 Division of Informatics, Imaging & Data Sciences, School of Health Sciences, Faculty of Biology, Medicine and Health, University of Manchester, Manchester M13 9PT, UK

5 Department of Surgery, King Edward VII's Hospital, London W1G6AA, UK

6 Clinical Trials and Statistics Unit, The Institute of Cancer Research, London SM25PT, UK

7 Department of Psychology, University Hospital of South Manchester NHS Trust, Wythenshawe, Manchester M23 9LT, UK

8 Manchester Centre for Genomic Medicine, Manchester University Hospitals NHS Foundation Trust, Manchester M23 9LT, UK

9 Division of Psychology and Mental Health, School of Health Sciences, Manchester Centre of Health Psychology, University of Manchester, Manchester M23 9LT, UK; david.french@manchester.ac.uk

10 NW Genomic Laboratory Hub, Manchester Centre for Genomic Medicine, Manchester University Hospitals NHS Foundation Trust, Manchester M13 9WL, UK

11 Faculty of Biology, Division of Evolution and Genomic Sciences, School of Biological Sciences, Medicine and Health, University of Manchester, Manchester Academic Health Science Centre, Manchester M23 9LT, UK

* Correspondence: anthony.howell@manchester.ac.uk (A.H.); anthony.maxwell@manchester.ac.uk (A.M.)

Simple Summary: This study reports the management of women at high risk for breast cancer over a 33 years period. The aim was to summarize the numbers seen and to report the results of our studies on gene testing, the outcomes of screening and the success of preventive methods including lifestyle change, chemoprevention and risk-reducing mastectomy. We also discuss how the clinical Family History Service may be improved in the future.

Abstract: Clinics for women concerned about their family history of breast cancer are widely established. A Family History Clinic was set-up in Manchester, UK, in 1987 in a Breast Unit serving a population of 1.8 million. In this review, we report the outcome of risk assessment, screening and prevention strategies in the clinic and propose future approaches. Between 1987–2020,

14,311 women were referred, of whom 6.4% were from known gene families, 38.2% were at high risk (≥30% lifetime risk), 37.7% at moderate risk (17–29%), and 17.7% at an average/population risk who were discharged. A total of 4168 (29.1%) women were eligible for genetic testing and 736 carried pathogenic variants, predominantly in *BRCA1* and *BRCA2* but also other genes (5.1% of direct referrals). All women at high or moderate risk were offered annual mammographic screening between ages 30 and 40 years old: 646 cancers were detected in women at high and moderate risk (5.5%) with a detection rate of 5 per 1000 screens. Incident breast cancers were largely of good prognosis and resulted in a predicted survival advantage. All high/moderate-risk women were offered lifestyle prevention advice and 14–27% entered various lifestyle studies. From 1992–2003, women were offered entry into IBIS-I (tamoxifen) and IBIS-II (anastrozole) trials (12.5% of invitees joined). The NICE guidelines ratified the use of tamoxifen and raloxifene (2013) and subsequently anastrozole (2017) for prevention; 10.8% women took up the offer of such treatment between 2013–2020. Since 1994, 7164 eligible women at ≥25% lifetime risk of breast cancer were offered a discussion of risk-reducing breast surgery and 451 (6.2%) had surgery. New approaches in all aspects of the service are needed to build on these results.

Keywords: family history; breast cancer; risk; genes; screening; prevention

---

1. Introduction

In the 1980s, the rising incidence of breast cancer (BC) and the introduction in the UK of the NHS National Health Service Breast Screening Programme (NHSBSP) led women with a family history of the disease to seek advice concerning management of their personal risk. In response to concerns expressed by primary care physicians and colleagues within our breast oncology service, we established a referral Family History Clinic (FHC) in Manchester, UK, in 1987 with a cancer genetics service (CGS) initiated in 1990 (DGRE, FL). The clinic serves a catchment population of 1.8 million, (just over half the population of Greater Manchester), although women at high-risk may be specifically referred to the centre from a population of approximately 5 million in North West England.

The aims of the FHC were to introduce a service for the estimation and management of BC risk for women with familial risk and to evaluate the short- and long-term effectiveness of the clinic. At presentation, an individual's risk was explained, annual breast screening initiated and advice given concerning diet and lifestyle factors which might affect risk. Later, chemoprevention (1992 as part of the IBIS I clinical trial), genetic testing (1994) and risk-reducing surgery (1994) were introduced. In 1994, we published local guidelines for the management of women with a family history of BC [1]. These were followed by national guidelines for the UK [2,3] and the USA [4,5].

Management was undertaken by a multi-disciplinary team. Following referral, each woman was sent a questionnaire to assess family history and breast factors and, if eligible, offered a clinic appointment. Women were initially seen by geneticists (DGRE, FL) or medical oncologists (AH, SJH). Breast examination was undertaken and advice given by specially trained nurses (RG, JW, AW) and annual mammography and MRIs performed by radiologists within the Breast Unit (represented by MW and AM). Risk-reducing surgery was performed by a team of surgeons (represented by AB, AG and LB). Quality of life aspects of risk communication, mutation testing and risk-reducing mastectomy (RRM) were an integrated part of the FHC clinical and research agenda provided by psycho-oncologists and a health psychologist (PH, JW, DF).

The aims of this paper were to present the results of each aspect of the service and to suggest potential future improvements. The results include the numbers of referrals, estimation of their BC risks and results of genetic testing, screening and uptake to lifestyle prevention, chemoprevention and risk-reducing surgery interventions. The main quality of life outcomes are also reported. The second half of this paper then suggests improvements to the service based on our own studies and those of others.

2. Results

2.1. Referrals to the Clinic

Over the period from September 1987 to September 2020, 14,311 women were referred to the clinic. Referrals were from primary care (GPs, 55.9%), from secondary care (mainly breast surgeons, 15.1%) and from the local Clinical Genetics Service for further follow up after risk assessment (20.9%). Women were also referred from a research study (notably, 3.1% from PROCAS—Prediction Risk Of Cancer At Screening, [6]) or from "other" sources such as relatives at risk attending with a proband (5.0%). The age at entry ranged from 16–81 years (median 39.9; interquartile range (IQR) 33.9–46.9, with 83% of women (11,878/14,311) below age 50 (Table 1). The number of referrals by year is shown in Figure 1 and ranged between approximately 300–700 per year following the initial 3 years lead in the period after the clinic was established.

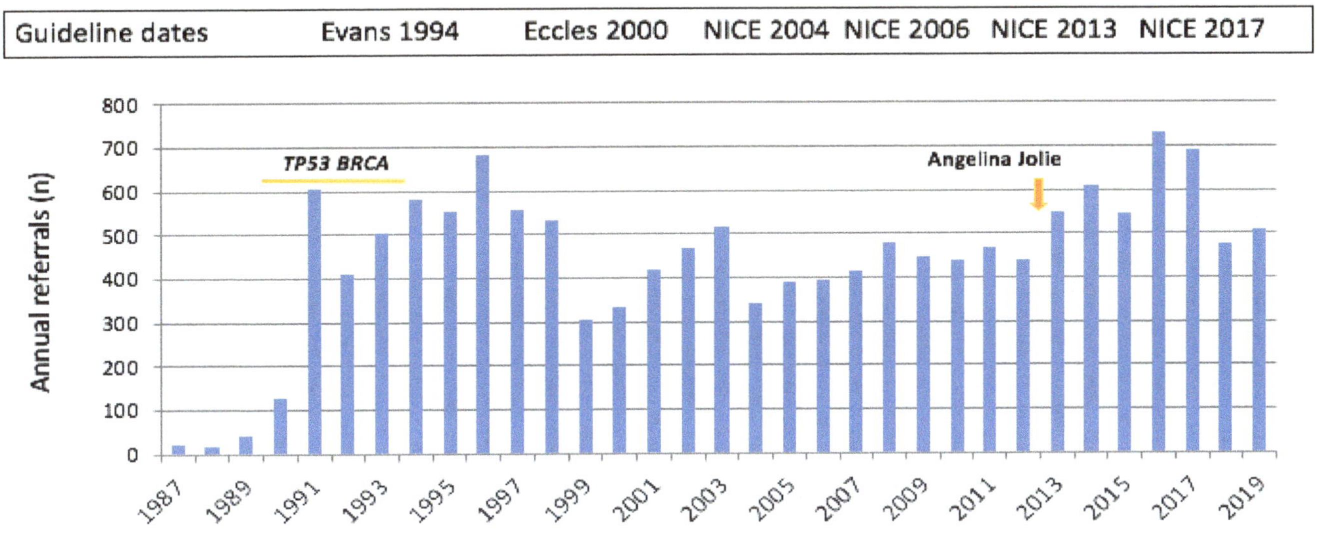

	1990-1994	1995-1999	2000-2004	2005-2009	2010-2014	2015-2019
BMI (kg/m²)	23.7	23.4	24.3	24.6	25.1	24.8
FFTP (years)	24	25	25	26	26	27

Figure 1. Annual referrals to the Manchester FHC between 1987 and 2020. Increases in referral were seen during the period when the first breast cancer genes, *TP53* and *BRCA1/2*, were identified and also related to the publicity surrounding Angelina Jolie when she indicated that she was a *BRCA1* PV carrier. The increase in median body mass index (BMI) and median age at first full-term pregnancy (FFTP) over this period are shown. Over the period of 33 years, lifetime risk of BC in the population increased from 1 in 12 to 1 in 8, an increase presumed to be associated with change in modifiable risk factors. These trends were apparent in the FHC. For example, the median age of first full-term pregnancy increased from 24 years to 27 years ($p < 0.001$), and median BMI at clinic entry increased from 23.7 to 24.8 kg/m^2 ($p < 0.001$).

Table 1. Number of referrals to the Family History Clinic (FHC) according to the source of referral, NICE guideline [3] risk category and *BCA1/2* status.

Group	Number	% of All Referrals	Known Gene in Family	%	High Risk	%	Moderate	%	Average	%	BRCA +v at Last Follow Up	%	Number
GP	8004	55.9%	165	2.1%	2646	33.1%	3542	44.3%	1651	20.6%	222	2.77%	8004
Surgery	2157	15.1%	38	1.8%	751	34.9%	831	38.6%	537	24.9%	55	2.55%	2157
Genetics	2868	20.0%	662	23.5%	1445	51.5%	594	21.2%	168	6.0%	406	14.16%	2868
PROCAS	448	3.1%	2	0.4%	311	69.4%	124	27.7%	11	2.5%	0	0.00%	448
Other	833	5.8%	54	6.5%	307	36.9%	299	35.9%	173	20.8%	53	6.36%	833
Totals	14,311		921	6.4%	5460	38.2%	5390	37.7%	2540	17.7%	736	5.14%	

GP, general practitioner; PROCAS, Prediction Risk Of Cancer At Screening.

2.2. Estimated Lifetime BC Risk

Risk was estimated initially by a modification of the Claus method with the addition of hormonal and lifestyle factors, such as age of first pregnancy and BMI, and by the Tyrer–Cuzick and BOADICEA models from 2004 [7–9]. We demonstrated that the modified Claus and the Tyrer–Cuzick models gave similar distributions of risk accurately, but the Gail model underpredicted risk [10,11].

Risk was reported as moderate (17–29% lifetime risk) and high (30%+) according to our original clinic guidelines (Evans 1994) and thereafter using the NICE Guidelines risk categories (2004) [1,3]. Overall, 44.6% of women were at high-risk (including 6.4% either with a pathogenic variant (PV) or a known PV in a close family member), 37.7% at moderate risk and 17.7% at average risk (Table 1). Following assessment of the referral questionnaire, women at average risk were referred back to primary care. It was clear that more higher risk women were referred to the Clinical Genetics Service reflecting a referral pathway from primary care to the Clinical Genetics Service for the highest risk women. (Table 1). After excluding referrals at average risk, 43.7% ($n = 3397$) of women directly referred to the clinic from primary and secondary care were estimated to be at high-risk and 56.7% ($n = 4373$) were at moderate risk.

2.3. Risk Perception and Cancer Worry

Risk was uniformly given as a proportion (e.g., 1 in 4 or 1 in 5). Our early studies reported that women had a relatively inaccurate perception of personal and population risk at presentation which improved when reassessed after risk counselling [12,13]. In another study, we demonstrated that the proportion of women with accurate personal risk perceptions significantly improved after risk counselling from 12% pre-counselling to 67% 3 months post-counselling ($p < 0.001$), which was maintained for 1 year [14]. Reassuringly, this improvement in accuracy of women's risk appraisal was not associated with increased anxiety. A subsequent analysis of questionnaire data from 500 FHC attendees over time indicated that BC risk counselling reduced self-reported cancer worry in women who initially overestimated their risk, with no significant change in levels for other risk perception groups, even if the risk was greater than they had estimated pre-counselling [15,16].

2.4. Genetic Testing

Genetic testing in the clinic began in 1991 just after the discovery of *TP53* and then the *BRCA1* (1994) and *BRCA2* (1995) genes [17–19]. Initially, testing was by single-strand confirmation polymorphism (SSCP) and protein truncation testing (PTT) [20], then, from 2001, Sanger sequencing all coding exons [20], and from 2013, next generation sequencing [21]. All samples, including retrospectively, were tested for large deletions and duplications by multiple ligation-dependent probe amplification (MLPA). All mutations detected by PTT or SSCP were confirmed by sequencing. From 2004, the probability of a *BRCA1* or *BRCA2* PV in the family was estimated using the Tyrer–Cuzick model [8] the BOADICEA model [9] or the Manchester Score [20,21]. The NICE Guidelines (2004) [3] initially indicated that the proband required the probability of a PV in BRCA1/2 of ≥20% for genetic testing in England and Wales [3]. In 2013, this was reduced to a ≥10% likelihood [22]. At present, gene testing in the UK is restricted to the *BRCA1*, *BRCA2*, and *PALB2* genes (National Genomic Test Directory (2020)) [23].

Of the 14,311 referrals to the FHC, *BRCA1* and *BRCA2* testing was completed for 4168 individuals (29.1%) or their affected family member. A total of 736 women (5.1% of the whole FHC cohort and 17.6% of those tested) were identified as *BRCA* PV carriers (*BRCA1* = 364, *BRCA2* = 372). However, only 2.5% of unaffected direct referrals to the FHC without a known gene in the family subsequently tested positive. No systematic approach to testing for PVs in other genes was undertaken. However, 35 potential BC and other risk genes were tested on a research basis in a subpopulation of 808 women unaffected by breast cancer representative of the risk distribution of direct referrals to the FHC [24]. Of the 808 tests there were 29 (3.6%) with PVs in other potentially actionable genes (*ATM* = 11, *CHEK2* = 11,

PALB2 = 7). These data indicate that approximately 6.1% of women directly referred to the FHC carry a PV in one of the actionable BC-associated genes.

2.5. Mammographic Screening

Annual mammography and clinical breast examination were offered from the inception of the clinic. Women were screened between the ages of 35 and 50 years (moderate risk) or 35 to 60 years (high risk), plus from 5 years younger than the earliest family diagnosis of BC. These screening periods were in accordance with an initial in-house protocol [25] and later, NICE guidelines [3,22]. Women with *BRCA1* and *BRCA2* PVs and others of equivalent high risk were screened by annual MRI between age 30 and 50 and annual mammography from age 30 to 70 according to NICE Guidelines [3,22].

Between 1987 and 2020, there were 129,119 women years of follow up; 646 BCs occurred prospectively, giving an annual incidence rate of 5.0 per 1000 which was approximately 1.7 times higher than the general population's annual rate of 3 per 1000 women aged 50–75 in the NHSBSP. Three hundred and ninety-four breast cancers occurred whilst on the screening programme or within 18 months of a screen. The majority of invasive cancers were lymph node negative (72.9%), small (≤20 mm, 73.2%) and stage 1 (61.4%). Cancers in women with *BRCA1* and *BRCA2* PVs were smaller overall with 75.0% and 85.4% being ≤20 mm, respectively, reflecting the benefits of MRI screening [26]. Breast cancer-specific survival at 10 years was 91.3% (87.4–94.0), compared with the current 10 year survival from BC in England, from 2013–2017, of 75.9% (74.9–77.0). Overall, 30.5% (92/322) of invasive cancers were oestrogen receptor negative (ER–) and 11/51 (21.5%) of carcinoma in situ (not assessed 21) were ER–.

2.6. Lifestyle Prevention

Excess weight, weight gain, sedentary lifestyle and high alcohol intake were established risk factors for BC before initiation to the FHC, and so verbal and standard written lifestyle advice was given to all women referred to the clinic. Lifestyle risk factors were common amongst high-risk women in the FHC with a similar prevalence of unhealthy lifestyles to women in the general population (57% are overweight/obese, 30% report <150 min moderate intensity physical activity/week and 45% have alcohol intakes of >14 units per week) [27]. Adult weight gain is a well-documented risk factor for BC (6% increased risk per 5 kg gain) [28]. We and others have reported that maintained weight loss of 5% or more before or after menopause in an unselected population cohort is associated with reductions of 39% and 23%, respectively, in the risk of post-menopausal BC [29]. Thus, women were advised to avoid weight gain if at a healthy weight and reduce weight by at least 5% if overweight/obese. Current guidelines include advising at least 150 min of moderate exercise per week and no more than 14 units of alcohol per week.

Since 2001 we conducted a series of randomised studies to determine the optimal methods for introducing and supporting weight control and other lifestyle changes amongst women in the FHC. These indicated that intermittent energy restriction (2 days of 50–60% energy restriction and 5 days of normal healthy eating/week) was associated with greater reductions in weight and insulin resistance than continuous energy restriction [30,31]. We also demonstrated that remotely supported (i.e., web and phone) weight loss/lifestyle behaviour change programmes are feasible and particularly effective amongst higher risk women producing ≥5% weight loss in approximately 60% of women at 12 months [32]. Uptake to these weight loss trials amongst moderate and high-risk women was between 14% and 27%.

2.7. Chemoprevention

Chemoprevention was not available at the inception of the FHC. However, women were randomised to tamoxifen or placebo in the IBIS-I trial (ISRCTN91879928). Between 1992 and 2001 and to anastrozole or placebo in the IBIS-II trial (SRCTN31488319). Between 2003 and 2012 [33,34]. Of the 7865 women invited to join these trials, 1003 women (12.8%) agreed (Table 2). These and other studies resulted in tamoxifen use being advised by NICE in the 2013 guidelines and anastrozole in the 2017 guidelines [22]. From 2013, 5121 women were invited to take either drug as part of management. To date, 282 have chosen chemoprevention and a further 284 in clinical trials so that overall 10.8% of eligible women have accepted treatment since 2013 (Table 2).

2.8. Risk-Reducing Mastectomy

Risk-reducing mastectomies were being performed, particularly in the USA, at the time of inception of the clinic. In 1994, we decided to offer this service in the FHC. Since then, 7164 women with a lifetime BC risk ≥25%, including *BRCA1/2* PV carriers, were offered a discussion concerning RRM according to a published protocol [35]. Of a total cohort of 7195 women at a ≥25% lifetime risk of BC, 451 (6.2%) without a current or previous breast cancer diagnosis elected to undergo RRM. Uptake of RRM was 49.3% in 479 *BRCA1/2* PV carriers and 5.2% in 6685 in non-carriers (9.4% for 1261 women at a ≥40% lifetime risk (non-BRCA), 4.9% in 3561 women at 30–39% risk and 3.0% in 1783 women at 25–29% lifetime risk).

In Cox regression analyses, factors which independently predicted risk-reducing mastectomy uptake included either the death of a sister with BC <50 years or mother <60 years, having children, having a breast biopsy or younger age at assessment (<30 years).

Of the 451 women who underwent RRM, four developed post-surgery BCs (all in *BRCA1/2* PV carriers) compared to 94 expected over a period of follow up of 7894 years, giving a risk reduction of 95.8%.

Twenty women (5.7%) had no reconstruction, whereas 352 (78%) had implant-based reconstruction (nipple sparing in 31% of these) and 63 (14%) flap-based reconstruction. The number of planned surgical procedures per patient was 2.41 ± 1.11 SD [36].

Two studies assessing psychological distress in our FHC patients undergoing risk-reducing mastectomy have been published [37,38]. Between 1995 and 1999, quality of life was assessed in 52 of 76 (79%) women undergoing surgery one-year post-operatively. At this point, 1 in 6 women had high scores for mental health problems on the General Health Questionnaire but for most, psychological distress appeared to be comparable with women at high risk who did not have surgery. Body image changes on the Body Image Scale were generally minor in degree with the most frequently reported changes reported in sexual attractiveness (55% responders), feeling less physically attractive (53%) and self-consciousness about appearance (53%). For the majority of women there was no evidence of significant mental health or body image problems in the first 3 years following RRM. Careful pre-operative preparation and long-term monitoring was advocated. In a second study, 79 women who chose to have surgery were compared with 64 women who declined surgery [38]. The main findings were that risk-reducing mastectomy reduced psychological morbidity and anxiety and did not have a significant detrimental impact on women's body image or sexual functioning.

Table 2. Number of women (A) randomised into the IBIS I or IBIS II trial 1992 and 2012; (B) number of women prescribed chemoprevention (CP) from 2013 either outside or as part of in-house trials.

		A						B			
Group	**Number Seen**	**Randomised to IBIS I/II Trial**	**Number Invited to Trial**	**% Joined Trial**	**Seen Since 2013**	**Prescribed Chemoprevention**	%	**Joined Chemoprevention Trial**	%	**Either Trial or CP**	
Known gene in family	921	11	554	1.99%	364	2	0.55%	2	0.55%	4	1.10%
High	5488	465	3178	14.63%	2604	162	6.22%	168	6.45%	323	12.40%
Moderate	5370	431	3200	13.47%	2221	118	5.31%	113	5.09%	226	10.18%
Average	2532	112	1188	9.43%	609	0		0		0	
Total	14,311	1019	8120	12.55%	5798	282	4.86%	283	4.88%	553	9.54%

3. Discussion

We summarised the developments that occurred since the inception of the clinic including updated models for risk and gene testing estimation (i.e., Tyrer-Cuzick v8 2017 [39], BOADICEA-V2019 [40], the Manchester Score [20,21] consistent use of mammography and MRI (NICE 2013 [22], a more po-active approach to lifestyle change [32], chemoprevention [41] and RRM [42]. We now suggest potential improvements to the service in each of the areas considered above based on our own studies and those of others.

3.1. Referrals

The numbers of referrals have remained relatively stable over the years and are still mainly instituted by women concerned about their family history and primary and secondary care clinicians who refer according the NICE familial breast FHC guidelines [3]. Our own and the reports of others indicate that approximately 10% of women in the UK have a first degree relative with BC; however, we estimate that <20% of these are referred [43]. It is interesting that referrals to FHCs and Clinical Genetics Services increased over two-fold after Angelina Jolie made her *BRCA1* PV carrier status and breast and ovarian surgery public [44,45]. This suggests that lack of awareness of the services may be an issue. Lack of uptake may also be related to a complex referral system which requires a visit to primary care for referral and the completion of extensive questionnaires. The latter is illustrated in our study of risk estimation in women undergoing breast screening. Thirty-seven percent of women invited completed a two-page questionnaire concerning their risk factors [6]. The cohort included 13% of women with a first-degree relative with breast cancer. Of 673 women found to be at high risk and invited for counselling and treatment at the FHC, 500 (74.3%) attended [46]. These data indicate a greater interest in risk management if the system is streamlined, suggesting that progress may best be made by more effort to align risk estimation with screening programmes. Referral would then be less dependent on health care professionals and would make it a more routine and streamlined service.

3.2. Risk Estimation

We demonstrated that the modified Claus model used in the clinic before 2004 gave similar results to the Tyrer–Cuzick model, suggesting consistent risk estimation for the duration of the clinic to date [10,11]. However, several studies indicate that the accuracy of risk estimation increases with the number of risk factors that are incorporated into the models used [47–50]. Recently, mammographic density (MD) and polygenic risk scores (PRS) based on single nucleotide polymorphism (SNP) results) have been added to risk models such as Tyrer–Cuzick (v8) and BOADICEA V [39,40]. In patients under follow up at the FHC, we assessed the effect on risk of incorporating the first 18 BC risk-associated SNPs discovered into the Tyrer–Cuzick model [51,52]. Adding SNP18 resulted in a change to the original given risk using Tyrer–Cuzick (version 6) in half the population of women: 25% had an increase in risk and 27% had a decrease in risk, indicating the potential importance of additional risk factors [53].

In the screening population we demonstrated that when both mammographic density and a PRS score were added to the Tyrer–Cuzick (v8), the proportion of women at elevated risk (>5% 10 years risk) increased from 12% to 18%. Ten percent of women changed from average to high risk and 4% from high to average [54,55]. These studies illustrate that using standard models may give erroneous risks and adding more risk factors may result in more appropriate management. However, more work is required to routinely apply optimal risk models in the clinic and deal with change in risk estimation over time.

3.3. Genes

Of the women directly referred to the FHC in which there was no currently known PVs, 2.5% were *BRCA1/2* PV carriers and 3.6% were found to have PVs in other genes after multigene panel testing [24]. This low pickup rate reflects that over 50% of referrals were at moderate risk and many of those at higher risk had undergone testing in themselves or their family (Table 1). At the FHC, much time was used to calculate the probability that the proband or her family are likely to carry a breast cancer gene PV. At present our Clinical Genetics Service forwards primary care referrals for women unlikely to carry a PV immediately to the FHC; conversely, we refer relatives of known PV carriers to the Clinical Genetics Service. A simple method where primary and secondary care physicians could estimate PV risk and refer appropriately would be invaluable. A more widespread use of the simple Manchester Score needs to be evaluated in this regard [20,21]. Currently, the NHS guidelines to the UK genetics departments allow estimation of *BRCA1/2* and *PALB2* (as well as syndromic genes where indicated such as *PTEN* in Cowden disease) [23]. The recent report illustrating the nine genes (*BRCA1, BRCA2, PALB2, CHEK2, ATM, CDH1, STK11, PTEN, TP53)* in which PVs more than doubles the risk of BC and three genes at the two-fold threshold (*RAD51C, RAD51D, BARD1)* might allow better selection for appropriate gene testing and a reduction in the need for multigene testing which, in the UK, is in the commercial sector [24].

3.4. Breast Screening

Mammographic screening in this at-risk population detects more cancers annually (5/1000 screened) than in the national programme (3/1000) as expected. It also results in the detection of smaller, better risk cancers. Three studies in the UK, one in our clinic and two in association with other clinics in the UK indicated that screening at-risk women results in a survival advantage compared (in non-randomised trials) with age matched populations [56–58]. The latest study was designed to assess the value of screening both moderate- and high-risk women from age 35–39 and confirmed a survival advantage even in the moderate-risk group [58].

Countries where national screening programmes begin at age 40 will already be screening in the high-risk groups. A review of the value of screening from age 40 in the general population concluded it was of equivocal value [59]. In the UK, screening is every 3 years for all from the age of 50, but a recent study now suggests a survival advantage in the general population when screening begins annually at the age of 40. This may lead to a change in UK policy [60]. The results of two randomised trials of risk adapted screening will inform a potential change in policy since they both screen women from age 40 onwards (WISDOM [61] MyPebs UNICANCER 2018 [62]). Further, a programme of work carried out in Manchester is considering how best to implement risk adapted screening to optimise the ratio of benefits and harms, including how to include ethnically minority women and to minimise harms of screening for women at low risk [63].

In countries where screening begins at 50 (e.g., the UK), consideration should be given to offering all women a one-off mammogram at age 40, together with risk estimation to determine future screening frequency. Mammographic density could be assessed automatically using artificial intelligence methods [64,65] and SNPs used only to determine precise risk where needed. The trials of risk and density-adapted screening and determination of the value of supplemental imaging techniques, such as whole breast ultrasound, contrast-enhanced mammography and abbreviated MRI, would further refine the management advice offered to women with high MD. Currently, at the FHC, women are offered an MRI if they carry a PV of a high-risk gene or if they have a 10 year risk of ≥8% aged 30 or ≥12% aged 40, based on the finding in trials that MRIs detect smaller tumours and may offer a survival advantage [66–70]. However, neither MRIs nor ultrasounds are routinely available (or proven) for a large group of women at increased risk outside those in very high-risk groups.

3.5. Lifestyle Advice

Women at high risk who have a high BMI [71], low physical activity levels, high alcohol intake [72] and smoke [73] have proportionately higher BC risks than similar women at population risk [71–73]. These potentially modifiable risk factors have also been associated in women at high risk due to the fact of family history or high PRS [72,73]. Thus, there is a rationale for focussing on lifestyle change in this higher risk group, and it is probable that the more avenues to promote change that are pursued, the greater the likelihood of success [74].

Women at high risk present a challenge for achieving lifestyle behaviour change. Firstly, some women can view their BC risk as unchangeable because of their family history [75]. This is consistent with a large body of literature that indicates education around disease risk does not alter behaviour by itself and that people require an appropriate level of support to achieve and sustain lifestyle behavioural change [76]. Lifestyle behaviour change programmes need to address the often complex psychological issues amongst women who have a high burden of cancer diagnoses and bereavements in their family. For many women, the majority of excess weight is acquired between the age of 18 and 35 years [76], indicating that lifestyle programmes should begin at younger ages. Interviews with young, high-risk women (under 35 years) in our FHC indicate that those women require a supportive weight control lifestyle programme that is remotely accessible, provides a point of contact within the high-risk service and promotes general wellbeing as well as cancer risk reduction [76]. There is a need for wider testing of low-cost programmes for lifestyle prevention which can reach and engage the maximum number of women across the network of UK FHCs.

3.6. Chemoprevention

The reduction of risk of BC by 30–50% by the use of SERMs and AIs such as tamoxifen, raloxifene and anastrozole are well known [77]. More recently, long-term follow up of the IBIS I and IBIS II trials indicate that risk reduction continues long after the usual five-year prescription period [41,78]. A recent analysis by NICE indicates that the use of anastrozole, in particular, is cost saving to the NHS in women at moderate to high risk of BC. However, whilst reduction of risk is of benefit, none of the trials to date have shown a survival benefit. This has led to the suggestion that premarin should be used for women at least 5 years post-menopausal and without a uterus, since in this group the Women's Health Initiative trial use was associated with a survival advantage [79].

Our report of recent uptake of chemoprevention being relatively low at 10% is consistent with many but not all studies [80,81]. Part of the reason for the low uptake concerns the side effects, although our own and other studies show that the observed frequency of side effects are comparable to controls [33,34,81–84]. We found four themes associated with low uptake: the perceived impact of side effects, the impact of others' experience on beliefs about tamoxifen, tamoxifen as a "cancer drug" and the daily reminder of cancer risk [80]. These reasons are understandable and consistent with other studies. Future developments require better communication of the pros and cons of therapy and alternative approaches including low dose or topical tamoxifen [85]. New agents such as antiprogestins [86], and denosumab [87] are currently being trialled in the FHC and elsewhere.

3.7. Risk-Reducing Surgery

Historically, our unit performed approximately 10–12 operations per year. With recent increases in publicity surrounding RRM [44], this has increased approximately three-fold in our own and other units [45]. The seminal paper by Hartmann [88] indicated BC a risk reduction of 92%, similar to our observed reduction of 95.8%. Over the years, our surgical approaches have evolved to reflect refinements in surgical technique and improved technology. Initially, mastectomy inevitably involved sacrifice of the nipple areolar complex, and immediate reconstructions relied exclusively on submuscular implant placement or use of the transverse rectus abdominus flap. In recent years, with the increasing appreciation of patient reported outcome measures in women undergoing risk reducing surgery [89], surgeons have sought more aesthetically focussed reconstruction options whilst not compromising risk-reduction principles. This has allowed the safe introduction of skin sparing and nipple sparing mastectomy [90] and autologous reconstruction with deep inferior epigastric perforator flaps [91] or single-stage prepectoral implant-based reconstruction [92]. The use of acellular dermal matrices has revolutionised implant-based reconstruction, allowing structural support of implants within a reconstruction to mimic natural breast ptosis [93]. Further improvements may come from the use of lipomodelling to improve aesthetics and thus patient satisfaction [94].

In *BRCA* PV carriers, RRM results in an improvement in survival, especially in women with *BRCA1* PVs, a result also found by others [95,96]. There may also be an improvement in women with *BRCA2* PVs with longer follow up [97]. Our previous studies indicated good acceptance and psychological health after RRM [37,38] More recent overviews have emphasised the enormous importance of excellent pre-surgical explanation, the presence of a psychologist in the multidisciplinary team and improved surgical techniques have been emphasised (Braude 2017) [98].

3.8. Summary

Here, we summarised the updated results from the Manchester FHC which spans the period from the inception of such clinics in the UK up to the present. A large proportion of these clinics in the UK are associated with Breast Units and work in conjunction with local Clinical Genetics Services.

The question remains regarding how their services may be improved (Table 3). At present, relatively small numbers of women are referred, partly because of the emphasis on family history for referral. Inclusion in FHCs of women at increased risk due to the presence of non-familial risk factors awaits the widespread introduction of MD and SNPs to risk prediction models. The introduction of new risk factors, such as MD and SNPs, is particularly important, as there is evidence that without them women are currently being given erroneous risk estimates that may result in imprecise treatment stratification. Clinical Genetics Services would be helped by more precise prediction of PVs. Consideration might be given to abandoning large panel tests and focussing on the nine genes in which the PVs are associated with a two-fold or more risk of BC [24].

Table 3. Summary of "current practice" and issues to be addressed for each of the interventions discussed.

Intervention	Current Practice	Issues to Be Addressed
Referral	Referrals from primary & secondary care established	Only 20% of women with FH referred Very few with 'other' risk factors
Risk estimation	Evolved to include more risk factors eg. mammographic density & SNPs	Using all factors approximately 20% of population at moderate & high risk
Gene testing	BRCA1/2 & PALB2 available in NHS 10% threshold for PV used (NICE)	New data suggest panel of 9 genes be should be used
Screening	Annual mammography & MRI established	Breast density & SNPs being tested in trials of risk & density adapted screening
Lifestyle change	Observational studies suggest introduction would be valuable	Mechanisms for general application being tested
Chemoprevention	Longer term risk and benefits established	Application suboptimal—consider assessment at home and primary care
Risk reducing surgery	Offer at appropriate risk levels established	Continue improvements in psychological and surgical techniques

We are currently testing the feasibility of introducing identification and referral of higher risk women as part of routine screening, i.e., research with a focus on implementation as part of routine care in a NHSBSP could bring about a "step change" if implemented [6]. There is already some evidence that communicating breast cancer risk estimates as part of routine screening does not produce the harms that have been anticipated [99]. For instance, communicating risk estimates in this setting did not produce adverse emotional effects or effects on screening uptake [100].

It appears that it is timely to consider introduction of the service into primary care as is seen in the USA [101]. A challenge to implementation is that the risk estimation and treatment algorithms have become more complex and efforts to introduce the two models we have focussed on here have led to legitimate difficulties amongst busy primary care physicians [102,103]. Even the mainstream estimation of cardiovascular risk on practice computer systems is apparently only applied to half of those in need and only half of these who need it are treated (Q-RISK; Hippisley-Cox 2017) [104] suggesting difficulties with the primary care approach.

A possible approach, pioneered in Melbourne, is to develop a simplified version of the Tyrer–Cuzick model, called iPrevent, and to make it widely available to all women. The model is user friendly and provides suggested treatment pathways in addition to an individual's risk. If made widely available this could lead to patient-initiated referral for initial screening and SNP estimation to define definitive management [105]. Other measures may be to establish one-off breast density assessment for all women at a certain age (e.g., 40 years, as suggested above) to estimate BC risk and introduce further screening and preventive measures for those found to be at high risk [99,106].

4. Conclusions

We reported the activity in a clinic designed for referral of women concerned about their family history of breast cancer. The long period of the clinic illustrates the changes in risk estimation and management over the years. The time span also allows for multiple studies on the effectiveness of management, for example, the effectiveness of breast screening. It also allows for the study of and introduction of preventive approaches such as use of tamoxifen and anastrozole.

A major aim of the clinic is to reduce the incidence of and deaths from breast cancer. These will be reduced by screening, lifestyle change and chemoprevention. Improvements in their effectiveness depends upon more widespread introduction not only into the current at-risk population but also into the large proportion of women unknowingly at high risk

Author Contributions: Conceptualisation, A.H. and D.G.E.; Data curation, D.G.E.; Formal analysis, E.H. and D.G.E.; Investigation, A.G., S.H., M.W., A.M. (Anthony Maxwell), S.A., M.H., M.P., L.B., A.B., E.H., P.H., J.W. (Julie Wisely), A.W., R.G., J.A., A.M. (Andrew Maurice), S.C., J.W. (Julia Wiseman), F.L., D.P.F. and D.G.E.; Project administration, A.H. and D.G.E.; Writing—original draft, A.H., A.G., S.H., M.W., A.W., S.A., M.H., M.P., L.B., E.H., P.H., J.W. (Julie Wisely), F.L., D.P.F. and D.G.E.; Writing—review and editing, A.H., A.G., S.H., M.W., A.M. (Anthony Maxwell), S.A., M.H., M.P., L.B., A.B., E.H., P.H., J.W. (Julie Wisely), A.W., R.G., J.A., A.M. (Andrew Maurice), J.W., (Julia Wiseman), F.L. and D.G.E. All authors have read and agreed to the published version of the manuscript.

Acknowledgments: D.G.E., E.F.H., S.J.H., D.P.F. and A.H. are supported by the National Institute for Health Research (NIHR) BRC Manchester (Grant Reference Number: 1215-200074). This work was also supported by Prevent Breast Cancer and Breast Cancer Now. We thank all the women referred to the clinic, the many unnamed individuals who have helped run the clinic over the years and the many investigators who have assisted with our clinical studies.We also thank Lorna McWilliam for comments on the manuscript.

References

1. Evans, D.G.; Fentiman, I.S.; McPherson, K.; Asbury, D.; Ponder, B.A.; Howell, A. Fortnightly review: Familial breast cancer. *BMJ* **1994**, *15*, 183–187. [CrossRef]
2. Eccles, D.M.; Evans, D.G.R.; Mackay, J. Guidelines for a genetic risk based approach to advising women with a family history of breast cancer. *J. Med. Genet.* **2000**, *37*, 203–209. [CrossRef]
3. McIntosh, A.; Shaw, C.; Evans, G.; Turnbull, N.; Bahar, N.; Barclay, M.; Easton, D.; Emery, J.; Gray, J.; Halpin, J.; et al. (2004 updated 2006 and 2013) Clinical Guidelines and Evidence Review for The Classification and Care of Women at Risk of Familial Breast Cancer, London: National Collaborating Centre for Primary Care/University of Sheffield. NICE Guideline CG164. Available online: https://www.nice.org.uk/Guidance/CG164 (accessed on 15 November 2020).
4. Hoskins, K.F.; Stopfer, J.E.; Calzone, K.A.; Merajver, S.D.; Rebbeck, T.R.; Garber, J.E.; Weber, B.L. Assessment and counseling for women with a family history of breast cancer. A guide for clinicians. *JAMA* **1995**, *15*, 577–585. [CrossRef]

5. Merajver, S.D.; Milliron, K. Breast cancer risk assessment: A guide for clinicians using the NCCN Breast Cancer Risk Reduction Guidelines. *J. Natl. Comp. Cancer Netw.* **2003**, *1*, 297–301. [CrossRef]
6. Evans, D.G.; Astley, S.; Stavrinos, P.; Harkness, E.; Donnelly, L.S.; Dawe, S.; Jacob, I.; Harvie, M.; Cuzick, J.; Brentnall, A.; et al. Improvement in Risk Prediction, Early Detection and Prevention of Breast Cancer in the NHS Breast Screening Programme and Family History Clinics: A Dual Cohort Study. *Southampt. (UK) NIHR J. Libr.* **2016**. [CrossRef]
7. Claus, E.B.; Risch, N.; Thompson, W.D. Genetic analysis of breast cancer in the cancer and steroid hormone study. *Am. J. Hum. Genet.* **1991**, *48*, 232–242.
8. Tyrer, J.; Duffy, S.W.; Cuzick, J. A breast cancer prediction model incorporating familial and personal risk factors. *Stat. Med.* **2004**, *23*, 1111–1130. [CrossRef]
9. Antoniou, A.C.; Pharoah, P.P.; Smith, P.; Easton, D.F. The BOADICEA model of genetic susceptibility to breast and ovarian cancer. *Br. J. Cancer* **2004**, *18*, 1580–1590. [CrossRef]
10. Amir, E.; Evans, D.G.; Shenton, A.; Lalloo, F.; Moran, A.; Boggis, C.; Wilson, M.; Howell, A. Evaluation of Breast Cancer Risk Assessment Packages in the Family History Evaluation and Screening Programme. *J. Med. Genet.* **2003**, *40*, 807–814. [CrossRef]
11. Evans, D.G.; Ingham, S.; Dawe, S.; Roberts, L.; Lalloo, F.; Brentnall, A.R.; Stavrinos, P.; Howell, A. Breast cancer risk assessment in 8,824 women attending a family history evaluation and screening programme. *FAM Cancer* **2014**, *13*, 189–196. [CrossRef]
12. Evans, D.G.R.; Burnell, L.; Hopwood, P.; Howell, A. Perception of risk in women with a family history of breast cancer. *Br. J. Cancer* **1993**, *67*, 612–614. [CrossRef] [PubMed]
13. Evans, D.G.R.; Blair, V.; Greenhalgh, R.; Hopwood, P.; Howell, A. The impact of genetic counselling on risk perception in women with a family history of breast cancer. *Br. J Cancer* **1994**, *70*, 934–938. [CrossRef] [PubMed]
14. Hopwood, P.; Keeling, F.; Long, A.; Pool, C.; Evans, G.; Howell, A. Psychological support needs for women at high genetic risk of breast cancer: Some preliminary indicators. *Psycho-Oncology* **1998**, *7*, 402–412. [CrossRef]
15. Hopwood, P.; Shenton, A.; Lalloo, F.; Evans, D.G.; Howell, A. Risk perception and cancer worry: An exploratory study of the impact of genetic risk counselling in women with a family history of breast cancer. *J. Med. Genet.* **2001**, *38*, 139. [CrossRef] [PubMed]
16. Hopwood, P.; Howell, A.; Lalloo, F.; Evans, G. Do women understand the odds? Risk perceptions and recall of risk information in women with a family history of breast cancer. *Community Genet.* **2003**, *6*, 214–223. [CrossRef]
17. Malkin, D.; Li, F.P.; Strong, L.C.; Fraumeni, J.F., Jr.; Nelson, C.E.; Kim, D.H.; Kassel, J.; Gryka, M.A.; Bischoff, F.Z.; Tainsky, M.A.; et al. Germ line p53 mutations in a familial syndrome of breast cancer, sarcomas, and other neoplasms. *Science* **1990**, *30*, 1233–1238. [CrossRef] [PubMed]
18. Miki, Y.; Swensen, J.; Shattuck-Eidens, D.; Futreal, P.A.; Harshman, K.; Tavtigian, S.; Liu, Q.; Cochran, C.; Bennett, L.M.; Ding, W.; et al. A strong candidate for the breast and ovarian cancer susceptibility gene BRCA1. *Science* **1994**, *266*, 66–71. [CrossRef]
19. Wooster, R.; Bignell, G.; Lancaster, J.; Swift, S.; Seal, S.; Mangion, J.; Collins, N.; Gregory, S.; Gumbs, C.; Micklem, G. Identification of the breast cancer susceptibility gene BRCA2. *Nature* **1995**, *378*, 789–792. [CrossRef]
20. Evans, D.G.; Eccles, D.M.; Rahman, N.; Young, K.; Bulman, M.; Amir, E.; Shenton, A.; Howell, A.; Lalloo, F. A new scoring system for the chances of identifying a BRCA1/2 mutation outperforms existing models including BRCAPRO. *J. Med. Genet.* **2004**, *41*, 474–480. [CrossRef]
21. Evans, D.G.; Harkness, E.F.; Plaskocinska, I.; Wallace, A.J.; Clancy, T.; Woodward, E.R.; Howell, A.; Tischkowitz, M.; Lalloo, F. Pathology update to the Manchester Scoring System based on testing in over 4000 families. *J. Med. Genet.* **2017**, *54*, 674–681. [CrossRef]
22. Familial Breast Cancer: Classification, care and Managing Breast Cancer and Related Risks in People with a Family History of Breast Cancer Clinical Guideline Published: 25 June 2013. Available online: www.nice.org.uk/guidance/cg164 (accessed on 12 October 2020).
23. NHS England. National Genomic Test Directory 2020. Available online: https://www.england.nhs.uk/publication/national-genomic-test-directories/ (accessed on 12 October 2020).

24. Dorling, L.; Carvalho, S.; Allen, J.; González-Neira, A.; Luccarini, C.; Wahlström, C.; Pooley, K.A.; Parsons, M.T.; Fortuno, C. Breast cancer risk genes: Association analysis of rare coding variants in 34 genes in 60,466 cases and 53,461 controls. *N. Engl. J. Med.* **2020**, *383*. in press.
25. Lalloo, F.; Boggis, C.R.; Evans, D.G.; Shenton, A.; Threlfall, A.G.; Howell, A. Screening by mammography, women with a family history of breast cancer. *Eur. J. Cancer* **1998**, *34*, 937–940. [CrossRef]
26. Leach, M.O.; Boggis, C.R.; Dixon, A.K.; Easton, D.F.; Eeles, R.A.; Evans, D.G.; Gilbert, F.J.; Griebsch, I.; Hoff, R.J.; Kessar, P.; et al. MARIBS study group. Screening with magnetic resonance imaging and mammography of a UK population at high familial risk of breast cancer: A prospective multicentre cohort study (MARIBS). *Lancet* **2005**, *365*, 1769–1778. [CrossRef] [PubMed]
27. Pegington, M.; Evans, D.G.; Howell, A.; Donnelly, L.S.; Wiseman, J.; Cuzick, J.M.; Harvie, M.N. Lifestyle behaviours and health measures of women at increased risk of breast cancer taking chemoprevention. *Eur. J. Cancer Prev.* **2019**, *28*, 500–506. [CrossRef] [PubMed]
28. World Cancer Research Fund. Diet, Nutrition, Physical Activity and Breast Cancer 2018. Available online: https://www.wcrf.org/sites/default/files/Breast-cancer-report.pdf (accessed on 12 October 2020).
29. Harvie, M.; Howell, A.; Vierkant, R.A.; Kumar, N.; Cerhan, J.R.; Kelemen, L.E.; Folsom, A.R.; Sellers, T.A. Association of gain and loss of weight before and after menopause with risk of postmenopausal breast cancer in the Iowa women's health study. *Cancer Epidemiol. Biomark. Prev.* **2005**, *14*, 656–661. [CrossRef]
30. Harvie, M.N.; Pegington, M.; Mattson, M.P.; Frystyk, J.; Dillon, B.; Evans, G.; Cuzick, J.; Jebb, S.A.; Martin, B.; Cutler, R.G.; et al. The effects of intermittent or continuous energy restriction on weight loss and metabolic disease risk markers: A randomized trial in young overweight women. *Int. J. Obes. (Lond.)* **2011**, *35*, 714–727. [CrossRef]
31. Harvie, M.; Wright, C.; Pegington, M.; McMullan, D.; Mitchell, E.; Martin, B.; Cutler, R.G.; Evans, G.; Whiteside, S.; Maudsley, S.; et al. The effect of intermittent energy and carbohydrate restriction v. daily energy restriction on weight loss and metabolic disease risk markers in overweight women. *Br. J. Nutr.* **2013**, *110*, 1534–1547. [CrossRef]
32. Harvie, M.; French, D.P.; Pegington, M.; Evans, D.G.R. Howell. Family History Lifestyle Study. *ISRCTN Regist.* **2020**, serial online.
33. Cuzick, J.; Forbes, J.; Edwards, R.; Baum, M.; Cawthorn, S.; Coates, A.; Hamed, A.; Howell, A.; Powles, T. IBIS investigators. First results from the International Breast Cancer Intervention Study (IBIS-I): A randomised prevention trial. *Lancet* **2002**, *360*, 817–824. [CrossRef]
34. Cuzick, J.; Sestak, I.; Forbes, J.F.; Dowsett, M.; Knox, J.; Cawthorn, S.; Saunders, C.; Roche, N.; Mansel, R.E.; von Minckwitz, G.; et al. Anastrozole for prevention of breast cancer in high-risk postmenopausal women (IBIS-II): An international, double-blind, randomised placebo-controlled trial. *Lancet* **2014**, *383*, 1041–1048. [CrossRef]
35. Lalloo, F.; Baildam ABrain, A.; Hopwood, P.; Evans, D.G.; Howell, A. A protocol for preventative mastectomy in women with an increased lifetime risk of breast cancer. *Eur. J. Surg. Oncol.* **2000**, *26*, 711–713. [CrossRef]
36. Gandhi, A.; Duxbury, P.; Murphy, J.; Foden, P.; Lalloo, F.; Clancy, T.; Wisely, J.; Howell, A.; Evans, D.G. Patient Reported Outcome Measures in a Cohort of Patients at High Risk of Breast Cancer Treated by Bilateral Risk Reducing Mastectomy and Breast Reconstruction. *Plast. Reconstr. Surg.*. in press.
37. Hopwood, P.; Lee, A.; Shenton, A.; Baildam, A.; Brain, A.; Lalloo, F.; Evans, G.; Howell, A. Clinical follow-up after bilateral risk reducing ('prophylactic') mastectomy: Mental health and body image outcomes. *Psychooncology* **2000**, *9*, 462–472. [CrossRef]
38. Hatcher, M.B.; Fallowfield, L.; A'Hern, R. The psychosocial impact of bilateral prophylactic mastectomy: Prospective study using questionnaires and semistructured interviews. *BMJ* **2001**, *322*, 76. [CrossRef] [PubMed]
39. Tyrer-Cuzick (IBIS) Risk Evaluation Tool. Available online: riskevaluator@ems-trials.org (accessed on 20 October 2020).
40. Lee, A.; Mavaddat, N.; Wilcox, A.N.; Cunningham, A.P.; Carver, T.; Hartley, S.; Babb de Villiers, C.; Izquierdo, A.; Simard, J.; Schmidt, M.K.; et al. Version 2.BOADICEA: A comprehensive breast cancer risk prediction model incorporating genetic and nongenetic risk factors. *Genet. Med.* **2019**, *21*, 1708–1718. [CrossRef] [PubMed]

41. Cuzick, J.; Sestak, I.; Forbes, J.F.; Dowsett, M.; Cawthorn, S.; Mansel, R.E.; Loibl, S.; Bonanni, B.; Evans, D.G.; Howell, A.; et al. Use of anastrozole for breast cancer prevention (IBIS-II): Long-term results of a randomised controlled trial. *Lancet* **2020**, *395*, 117–122. [CrossRef]
42. Evans, D.G.; Lalloo, F.; Ashcroft, L.; Shenton, A.; Clancy, T.; Baildam, A.D.; Brain, A.; Hopwood, P.; Howell, A. Uptake of risk-reducing surgery in unaffected women at high risk of breast and ovarian cancer is risk, age, and time dependent. *Cancer Epidemiol. Biomark. Prev.* **2009**, *18*, 2318–2324. [CrossRef]
43. Evans, D.G.; Brentnall, A.R.; Harvie, M.; Dawe, S.; Sergeant, J.C.; Stavrinos, P.; Astley, S.; Wilson, M.; Ainsworth, J.; Cuzick, J.; et al. Breast cancer risk in young women in the national breast screening programme: Implications for applying NICE guidelines for additional screening and chemoprevention. *Cancer Prev. Res. (Phila.)* **2014**, *7*, 993–1001. [CrossRef]
44. Evans, D.G.; Barwell, J.; Eccles, D.M.; Collins, A.; Izatt, L.; Jacobs, C.; Donaldson, A.; Brady, A.F.; Cuthbert, A.; Harrison, R.; et al. The Angelina Jolie effect: How high celebrity profile can have a major impact on provision of cancer related services. *Breast Cancer Res.* **2014**, *16*, 442. [CrossRef]
45. Evans, D.G.; Wisely, J.; Clancy, T.; Lalloo, F.; Wilson, M.; Johnson, R.; Duncan, J.; Barr, L.; Gandhi, A.; Howell, A. Longer term effects of the Angelina Jolie effect: Increased risk-reducing mastectomy rates in BRCA carriers and other high-risk women. *Breast Cancer Res.* **2015**, *17*, 143. [CrossRef]
46. Evans, D.G.; Donnelly, L.S.; Harkness, E.F.; Astley, S.M.; Stavrinos, P.; Dawe, S.; Watterson, D.; Fox, L.; Sergeant, J.C.; Ingham, S.; et al. Breast cancer risk feedback to women in the UK NHS breast screening population. *Br. J. Cancer* **2016**, *114*, 1045–1052. [CrossRef] [PubMed]
47. Vachon, C.M.; Pankratz, V.S.; Scott, C.G.; Haeberle, L.; Ziv, E.; Jensen, M.R.; Brandt, K.R.; Whaley, D.H.; Olson, J.E.; Heusinger, K.; et al. The contributions of breast density and common genetic variation to breast cancer risk. *J. Natl. Cancer Inst.* **2015**, *107*, dju397. [CrossRef] [PubMed]
48. Zhang, X.; Rice, M.; Tworoger, S.S.; Rosner, B.A.; Eliassen, A.H.; Tamimi, R.M.; Joshi, A.D.; Lindstrom, S.; Qian, J. Addition of a polygenic risk score, mammographic density, and endogenous hormones to existing breast cancer risk prediction models: A nested case-control study. *PLoS Med.* **2018**, *15*, e1002644. [CrossRef] [PubMed]
49. Terry, M.B.; Liao, Y.; Whittemore, A.S.; Leoce, N.; Buchsbaum, R.; Zeinomar, N.; Dite, G.S.; Chung, W.K.; Knight, J.A.; Southey, M.C.; et al. 10-year performance of four models of breast cancer risk: A validation study. *Lancet Oncol.* **2019**, *20*, 504–517. [CrossRef]
50. Pal, C.P.; Wilcox, A.N.; Brook, M.N.; Zhang, Y.; Ahearn, T.; Orr, N.; Coulson, P.; Schoemaker, M.J.; Jones, M.E.; Gail, M.H.; et al. Comparative Validation of Breast Cancer Risk Prediction Models and Projections for Future Risk Stratification. *J. Natl. Cancer Inst.* **2020**, *112*, 278–285. [CrossRef]
51. Easton, D.F.; Pooley, K.A.; Dunning, A.M.; Pharoah, P.D.; Thompson, D.; Ballinger, D.G.; Struewing, J.P.; Morrison, J.; Field, H.; Luben, R.; et al. Genome-wide association study identifies novel breast cancer susceptibility loci. *Nature* **2007**, *447*, 1087–1093. [CrossRef]
52. Turnbull, C.; Ahmed, S.; Morrison, J.; Pernet, D.; Renwick, A.; Maranian, M.; Seal, S.; Ghoussaini, M.; Hines, S.; Healey, C.S.; et al. Genome-wide association study identifies five new breast cancer susceptibility loci. *Nat. Genet.* **2010**, *42*, 504–507. [CrossRef]
53. Evans, D.G.; Brentnall, A.; Byers, H.; Harkness, E.; Stavrinos, P.; Howell, A.; FH-risk study Group; Newman, W.G.; Cuzick, J. The impact of a panel of 18 SNPs on breast cancer risk in women attending a UK familial screening clinic: A case-control study. *J. Med. Genet.* **2017**, *54*, 111–113. [CrossRef]
54. Van Veen, E.M.; Brentnall, A.R.; Byers, H.; Harkness, E.F.; Astley, S.M.; Sampson, S.; Howell, A.; Newman, W.G.; Cuzick, J.; Evans, D.G.R. Use of Single-Nucleotide Polymorphisms and Mammographic Density Plus Classic Risk Factors for Breast Cancer Risk Prediction. *JAMA Oncol.* **2018**, *4*, 476–482. [CrossRef]
55. Brentnall, A.R.; van Veen, E.M.; Harkness, E.F.; Rafiq, S.; Byers, H.; Astley, S.M.; Sampson, S.; Howell, A.; Newman, W.G.; Cuzick, J.; et al. A case-control evaluation of 143 single nucleotide polymorphisms for breast cancer risk stratification with classical factors and mammographic density. *Int. J. Cancer* **2020**, *146*, 2122–2129. [CrossRef]
56. Maurice, A.R.; Evans, D.G.R.; Shenton, A.; Ashcroft, L.; Baildam, A.; Barr, L.; Byrne, G.; Bundred, N.; Boggis, C.; Wilson, M.; et al. Howell A Screening younger women with a family history of breast cancer-does early detection improve outcome? *Eur. J. Cancer* **2006**, *42*, 1385–1390. [CrossRef] [PubMed]

57. Duffy, S.W. FH01 collaborative teams. Mammographic surveillance in women younger than 50 years who have a family history of breast cancer: Tumour characteristics and projected effect on mortality in the prospective, single-arm, FH01 study. *Lancet Oncol.* **2010**, *11*, 1127–1134. [CrossRef]
58. Evans, D.G.; Thomas, S.; Caunt, J.; Burch, A.; Brentnall, A.R.; Roberts, L.; Howell, A.; Wilson, M.; Fox, R.; Hillier, S.; et al. Final Results of the Prospective FH02 Mammographic Surveillance Study of Women Aged 35-39 at Increased Familial Risk of Breast Cancer. *EClinicalMedicine* **2019**, *7*, 39–46. [CrossRef]
59. Van den Ende, C.; Oordt-Speets, A.M.; Vroling, H.; van Agt, H.M.E. Benefits and harms of breast cancer screening with mammography in women aged 40-49 years: A systematic review. *Int. J. Cancer* **2017**, *141*, 1295–1306. [CrossRef] [PubMed]
60. Duffy, S.W.; Vulkan, D.; Cuckle, H.; Parmar, D.; Sheikh, S.; Smith, R.A.; Evans, A.; Blyuss, O.; Johns, L.; Ellis, I.O.; et al. Effect of mammographic screening from age 40 years on breast cancer mortality (UK Age trial): Final results of a randomised, controlled trial. *Lancet Oncol.* **2020**, *21*, 1165–1172. [CrossRef]
61. Shieh, Y.; Eklund, M.; Madlensky, L.; Sawyer, S.D.; Thompson, C.K.; Stover Fiscalini, A.; Ziv, E.; Van't Veer, L.J.; Esserman, L.J.; Tice, J.A.; et al. Breast Cancer Screening in the Precision Medicine Era: Risk-Based Screening in a Population-Based Trial. *J. Natl. Cancer Inst.* **2017**, *109*. [CrossRef]
62. UNICANCER (2018) My Personalized Breast Screening (myPeBS). Available online: https://clinicaltrials.gov/ct2/show/NCT0367233 (accessed on 12 October 2020).
63. Williams, M.; Woof, V.G.; Donnelly, L.S.; Howell, A.; Evans, D.G.; French, D.P. Risk stratified breast cancer screening: UK healthcare policy decision-making stakeholders' views on a low-risk breast screening pathway. *BMC Cancer* **2020**, *20*, 680. [CrossRef]
64. Ionescu, G.V.; Fergie, M.; Berks, M.; Harkness, E.F.; Hulleman, J.; Brentnall, A.R.; Cuzick, J.; Evans, D.G.; Astley, S.M. Prediction of reader estimates of mammographic density using convolutional neural networks. *J. Med. Imaging (Bellingham)* **2019**, *6*, 031405. [CrossRef]
65. Hopper, J.L.; Nguyen, T.L.; Schmidt, D.F.; Makalic, E.; Song, Y.M.; Sung, J.; Dite, G.S.; Dowty, J.G.; Li, S. Going Beyond Conventional Mammographic Density to Discover Novel Mammogram-Based Predictors of Breast Cancer Risk. *J. Clin. Med.* **2020**, *9*, 627. [CrossRef]
66. Evans, D.G.; Kesavan, N.; Lim, Y.; Gadde, S.; Hurley, E.; Massat, N.J.; Maxwell, A.J.; Ingham, S.; Eeles, R.; Leach, M.O.; et al. MRI breast screening in high-risk women: Cancer detection and survival analysis. *Breast Cancer Res. Treat.* **2014**, *145*, 663–672. [CrossRef]
67. Kuhl, C.K.; Schrading, S.; Leutner, C.C.; Morakkabati-Spitz, N.; Wardelmann, E.; Fimmers, R.; Kuhn, W.; Schild, H.H. Mammography, breast ultrasound, and magnetic resonance imaging for surveillance of women at high familial risk for breast cancer. *J. Clin. Oncol.* **2005**, *23*, 8469–8476. [CrossRef] [PubMed]
68. Kriege, M.; Brekelmans, C.T.; Boetes, C.; Besnard, P.E.; Zonderland, H.M.; Obdeijn, I.M.; Manoliu, R.A.; Kok, T.; Peterse, H.; Tilanus-Linthorst, M.M.; et al. Efficacy of MRI and mammography for breast-cancer screening in women with a familial or genetic predisposition. *N. Engl. J. Med.* **2004**, *351*, 427–437. [CrossRef] [PubMed]
69. Warner, E.; Plewes, D.B.; Hill, K.A.; Causer, P.A.; Zubovits, J.T.; Jong, R.A.; Cutrara, M.R.; DeBoer, G.; Yaffe, M.J.; Messner, S.J.; et al. Surveillance of BRCA1 and BRCA2 mutation carriers with magnetic resonance imaging, ultrasound, mammography, and clinical breast examination. *JAMA* **2004**, *292*, 1317–1325. [CrossRef] [PubMed]
70. Evans, D.G.; Harkness, E.; Howell, A.; Wilson, M.; Hurley, E.; Lim, Y.; Maxwell, A.; Moller, P. Intensive breast screening in BRCA2 mutation carriers is associated with reduced breast cancer specific and all cause mortality. *Hered. Cancer Clin. Pract.* **2016**, *14*, 8. [CrossRef]
71. Hopper, J.L.; Dite, G.S.; MacInnis, R.J. Age-specific breast cancer risk by body mass index and familial risk: Prospective family study cohort (ProF-SC). *Breast Cancer Res.* **2018**, *20*, 132. [CrossRef]
72. Arthur, R.S.; Wang, T.; Xue, X.; Kamensky, V.; Rohan, T.E. Genetic factors, adherence to healthy lifestyle behavior, and risk of invasive breast cancer among women in the UK Biobank. *J. Natl. Cancer Inst* **2020**, 893–901. [CrossRef]
73. Maas, P.; Barrdahl, M.; Joshi, A.D. Breast Cancer Risk from Modifiable and Nonmodifiable Risk Factors among White Women in the United States. *JAMA Oncol.* **2016**, *2*, 1295–1302. [CrossRef]
74. Behaviour Change Guidance PH6. 2007. Available online: https://www.nice.org.uk/Guidance/PH6 (accessed on 12 October 2020).

75. Wright, C.E.; Harvie, M.; Howell, A.; Evans, D.G.; Hulbert-Williams, N.; Donnelly, L.S. Beliefs about weight and breast cancer: An interview study with high risk women following a 12 month weight loss intervention. *Hered Cancer Clin. Pract* **2015**, *13*, 1. [CrossRef]
76. French, D.P.; Cameron, E.; Benton, J.S.; Deaton, C.; Harvie, M. Can Communicating Personalised Disease Risk Promote Healthy Behaviour Change? A Systematic Review of Systematic Reviews. *Ann. Behav. Med.* **2017**, *51*, 718–729. [CrossRef]
77. Cuzick, J.; Sestak, I.; Bonanni, B.; Costantino, J.P.; Cummings, S.; DeCensi, A.; Dowsett, M.; Forbes, J.F.; Ford, L.; LaCroix, A.Z.; et al. Selective oestrogen receptor modulators in prevention of breast cancer: An updated meta-analysis of individual participant data. *Lancet* **2013**, *381*, 1827–1834. [CrossRef]
78. Cuzick, J.; Sestak, I.; Cawthorn, S.; Hamed, H.; Holli, K.; Howell, A.; Forbes, J.F.; IBIS-I Investigators. Tamoxifen for prevention of breast cancer: Extended long-term follow-up of the IBIS-I breast cancer prevention trial. *Lancet Oncol.* **2015**, *16*, 67–75. [CrossRef]
79. Chlebowski, R.T.; Anderson, G.L.; Aragaki, A.K.; Manson, J.E.; Stefanick, M.L.; Pan, K.; Barrington, W.; Kuller, L.H.; Simon, M.S.; Lane, D.; et al. Association of Menopausal Hormone Therapy With Breast Cancer Incidence and Mortality During Long-term Follow-up of the Women's Health Initiative Randomized Clinical Trials. *JAMA* **2020**, *324*, 369–380. [CrossRef] [PubMed]
80. Donnelly, L.S.; Evans, D.G.; Wiseman, J.; Fox, J.; Greenhalgh, R.; Affen, J.; Juraskova, I.; Stavrinos, P.; Dawe, S.; Cuzick, J.; et al. Uptake of tamoxifen in consecutive premenopausal women under surveillance in a high-risk breast cancer clinic. *Br. J. Cancer* **2014**, *110*, 1681–1687. [CrossRef] [PubMed]
81. Smith, S.G.; Sestak, I.; Forster, A.; Partridge, A.; Side, L.; Wolf, M.S. Factors affecting uptake and adherence to breast cancer chemoprevention: A systematic review and meta-analysis. *Ann. Oncol.* **2016**, *27*, 575–590. [CrossRef]
82. Fallowfield, L.; Fleissig, A.; Edwards, R.; West, A.; Powles, T.J.; Howell, A.; Cuzick, J. Tamoxifen for the prevention of breast cancer: Psychosocial impact on women participating in two randomized controlled trials. *J. Clin. Oncol.* **2001**, *19*, 1885–1892. [CrossRef]
83. Smith, S.G.; Sestak, I.; Howell, A.; Forbes, J.; Cuzick, J. Participant-Reported Symptoms and Their Effect on Long-Term Adherence in the International Breast Cancer Intervention Study I (IBIS I). *J. Clin. Oncol.* **2017**, *35*, 2666–2673. [CrossRef]
84. Sestak, I.; Smith, S.G.; Howell, A.; Forbes, J.F.; Cuzick, J. Early participant-reported symptoms as predictors of adherence to anastrozole in the International Breast Cancer Intervention Studies II. *Ann. Oncol.* **2018**, *29*, 504–509. [CrossRef]
85. DeCensi, A.; Puntoni, M.; Guerrieri-Gonzaga, A.; Caviglia, S.; Avino, F.; Cortesi, L.; Taverniti, C.; Pacquola, M.G.; Falcini, F.; Gulisano, M.; et al. Randomized Placebo Controlled Trial of Low-Dose Tamoxifen to Prevent Local and Contralateral Recurrence in Breast Intraepithelial Neoplasia. *J. Clin. Oncol.* **2019**, *37*, 1629–1637. [CrossRef]
86. Robertson, J.F.; Willsher, P.C.; Winterbottom, L.; Blamey, R.W.; Thorpe, S. Onapristone, a progesterone receptor antagonist, as first-line therapy in primary breast cancer. *Eur. J. Cancer* **1999**, *35*, 214–218. [CrossRef]
87. Nolan, E.; Vaillant, F.; Branstetter, D.; Pal, B.; Giner, G.; Whitehead, L.; Lok, S.W.; Mann, G.B.; Kathleen Cuningham Foundation Consortium for Research into Familial Breast Cancer (kConFab); Rohrbach, K.; et al. RANK ligand as a potential target for breast cancer prevention in BRCA1-mutation carriers. *Nat. Med.* **2016**, *22*, 933–939. [CrossRef]
88. Hartmann, L.C.; Schaid, D.J.; Woods, J.E.; Crotty, T.P.; Myers, J.L.; Arnold, P.G.; Petty, P.M.; Sellers, T.A.; Johnson, J.L.; McDonnell, S.K.; et al. Efficacy of bilateral prophylactic mastectomy in women with a family history of breast cancer. *N. Engl. J. Med.* **1999**, *340*, 77–84. [CrossRef] [PubMed]
89. Razdan, S.N.; Patel, V.; Jewell, S.; McCarthy, C.M. Quality of life among patients after bilateral prophylactic mastectomy: A systematic review of patient-reported outcomes. *Qual. Life Res.* **2016**, *25*, 1409–1421. [CrossRef] [PubMed]
90. Jakub, J.W.; Peled, A.W.; Gray, R.J.; Greenup, R.A.; Kiluk, J.V.; Sacchini, V.; McLaughlin, S.A.; Tchou, J.C.; Vierkant, R.A.; Degnim, A.C.; et al. Oncologic Safety of Prophylactic Nipple-Sparing Mastectomy in a Population With BRCA Mutations: A Multi-institutional Study. *JAMA Surg.* **2018**, *153*, 123–129. [CrossRef] [PubMed]
91. Shay, P.; Jacobs, J. Autologous reconstruction following nipple sparing mastectomy: A comprehensive review of the current literature. *Gland Surg.* **2018**, *7*, 316–324. [CrossRef] [PubMed]

92. Dave, R.V.; Vucicevic Al Highton, L.; Harvey, J.R.; Johnson, R.; Kirwan, C.C.; Murphy, J. Medium term outcomes following immediate prepectoral implant based breast reconstruction using acellular dermal matrix. *Br. J. Surg.* **2020**. [CrossRef]
93. Gandhi, A.; Barr, L.; Johnson, R. Bioprosthetics: Changing the landscape for breast reconstruction. *Eur. J. Surg. Oncol.* **2013**, *39*, 24–25. [CrossRef] [PubMed]
94. Groen, J.W.; Negenborn, V.L.; Twisk, D.J.W.R.; Rizopoulos, D.; Ket, J.C.F.; Smit, J.M.; Mullender, M.G. Autologous fat grafting in onco-plastic breast reconstruction: A systematic review on oncological and radiological safety, complications, volume retention and patient/surgeon satisfaction. *J. Plast. Reconstr. Aesthet. Surg.* **2016**, *69*, 742–764. [CrossRef]
95. Ingham, S.L.; Sperrin, M.; Baildam, A.; Ross, G.L.; Clayton, R.; Lalloo, F.; Buchan, I.; Howell, A.; Evans, D.G. Risk-reducing surgery increases survival in BRCA1/2 mutation carriers unaffected at time of family referral. *Breast Cancer Res. Treat.* **2013**, *142*, 611–618. [CrossRef]
96. Heemskerk-Gerritsen, B.A.M.; Jager, A.; Koppert, L.B.; Obdeijn, A.I.; Collée, M.; Meijers-Heijboer, H.E.J.; Jenner, D.J.; Oldenburg, H.S.A.; van Engelen, K.; de Vries, J.; et al. Survival after bilateral risk-reducing mastectomy in healthy BRCA1 and BRCA2 mutation carriers. *Breast Cancer Res. Treat.* **2019**, *177*, 723–733. [CrossRef]
97. Evans, D.G.; Howell, S.J.; Howell, A. Should unaffected female *BRCA2* pathogenic variant carriers be told there is little or no advantage from risk reducing mastectomy? *Fam. Cancer* **2019**, *18*, 377–379. [CrossRef]
98. Braude, L.; Kirsten, L.; Gilchrist, J.; Juraskova, I. A systematic review of women's satisfaction and regret following risk-reducing mastectomy. *Patient Educ. Couns.* **2017**, *100*, 2182–2189. [CrossRef] [PubMed]
99. French, D.P.; Astley, S.; Brentnall, A.R.; Cuzick, J.; Dobrashian, R.; Duffy, S.W.; Gorman, L.S.; Harkness, E.F.; Harrison, F.; Harvie, M.; et al. What are the benefits and harms of risk stratified screening as part of the NHS Breast Screening Programme? Study protocol for a multi-site non-randomised comparison of BC-Predict versus usual screening. *BMC Cancer* **2020**, *20*, 570. [CrossRef] [PubMed]
100. French, D.P.; Southworth, J.; Howell, A.; Harvie, M.; Stavrinos, P.; Watterson, D.; Sampson, S.; Evans, D.G.; Donnely, L.S. Psychological impact of providing women with personalized ten-year breast cancer risk estimates. *Br. J. Cancer* **2018**, *118*, 1648–1657. [CrossRef] [PubMed]
101. Sabatino, S.A.; McCarthy, E.P.; Phillips, R.S.; Burns, R.B. Breast cancer risk assessment and management in primary care: Provider attitudes, practices, and barriers. *Cancer Detect Prev.* **2007**, *31*, 375–383. [CrossRef] [PubMed]
102. Keogh, L.A.; Steel, E.; Weideman, P.; Butow, P.; Collins, I.M.; Emery, J.D.; Mann, G.B.; Bickerstaffe, A.; Trainer, A.H.; Hopper, L.J.; et al. Consumer and clinician perspectives on personalising breast cancer prevention information. *Breast* **2019**, *43*, 39–47. [CrossRef] [PubMed]
103. Archer, S.; Babb de Villiers, C.; Scheibl, F.; Carver, T.; Hartley, S.; Lee, A.; Cunningham, A.P.; Easton, D.F.; McIntosh, J.G.; Emery, J.; et al. Evaluating clinician acceptability of the prototype CanRisk tool for predicting risk of breast and ovarian cancer: A multi-methods study. *PLoS ONE* **2020**, *15*, e0229999. [CrossRef]
104. Hippisley-Cox, J.; Coupland, C. Development and validation of QMortality risk prediction algorithm to estimate short term risk of death and assess frailty: Cohort study. *BMJ* **2017**, *358*, j4208. [CrossRef]
105. Lo, L.L.; Collins, I.M.; Bressel, M.; Butow, P.; Emery, J.; Keogh, L.; Weideman, P.; Steel, E.; Hopper, J.L.; Trainer, A.H.; et al. The iPrevent Online Breast Cancer Risk Assessment and Risk Management Tool: Usability and Acceptability Testing. *JMIR Form Res.* **2018**, *2*, e24. [CrossRef]
106. Howell, A.; Anderson, A.S.; Clarke, R.; Duffy, S.W.; Evans, D.G.; Garcia–Closas, M.; Gescher, A.J.; Key, T.J.; Saxton, J.M.; Harvie, M.N. Risk Determination and Prevention of Breast Cancer. *Breast Cancer Res.* **2014**, *16*, 446. [CrossRef]

5

Women's Intentions to Engage in Risk-Reducing Behaviours after Receiving Personal Ovarian Cancer Risk Information: An Experimental Survey Study

Ailish Gallagher [1], Jo Waller [2], Ranjit Manchanda [3,4], Ian Jacobs [5] and Saskia Sanderson [1,6,*]

1 Research Department of Behavioural Science and Health, University College London, Gower Street, London WC1E 6BT, UK; Ailish.gallagher@gstt.nhs.uk
2 Cancer Prevention Group, School of Cancer & Pharmaceutical Sciences, King's College London, Guy's Hospital, Great Maze Pond, London SE1 9RT, UK; jo.waller@kcl.ac.uk
3 Wolfson Institute of Preventive Medicine, Barts Cancer Institute, Queen Mary University of London, Charterhouse Square, London EC1M 6BQ, UK; r.manchanda@qmul.ac.uk
4 Department of Gynaecological Oncology, Barts Health NHS Trust, London EC1A 7BE, UK
5 Department of Women's Health, University of New South Wales, Australia, Level 1, Chancellery Building, Sydney 2052, Australia; i.jacobs@unsw.edu.au
6 Early Disease Detection Research Project UK (EDDRP UK), 2 Redman Place, London E20 1JQ, UK
* Correspondence: saskia.sanderson@ucl.ac.uk

Simple Summary: Risk stratification using genetic testing to identify women at increased risk of ovarian cancer may increase the number of patients to whom risk-reducing surgery (e.g., salpingo-oophorectomy) may be offered. However, little is known about public acceptability of such approaches. Our online experimental survey aimed to explore whether women aged 45–75 in the general population are willing to undergo ovarian cancer risk assessment, including genetic testing, and whether women's potential acceptance of risk-reducing surgery differs depending on their estimated risk. We looked at whether psychological and cognitive factors mediated women's decision-making. The majority of participants would be interested in having genetic testing. In response to our hypothetical scenarios, a substantial proportion of participants were open to the idea of surgery to reduce risk of ovarian cancer, even if their absolute lifetime risk is only increased from 2% to 5 or 10%.

Abstract: Risk stratification using genetic and/or other types of information could identify women at increased ovarian cancer risk. The aim of this study was to examine women's potential reactions to ovarian cancer risk stratification. A total of 1017 women aged 45–75 years took part in an online experimental survey. Women were randomly assigned to one of three experimental conditions describing hypothetical personal results from ovarian cancer risk stratification, and asked to imagine they had received one of three results: (a) 5% lifetime risk due to single nucleotide polymorphisms (SNPs) and lifestyle factors; (b) 10% lifetime risk due to SNPs and lifestyle factors; (c) 10% lifetime risk due to a single rare mutation in a gene. Results: 83% of women indicated interest in having ovarian cancer risk assessment. After receiving their hypothetical risk estimates, 29% of women stated they would have risk-reducing surgery. Choosing risk-reducing surgery over other behavioural responses was associated with having higher surgery self-efficacy and perceived response-efficacy, but not with perceptions of disease threat, i.e., perceived risk or severity, or with experimental condition. A substantial proportion of women age 45–75 years may be open to the idea of surgery to reduce risk of ovarian cancer, even if their absolute lifetime risk is only increased to as little as 5 or 10%.

Keywords: risk stratification; genomics; questionnaires; attitudes

1. Introduction

Ovarian cancer is the sixth most common cancer among women in the UK. The general population lifetime risk of developing ovarian cancer is approximately 2%, and incidence is predicted to rise by 26% in the UK, 14% in Europe, and by 55% worldwide over the next two decades [1]. The risk of ovarian cancer rises with age, increasing significantly in women over 45 years [2]. DNA variants in a number of cancer susceptibility genes are known to be associated with ovarian cancer: women with a high penetrance genetic variant, such as a *BRCA1* or *BRCA2* mutation, are considered to be at high risk for developing breast and ovarian cancer [3–5]. Historically, genetic testing for ovarian cancer risk has been clinically indicated only for women with a strong family history of breast and/or ovarian cancer. However, using a family history based approach misses over half the cancer susceptibility gene (CSG) carriers at risk [6,7], and is associated with restricted access and limited utilization of genetic testing [8]. Additionally, the majority of cases of ovarian cancer do not occur in affected families [9]. There is increasing interest in the idea of adopting a risk-stratified approach to ovarian cancer prevention by offering genetic testing to all women regardless of family history [10–12].

In addition to rare variants of high penetrance, genome-wide association studies have to date identified a number of common single nucleotide polymorphisms (SNPs) associated with slightly increased risk of ovarian cancer [13]. SNP-based information and certain lifestyle factors each increase ovarian cancer risk by a small amount individually, but this becomes clinically significant when the information is combined, e.g., from 2% to between 5% and 10% lifetime risk [9,14,15]. Surgical prevention has been shown to be cost-effective at the 4–5% ovarian cancer risk threshold [16,17]. Newer risk models and recently validated intermediate risk genes can identify individuals at these risk thresholds. Risk stratification using multigene testing to identify women at increased risk of ovarian cancer is potentially more cost- and time-effective than single gene testing and increases the number of patients to whom risk-reducing surgery (e.g., salpingo-oophorectomy) may be offered [18]. While clinical practice has gradually begun to change [19], data on public acceptability of such approaches are limited.

An initial quantitative study assessing attitudes towards population-based genetic testing for ovarian cancer risk in a general population sample found high levels of support for risk-stratified ovarian cancer screening based on prior genetic risk assessment [20]. There is good evidence to suggest that population-wide genetic testing for ovarian cancer is acceptable, feasible and cost-effective amongst Ashkenazi Jewish populations [6,7,21–23]. Preliminary data from the general population also indicate that population-based personalised ovarian cancer risk stratification is feasible, acceptable, has high satisfaction, reduces cancer worry/risk perception, and does not negatively impact psychological health or quality of life [12].

Bilateral risk-reducing salpingo-oophorectomy (surgical removal of the ovaries and fallopian tubes, hereafter referred to as "risk-reducing salpingo-oophorectomy" or "RRSO") is currently recommended as the main and most effective preventative strategy for ovarian cancer in women at increased risk of ovarian cancer such as *BRCA* mutation carriers. RRSO can reduce ovarian cancer risk by 85–90% [24]. Traditionally the most common group of women undergoing surgical prevention have been *BRCA* carriers, who have a 17–44% lifetime risk of ovarian cancer [5,25]. In the UK, women with an estimated lifetime ovarian cancer risk of greater than 10%, who have completed their families, have traditionally been offered risk-reducing surgery [15]. Undertaking surgery on the basis of family history alone in the absence of a known mutation (at lower than *BRCA* levels of risk) has thus been clinical practice in the UK and other countries for many years [25,26]. Recently, the 10% threshold was relaxed to 4–5% [14,15]. A number of new ovarian cancer risk genes have been identified, such as *RAD51C* (lifetime risk 11%) [27], *RAD51D* (lifetime risk 13%), *PALB2* (lifetime risk 5%) [28], and *BRIP1* (lifetime risk 5.8%) [29], testing for which is part of routine clinical practice. RRSO is now offered and being undertaken for these CSGs too. Thus a number of clinical teams now offer RRSO to women in the "intermediate" risk category (5–10%) as well as those in the "high" risk category (over 10%) [15]. Additionally, more complex models using SNP profiles, in combination with other epidemiological and genetic risk factors, are being validated, which will provide absolute lifetime risk estimates in these ranges in the not too distant future [12].

National screening programmes for ovarian cancer are unavailable. In a large randomised control trial designed to establish the effect of early detection by ovarian screening in the general low-risk population, no conclusive significant impact on mortality from ovarian cancer was found [30], and definitive mortality data are awaited in 2021. Surveillance for those identified as high-risk (or in some cases moderate-to-high-risk) for ovarian cancer currently consists of serial 3–4 monthly serum CA125 (Cancer Antigen 125 protein; a tumour marker) measurement (and annual transvaginal ultrasound) aiming to detect pre-symptomatic cancer in the earlier stages and/or low volume disease where treatment is more effective [31]. This 4 monthly longitudinal CA125 biomarker driven surveillance strategy, using the risk of the ovarian cancer (ROCA) algorithm, may be beneficial in women at high risk of ovarian cancer [31]. We have shown that this is associated with a significant stage shift, which can be a surrogate for improved survival [31]. Identifying those at increased risk using a population wide risk-stratified approach may result in more timely risk reduction options and could have a significant impact on disease burden: modelling suggests that 13% of the female UK population have greater than 4% lifetime risk and 9% have greater than 5% lifetime risk [15]. Manchanda et al. (2018) suggest that, based on National Institute for Health and Care Excellence (NICE) cost-effectiveness guidelines, risk-reducing surgery may be cost effective for postmenopausal women over the age of 50, with a lifetime ovarian cancer risk of ≥5%. Wider implementation of targeted surgical prevention for women at greater than 4–5% lifetime risk threshold provides a huge opportunity for cost-effective targeted primary prevention.

Offering risk stratification to women in the general population, including communicating personal ovarian cancer risk information and offering risk-reducing surgery, has the potential to be a feasible way to reduce ovarian cancer mortality and reduce the population burden of the disease. However, risk stratification will only lead to improved ovarian cancer prevention and early diagnosis if women whose results indicate increased risk take action to reduce their risk. Women with a family history of breast and ovarian cancer have been found to opt for risk reduction surgery, e.g., among *BRCA1* and *BRCA2* mutation carriers, the majority underwent risk-reducing surgery (salpingo-oophorectomy) after their risk was communicated to them [25,32]. However, although quite a lot is known about how genetic risk information impacts psychological wellbeing and behaviours among women from families affected with ovarian (and/or breast) cancer, less is known about how women in the wider non-Jewish population might react to being informed they have an increased genetic risk of ovarian cancer [33–37]. Further research is needed to determine how women in the general population might respond if presented with ovarian cancer risk information indicating they are at high risk based on genetic as well as other risk factors.

Based on research prior to 2016, the evidence does not support the hypothesis that communicating CSG-based risk estimates motivates lifestyle behaviour changes [33,38]. CSG-based risk information also has not been associated with negative psychological outcomes [7,33,38,39]. More recently, a nested study within the Predicting Risk of Cancer at Screening (PROCAS) study was conducted comparing the psychological impact of providing women with personalised breast cancer risk estimates based on: (a) the Tyrer–Cuzick (T–C) risk algorithm including breast density, or (b) T–C including breast density plus SNPs, versus (c) comparison women awaiting results. This study found little evidence of either psychological harm or of differences between women provided with risk estimates based on SNPs versus others. However, women categorised as high-risk were excluded from the study, so no conclusions could be drawn regarding high-risk results specifically. It remains to be seen whether the source of the risk may have impacted psychological factors or if it had an effect on acceptance of the risk information in this study [40]. In another recent study that examined the impact of returning secondary findings (including *BRCA1/2*) from genomic sequencing to unselected populations, few adverse psychological effects were found [41].

As an initial step to providing some empirical data on the question of how women in the general population might respond to personal ovarian cancer risk information indicating increased risk (as against moderate risk [40]), we conducted an experimental survey study with women in the general population, using the Extended Parallel Process Model (EPPM) [42] as our theoretical framework, and to inform our selection of variables and measures. The EPPM is a social cognition model of information processing and behaviour: it posits that how individuals react to threatening information is informed by (a) their perceptions of the threat (perceived risk or susceptibility, and perceived severity), and (b) their perceptions of the recommended action to reduce the threat (self-efficacy, i.e., their confidence in their ability to carry out the recommended behaviour, and perceived response efficacy, i.e., their confidence that the recommended behaviour will effectively reduce the threat to their health).

Our specific aims were to: (1) explore whether women in the general population are willing to undergo ovarian cancer risk assessment which includes genetic testing; (2) examine whether women's potential acceptance of risk-reducing surgery differs depending on whether their estimated risk is 5% or 10%; (3) examine whether women's potential acceptance of risk-reducing surgery differs depending on whether their estimated risk is based on a single rare genetic variant of high penetrance or a more complex combination of genetic and non-genetic factors. We also explored whether threat and efficacy cognitions mediated any observed between-group differences, and examined the associations between these cognitions (threat, efficacy) and acceptance of risk-reducing surgery in the sample overall.

2. Results

2.1. Sample Characteristics

Table 1 provides an overview of the participant characteristics. Age ranged from 45 to 75 years with a mean of 57.50 (SD = 8.13). The majority were White (95.6%) with 3.8% from other ethnic backgrounds. Educational attainment was fairly evenly split between General Certificate of Secondary Education (GCSE) or equivalent (34.6%), A levels or equivalent (23.8%), and undergraduate degree or equivalent (24.1%). The majority (85.2%) of women were either perimenopausal (beginning menopause) or post-menopausal. See Figure 1 for the Consolidated Standards of Reporting Trials (CONSORT) flow diagram of participants throughout the study.

Table 1. Sample characteristics and interest in genetic testing overall and in each randomised experimental group (total $n = 1017$).

Variables	Group 1: 5% SNPs and Lifestyle ($n = 340$)	Group 2: 10% SNPs and Lifestyle ($n = 343$)	Group 3: 10% Rare Genetic Variant ($n = 334$)
Demographics		n (%)	
Age Mean (SD)	57.43 (8.32)	57.37 (7.78)	58.08 (8.19)
Age group			
45–50	89 (26.2)	82 (23.9)	73 (21.9)
51–55	71 (20.9)	66 (19.2)	67 (20.1)
56–60	59 (17.4)	70 (20.4)	65 (19.5)
61–65	53 (15.6)	70 (20.4)	61 (18.3)
66–70	42 (12.4)	34 (9.9)	38 (11.4)
71–75	26 (7.6)	21 (6.1)	30 (9.0)
Ethnicity			
White (Any background)	327 (96.2)	324 (94.5)	321 (96.1)
Other ethnic group	11 (3.2)	17 (5.0)	11 (3.3)
Educational Attainment			
No Formal Qualification	26 (7.6)	23 (6.7)	17 (5.1)
GCSE or equivalent	115 (33.8)	126 (36.7)	111 (33.2)
A-Levels or equivalent	75 (22.1)	80 (23.3)	87 (26.0)
Undergraduate degree/equivalent	89 (26.2)	77 (22.4)	79 (23.7)
Postgraduate degree/equivalent	31 (9.1)	30 (8.7)	31 (9.3)
Other	4 (1.2)	7 (2.0)	9 (2.7)

Table 1. *Cont.*

Variables	Group 1: 5% SNPs and Lifestyle (n = 340)	Group 2: 10% SNPs and Lifestyle (n = 343)	Group 3: 10% Rare Genetic Variant (n = 334)
Relationship Status			
Married/Cohabiting/In a relationship	245 (72.1)	232 (67.6)	233 (69.8)
Single/Separated/divorced/widowed	93 (27.4)	111 (32.4)	99 (29.6)
Health Characteristics			
Menopause status			
Premenopausal	41 (12.1)	37 (10.8)	43 (12.9)
During/post menopause	283 (83.2)	298 (86.9)	285 (85.3)
Personal History of Cancer			
Yes	17 (5.0)	16 (4.7)	17 (5.1)
No/Not sure	323 (95.0)	327 (95.3)	317 (94.9)
Family History of Cancer			
Yes	214 (62.4%)	206 (59.7%)	201 (58.8%)
No/Not sure	129 (37.6%)	139 (40.3%)	141 (41.2%)
Cervical Screening			
Regular	192 (72.7)	214 (76.7)	179 (67.8)
Irregular	72 (27.3)	65 (23.3)	85 (32.2)
Not eligible	58 (17.1)	44 (12.8)	62 (18.6)
Breast Screening			
Regular	196 (81.0)	201 (79.4)	196 (79.7)
Irregular	46 (19.0)	52 (20.6)	50 (20.3)
Not eligible	72 (21.2)	59 (17.2)	61 (18.3)
Interest in ovarian cancer risk assessment			
Yes Definitely	139 (40.9)	122 (35.6)	125 (37.4)
Yes Probably	151 (44.4)	156 (45.5)	153 (45.8)
No Probably not	36 (10.6)	46 (13.4)	46 (13.8)
No definitely not	14 (4.1)	19 (5.5)	10 (3.0)

SNPs: single nucleotide polymorphisms; SD: standard deviation; GCSE: General Certificate of Secondary Education.

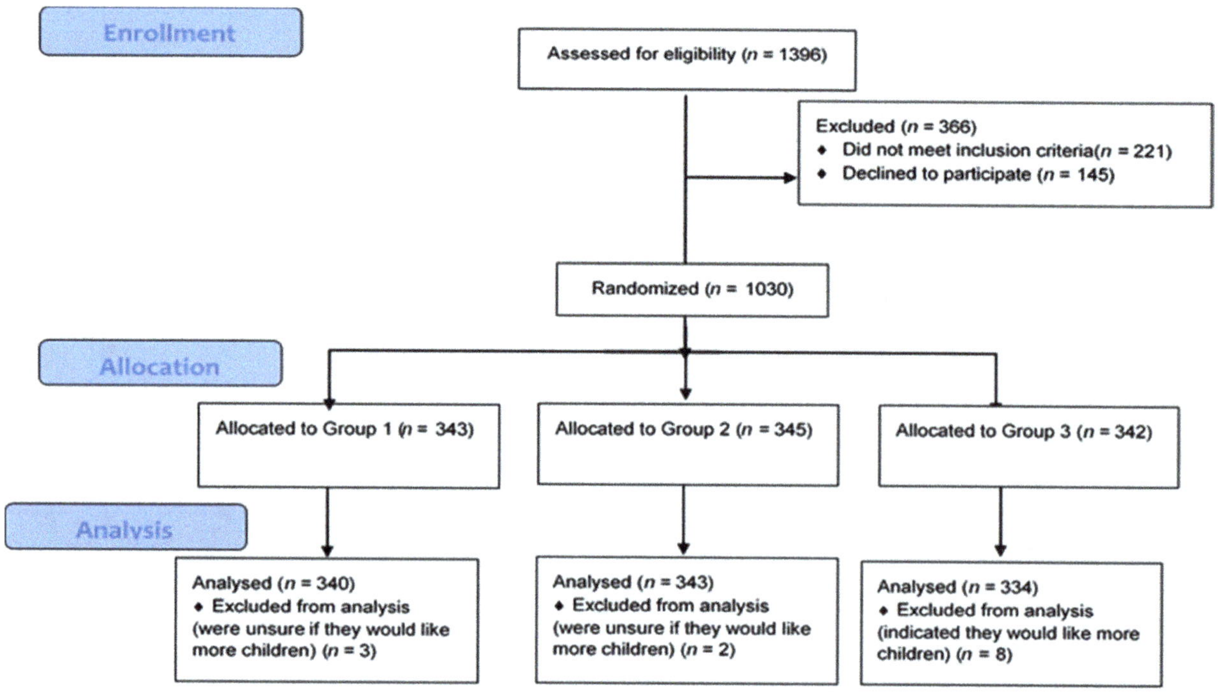

Figure 1. CONSORT 2010 Flow Diagram.

2.2. Interest in Ovarian Cancer Risk Assessment

Overall, 83.2% of women indicated they would "yes definitely" (38.0%) or "yes probably" (45.2%) have an ovarian cancer risk assessment if it was offered to them by their general practitioner (GP) on the National Health Service (NHS) (see Table 1 and Figure 2).

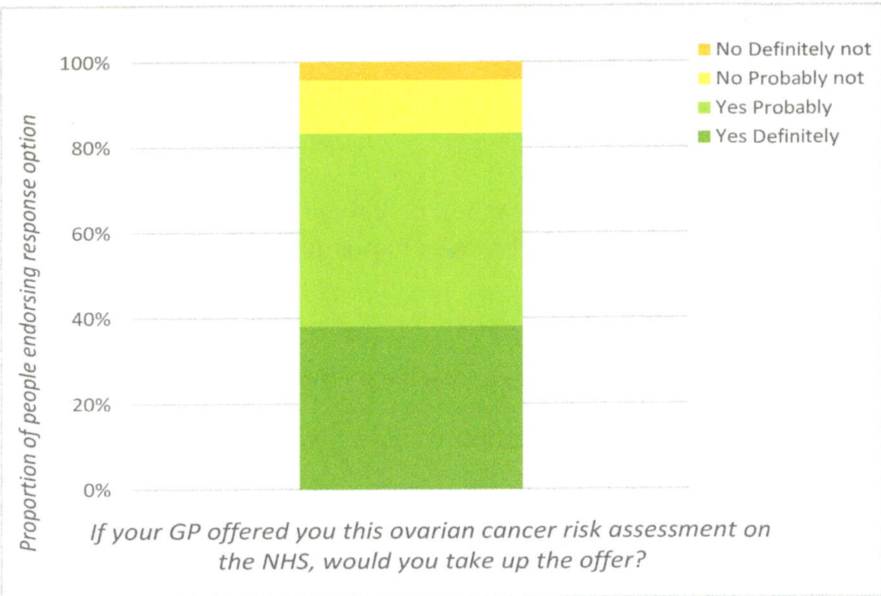

Figure 2. Interest in ovarian cancer risk assessment.

2.3. Behavioural Response to Personalised Ovarian Cancer Risk Information

After receiving their hypothetical risk result, 28.5% of women said they would opt for risk-reducing surgery, 33.9% for increased surveillance (transvaginal ultrasound), and 20.9% would make lifestyle changes (e.g., quitting smoking, maintaining a healthy weight; see Figure 3 and Table S1).

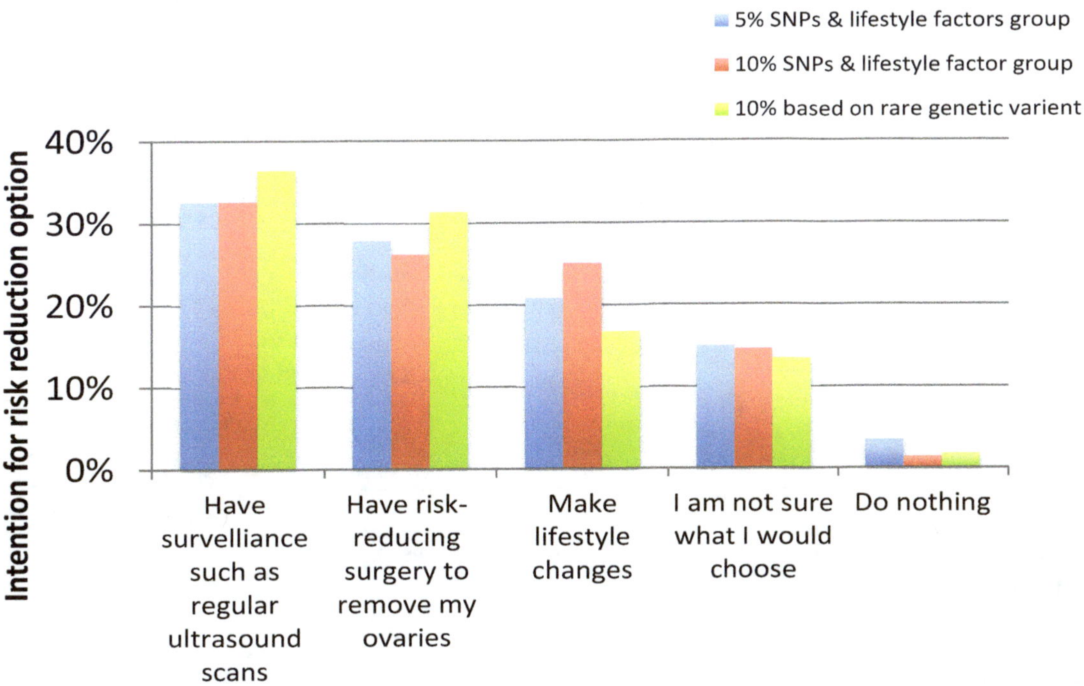

Figure 3. Behavioural intentions after exposure to hypothetical risk scenario compared between groups.

2.4. Differences by Experimental Condition

Women's intentions to have risk-reducing surgery did not differ significantly between the 5% and 10% multifactorial SNPs + lifestyle groups (27.9% vs. 26.2%, respectively) ($\chi^2(1) = 0.314$, $p = 0.61$). Women who received a 10% risk result based on a rare genetic variant were no more likely to opt for RRSO over other risk-reducing options than women who received a 10% risk result based on multifactorial SNPs + lifestyle factors (31.4% vs. 26.2%, respectively) ($\chi^2(1) = 2.512$, $p = 0.13$).

2.5. EPPM Variables

The mean (M) and standard deviation (SD) of the EPPM variables were: perceived risk (M = 3.51, SD = 0.82), perceived severity (M = 4.52, SD = 0.58), perceived response-efficacy (M = 4.03, SD = 0.78), perceived self-efficacy (M = 2.98, SD = 1.34). Means by exposure group are shown in the Supplementary Materials (Table S2).

2.6. Intention to Have Risk-Reducing Surgery (RRSO) versus Other Risk-Management Options

A binary logistic regression was conducted to investigate what factors were associated with hypothetical intention to have risk-reducing surgery vs. other behavioural options. Independent variables included in the model were age, ethnicity, educational attainment, previous breast and cervical screening participation, experimental group and EPPM variables (perceived risk, perceived severity, self-efficacy, perceived response-efficacy). In unadjusted analyses, women reporting higher perceived risk of ovarian cancer and higher perceived severity of ovarian cancer (i.e., the perceived threat variables), and higher surgery self-efficacy and perceived response-efficacy (i.e., variables relating to perceptions of the risk-reducing behaviour) were more likely than other women to opt for risk-reducing surgery. In the multivariable model, perceived response-efficacy (odds ratio (OR) = 2.22; 95% confidence interval (CI): 1.64–3.00) and self-efficacy (OR = 1.90; 95% CI: 1.63–2.22) remained significantly associated, whereas the perceived threat variables were no longer significantly associated, with choosing risk-reducing surgery over other behavioural options. None of the measured socio-demographic or health-related factors were significantly associated with intention to have surgery (see Table 2).

Table 2. Logistic regression predicting likelihood of intending to have risk-reducing surgery vs. other behavioural response (n = 1017).

Variable	Intention to Have Risk-Reducing Surgery	Odds Ratios (95% CI)	
Demographic Factors	n (%)	Unadjusted	Adjusted
Age			
45–50	74 (30.3)	Ref	Ref
51–55	65 (31.9)	1.07 (0.72–1.61)	0.94 (0.51–1.74)
56–60	60 (30.9)	1.03 (0.68–1.55)	1.00 (0.53–1.87)
61–65	49 (26.6)	0.83 (0.55–1.28)	0.62 (0.32–1.19)
66–70	27 (23.7)	0.71 (0.43–1.19)	0.48 (0.14–1.65)
71–75	15 (19.5)	0.56 (0.30–1.04)	0.29 (0.06–1.50)
Ethnicity			
White (Any background)	278 (28.6)	Ref	Ref
Other ethnic group	11 (28.2)	0.98 (0.48–2.00)	1.16 (0.38–3.50)
Educational Attainment			
No formal qualifications	16 (24.2)	Ref	
GCSE/O Levels	111 (31.5)	1.44 (0.79–2.64)	
A-Levels or Equivalent	68 (28.1)	1.22 (0.68–2.29)	
Undergraduate degree	59 (24.1)	0.99 (0.53–1.87)	
Postgraduate degree	28 (30.4)	1.37 (0.67–2.80)	
Other	8 (40.0)	2.08 (0.72–6.00)	

Table 2. *Cont.*

Variable	Intention to Have Risk-Reducing Surgery	Odds Ratios (95% CI)	
		Unadjusted	Adjusted
Demographic Factors	*n* (%)		
Relationship Status			
Not married/in a relationship	82 (27.1)	Ref	
Married/in a relationship	207 (29.2)	1.11 (0.82–1.50)	
Health history			
Cervical Screening Attendance (*n* = 807)			
Regular	200 (34.2)	Ref	Ref
Irregular	49 (22.1)	0.59 (0.41–0.85) *	0.67 (0.41–1.11)
Breast Screening Attendance (*n* = 741)			
Regular	205 (34.6)	Ref	Ref
Irregular	35 (23.6)	0.53 (0.36–0.80) *	0.67 (0.38–1.17)
Menopause status			
Pre-menopause	35 (28.9)	Ref	Ref
Peri/Post-menopause	243 (28.1)	0.96 (0.63–1.46)	
Extended Parallel Processing Model Variables			
Perceived Risk		1.43 (1.19–1.71) **	1.14 (0.90–1.45)
Perceived Severity		1.42 (1.11–1.82) *	1.08 (0.74–1.57)
Self-Efficacy		2.19 (1.94–2.47) **	1.90 (1.63–2.22) **
Perceived Response Efficacy		3.15 (2.50–3.96) **	2.22 (1.64–3.00) **
Experimental condition			
5% SNPs & Lifestyle	95 (32.8)	Ref	Ref
10% SNPS & Lifestyle	90 (31.0)	0.92 (0.66–1.29)	1.08 (0.67–1.73)
10% rare genetic variant	105 (36.2)	1.18 (0.85–1.65)	1.87 (1.17–3.00) **

** Predictor significant at the 0.01 level (2-tailed), * Predictor significant at the 0.05 level (2-tailed), CI = Confidence Interval. Ref = reference category.

3. Discussion

A high proportion (83%) of women in this sample indicated they would be interested in having an ovarian cancer risk assessment if offered by their GP on the NHS. This is consistent with previous research by Meisel et al. (2016), who found that 88% of a general population sample of women in the UK would be interested in genetic testing for ovarian cancer risk if it were offered by the NHS, and included information about breast cancer risk, echoing previous support from qualitative research for the availability of genetic testing and risk-stratified screening [43]. It is also consistent with uptake of genetic testing in our population-based studies [12,21].

We also found that a substantial proportion of British women over the age of 45 years might be open to the idea of having RRSO, even if their absolute lifetime risk were increased from a general population risk of 2% to as little as 5% or 10%. In addition, we also demonstrated in multivariable analyses that perceptions of risk-reducing surgery (self-efficacy and perceived response-efficacy) were independently associated with choosing surgery over other options, whereas the perceived threat of ovarian cancer (perceived risk and perceived severity) was not.

Although over a quarter (29%) of women opted for RRSO, slightly more women opted for surveillance (34%). The observed preference for surveillance may be due to the invasiveness of surgery, and could also potentially be due to the generally positive attitude towards cancer screening in the UK [44]. Lack of detailed information on the efficacy of each risk management option due to the hypothetical nature of this study may have resulted in participants deciding on the less invasive option, i.e., surveillance. Research suggests perceptions about risk-reducing surgery and surveillance are potentially modifiable: Mai et al. (2017) identified misperceptions about ovarian cancer risk and benefits of screening as important factors influencing decisions about risk-reducing surgery versus surveillance [45]. The concept of common genetic variants of low penetrance single nucleotide polymorphisms (SNPs) may be unfamiliar to the majority of individuals in the general public. For example, in a study by French et al. (2018), there was considerable variation in understanding of test results. The role of SNPs in cancer risk may be less familiar to individuals than more widely publicised rare genetic variants such as those in the *BRCA* genes [40]. Additionally, lifestyle factors may be perceived as being under greater personal control and, therefore, less serious than rare genetic variants.

Our study findings suggest that individuals interpreted the two levels of risk (5% vs. 10%) similarly, with the difference in communicated risk having a non-significant impact on participants' intentions to have RRSO. This supports previous research exploring the effect of risk information on behaviour, suggesting there is not a simple linear relationship between increments in risk and risk perception [39,40].

In addition to the lack of impact on perceived risk of ovarian cancer, we similarly found that different presentations of risk in the hypothetical scenarios (5% SNPs + lifestyle vs. 10% SNPs + lifestyle risk; 10% rare genetic variant vs. 10% SNPs + lifestyle) did not lead to differences in any other cognitive factors considered in the EPPM framework (i.e., perceived severity of ovarian cancer, perceived response-efficacy of risk-reducing surgery, self-efficacy to undertake risk-reducing surgery).

In contrast, we found that, in the sample overall, opting for risk-reducing surgery was associated with higher self-efficacy and higher perceived response-efficacy of risk-reducing surgery. According to the Extended Parallel Processing Model [46], higher perceptions of self-efficacy and/or response-efficacy relating to the recommended behaviour are associated with greater likelihood that systematic processing of threatening (risk) information will occur. Conversely, when perceptions of efficacy are low, people are more likely to avoid threatening risk information. Together, our findings suggest that if women perceive or believe that RRSO is being recommended to them clinically, this may have a greater impact on their decision-making than the details of their risk result (i.e., whether their risk is 5% or 10%, and whether that risk is based on a single rare genetic variant or a more complex combination of SNPs and lifestyle factors). The observation that psychological variables had a greater impact on intentions than the absolute risk numbers suggest that this might be important to consider in any potential future national rollouts. Offering psychological support for those who need it as part of the RRSO discussion and decision-making process is part of routine clinical practice in many centres today. Our study highlights the importance of incorporating this into future national guidelines.

In previous research using hypothetical scenarios, there has been some evidence to suggest that genetic information leads to more deterministic responses than non-genetic information [33,38,47–49]. Our study did not include a non-genetic condition and so does not speak to this aspect of how people respond to personal genetic versus non-genetic information.

The present study had several limitations. The cross-sectional design of the study did not allow for causation to be inferred. However, exploratory experimental studies such as this one can be valuable in informing hypotheses before moving on to study designs designed to trial real risk assessments. The use of hypothetical scenarios was both a strength and a limitation. This study attempted to model a "real life" scenario in which genetic risk information was provided to the general population. However, many of the contextual details and additional resources that accompany risk information are not available in hypothetical scenarios, which may limit the ecological validity of the study. This study was concerned with behavioural intention, as ovarian cancer population surveillance or population-wide genetic testing is not currently clinically available, so actual behaviour could not be measured. The presence of a potential intention behaviour gap is well established for other clinical interventions and cannot be excluded here.

The measures used in this study are adapted from previous research; however, they were almost all single-item measures, which may not be sensitive enough to adequately represent the underlying construct being measured due to the lack of psychometric information (e.g., test-retest reliability, discriminant or convergent validity). Prior knowledge may have an influence on how individuals appraise threatening health information [50]: this study did not measure previous ovarian cancer and genetic risk knowledge or previous genetic testing, which may have had an impact on behavioural intention (however this may be unlikely given this type of genetic testing is not widely available in the UK). In addition, we did not assess understanding of the information provided, and it is possible that some concepts (e.g., SNPs) may not have been well understood.

The sample was predominately White British and, therefore, may not be generalisable to other ethnic groups, given decisions about risk-reducing surgery and psychological effects may differ cross-culturally. In addition, the restricted age-range of the sample limits the generalisability of the findings (e.g., to younger women age 35 years and over who may also be offered risk-reducing surgery if they are at high risk). However, most women from the general population who are at increased risk of ovarian cancer will fall in the intermediate risk (5–10% lifetime risk) category [9]. RRSO at intermediate ovarian cancer risk levels (including for moderate penetrance CSGs) is recommended to be undertaken over the age of 45–50 years [15]. The sample was self-selected and may have had greater interest in the topic than the wider general population; the generalizability of the findings is therefore uncertain. Finally, as with any experimental study, we are unable to rule out the possibility of demand characteristics, i.e., participants responding in a way they think is expected according to their perceptions of the aim of the study. Despite the limitations, this study provides insights on the effects of experimentally manipulating genetic risk information for ovarian cancer on outcomes, comparing different sources and levels of risk on risk management behavioural intentions and psychological variables in the general population.

The information provided before being exposed to the hypothetical risk scenario on ovarian cancer, risk factors, and the efficacy of risk management was necessarily basic and brief, which may be an additional limitation. However, previous research did not find any difference in behavioural outcomes between use of gist and extended versions of decision aids in relation to ovarian cancer risk management [51]. Future research might usefully provide more detailed information containing details about the efficacy of a particular risk management behaviour to encourage "danger control" cognitive processing. This may aid in changing risk management preferences.

Future research might also benefit from including measures of other psychological and cognitive factors as potential predictors of risk management, e.g., causal beliefs. In addition, further research is needed on communicating risk information incorporating genetics to people in the general population outside of traditional clinical genetics department settings. Furthermore, a control group where participants are given a general population-based risk estimate would be useful for future research, as we were unable to compare between the general population risk and increased risk in this study.

The mean age of participants in this study was 57 years, with the majority of participants having completed having children and/or being past childbearing age, with most participants reporting they had begun menopause or were post-menopausal. Future research should explore the psychological and cognitive effects of ovarian cancer risk information being offered to younger women. In addition, there were relatively few women in the oldest age group (71–75 years) in this study, and so it is possible the apparent trend of increasing age being less associated with interest in surgery was due to the study being underpowered. This could also be a topic of investigation in future research.

Risk-reducing surgery, specifically RRSO, is at present the most effective risk management option available to women at increased risk of ovarian cancer. Our findings suggest there are a number of cognitive factors that influence intention to have ovarian cancer risk-reducing clinical interventions, beyond perceptions of risk. Future research should explore other possible factors that may have an impact on decision-making about risk management strategies. It is imperative to identify whether and/or how genetic risk information about common complex diseases will be translated into public health benefit: this is arguably especially urgent for diseases, such as ovarian cancer, which are characterised by being notoriously difficult to detect early and by having a high prevalence of late-stage diagnosis. Combined testing for multiple genetic factors together with lifestyle and other risk factors may lead to the ability to stratify the population for ovarian cancer risk for targeted prevention thus potentially saving lives.

Population testing provides a new paradigm for ovarian cancer prevention and can prevent thousands more cancers than the current clinical approach [52]. Jewish population studies support population testing for CSGs [53]. Our pilot study shows that population testing for lifetime risk of ovarian cancer is feasible, acceptable and has high satisfaction in general population women [12].

However, there is now need for large implementation studies, with long term outcomes, to provide real world evidence and develop context-specific models for implementing this approach for women in the general population. This will valuably inform future policy decisions regarding population-wide risk stratified approaches for risk-adapted ovarian cancer screening and prevention.

4. Materials and Methods

4.1. Overview

Participants (n = 1017) were women aged 45–75 years recruited via online survey company Survey Sampling International (SSI) in July 2017. An email containing a web link was sent to SSI panellists who fit the study criteria with respect to gender and age, inviting them to take part. The email did not contain information about the topic of the study. Those responding were directed to a short screening questionnaire. Eligible participants were then presented with a consent form. Incentive points, which can be exchanged for shopping vouchers, were awarded to SSI panellists for their time (equivalent to ~£0.50 for this 10 min study).

All participants were given information about ovarian cancer, including that on average around 2% of women will develop ovarian cancer in their lifetime; asked to imagine that they had had an ovarian cancer risk assessment via the NHS; and asked to imagine they had received a result indicating they were at increased risk of ovarian cancer (see Appendix A).

Women were randomly assigned to one of three experimental conditions using a software algorithm (See Figure 1). They were asked to imagine they had undergone an ovarian cancer risk assessment and had received this personalised risk estimate from their GP: (a) 5% ovarian cancer risk due to common genetic variants and lifestyle factors; (b) 10% ovarian cancer risk due to common genetic variants and lifestyle factors; or (c) 10% ovarian cancer risk due to a single rare variant in a cancer susceptibility gene such as *BRCA2* (see Appendix B).

The study was approved by the University College London ethics committee (Project ID Number: 10251/001).

4.2. Inclusion Criteria

Eligible participants were women aged 45–75 years, with no previous history of breast or ovarian cancer diagnosis. Women who indicated they were unsure of, or had not completed childbearing, were excluded from analyses (n = 13).

4.3. Measures

All measures are shown in Appendix C.

4.3.1. Interest in Ovarian Cancer Risk Assessment

Interest was assessed before exposure to the hypothetical test results, with the item, "If your GP offered you this ovarian cancer risk assessment on the NHS, would you take up the offer?" (adapted from [20]. Response options were "no, definitely not"; "no probably not"; "yes, probably" and "yes, definitely". The information women read before answering the question explained that the risk assessment would involve providing lifestyle information as well as a blood sample for genetic testing (see Appendix A).

4.3.2. Perceived Risk of Ovarian Cancer

Perceived risk was measured using a single item, "If I had just received this personal ovarian cancer risk result, I would feel that my risk of developing ovarian cancer was" adapted from [54]. Responses for these questions were recorded on a 5-point Likert scale with response options ranging from "much lower than other women of my age" to "much higher than women of my age". A higher score on the 5-point scale indicated greater perceived risk.

4.3.3. Perceived Severity of Ovarian Cancer

Perceived severity was measured using two questions adapted from [55]: "Developing ovarian cancer would have major consequences on my life" and "ovarian cancer is a serious condition" with five response options ranging from "strongly agree" to "strongly disagree". A higher score on the (possible scores 1–5) scale indicated greater perceived severity.

4.3.4. Self-Efficacy for Risk-Reducing Surgery

One item, adapted from [56], assessed participants' confidence in their ability to have risk-reducing surgery. Individuals were asked "How confident are you that you would go through with risk-reducing surgery if you were motivated to do so". The response options ranged from "not at all confident" to "extremely confident". A higher score on the scale indicated greater perceived self-efficacy.

4.3.5. Perceived Response-Efficacy of Risk-Reducing Surgery

For perceived response-efficacy of risk-reducing surgery, participants were asked to indicate how effective they felt risk-reducing surgery would be in lowering their ovarian cancer risk using a single item adapted from [56]: "Having surgery to remove your ovaries and fallopian tubes is an effective way to lower your risk of ovarian cancer". The response options were "strongly agree" to "strongly disagree". Items were reverse coded: a higher score on the (possible scores 1–5) scale indicated greater perceived response-efficacy.

4.3.6. Behavioural Intention

To assess women's potential behavioural reactions to their risk results, they were asked: "If I had just received this personal ovarian cancer risk result, I would choose to...". The response options were: "have risk-reducing surgery to remove my ovaries"; "have surveillance such as regular ultrasound scans"; "make lifestyle changes"; "do nothing"; and "I am not sure what I would do".

4.3.7. Demographic and Health Characteristic Measures

Information on demographics was collected from all participants including: age, ethnicity, educational attainment, relationship status, health characteristics, family history of cancer, personal history of cancer, menopause status, and breast and cervical screening attendance. Ethnicity (White vs. other ethnic group), menopause status (pre-menopausal vs. peri/post-menopause) and breast and cervical screening attendance (regular vs. irregular or not yet eligible) were dichotomised.

4.4. Data Analyses

A power calculation based on the primary binary outcome, intention to have risk-reducing surgery, taking into account group comparisons of three groups, suggested a sample size of 782 was required (medium effect size, power of 90%, alpha of 0.05). All statistical analyses of the data were carried out using SPSS 24. Analyses of variance (ANOVAs) and chi-square tests were conducted to explore between-group differences. Logistic regression was used to explore predictors of willingness to have risk-reducing surgery (vs. other behavioural responses to the risk information). Unadjusted and adjusted models were examined to explore the predictive effect of the experimental group and psychological variables on intention to have surgery and address possible demographic and health-related covariates.

5. Conclusions

The findings of this study contribute to a growing body of risk stratification research exploring the potential usefulness and clinical utility of population-wide risk assessment incorporating genetic testing alongside other risk factors. The need for risk stratification is perhaps particularly urgent for diseases, such as ovarian cancer, where survival outcomes are poor and population-wide screening for the disease is not currently recommended. We provide initial evidence, suggesting that a substantial proportion of women aged 45 years and over are open to the idea of risk stratification and having surgery to reduce their risk of ovarian cancer in response to increased risk results, even if their absolute lifetime risk is only increased by a few percentage points in absolute terms. Our findings do not speak to other barriers that might prevent women's behavioural intentions or preferences being translated into actions—barriers such as lack of timely access to healthcare services.

Author Contributions: Conceptualization, S.S. and J.W.; methodology, J.W., A.G., S.S., R.M.; formal analysis, A.G., J.W., S.S.; resources, I.J., R.M., J.W.; data curation, A.G., S.S., J.W.; writing—original draft preparation, A.G.; writing—review and editing, J.W., S.S., I.J., R.M.; visualization, A.G., J.W., S.S.; supervision, J.W., S.S., I.J., R.M.; project administration, A.G.; funding acquisition, J.W. All authors have read and agreed to the published version of the manuscript.

Acknowledgments: We are grateful to the women who took part in the study.

Appendix A

Ovarian cancer and risk information

Section 1: Hypothetical scenario

Please imagine that you have gone to your GP, and they have offered you a new approach to assessing your risk of developing ovarian cancer in the future. When your GP offered this to you, they gave you some written information to help you decide whether or not you want to have the risk assessment done. This information is below. Please read the information, and then answer the question that follows.

Assessing ovarian cancer risk

Ovarian cancer is the sixth most common cancer among women in the UK: 2% of women will be diagnosed with ovarian cancer during their lifetime. Ovarian cancer is caused by many genetic and non-genetic factors. Currently, ovarian cancer is often detected at a late stage because symptoms are hard to spot. This means that it is often very hard to treat effectively.

A new ovarian cancer risk assessment has been developed. This risk assessment combines lots of different types of information about you to estimate how likely you are to develop ovarian cancer in your lifetime. The types of information included in the risk assessment include lifestyle factors, rare genetic variants, and common genetic variants.

Lifestyle factors: Lifestyle factors that may increase a woman's risk of ovarian cancer include tobacco smoking and being overweight.

Common genetic variants: Single nucleotide polymorphisms, frequently called SNPs (pronounced "snips"), are the most common type of genetic variation among people. SNPs occur normally throughout a person's DNA. Most SNPs have no effect on health, but some are important to a person's health. Some SNPs can influence a woman's risk of developing ovarian cancer. Individually, each one of these SNPs only influences ovarian cancer risk by a tiny amount, but if a woman has a large number of these SNPs then her risk of ovarian cancer may be increased.

Rare genetic variants: Some ovarian cancers are caused by a rare variant in a person's DNA. These rare variants can have quite a strong effect on a woman's risk of developing ovarian cancer. For example, variants in the *BRCA2* gene can increase a woman's lifetime risk of ovarian cancer up to between 10% and 20%.

If you want to have this ovarian cancer risk assessment carried out, you will need to provide your GP with the information they request, including about your lifestyle. You will also need to have a blood test, so that the scientists can see whether you have any of the genetic variants that increase your risk.

Appendix B

Generic Risk Scenarios

Next, regardless of how you answered in the previous question, please imagine that you have had the ovarian cancer risk assessment done, and your GP has now given you the result from the assessment. Please read your hypothetical result below.

Your personal ovarian cancer risk assessment: results [Group 1 only]

Your result indicates that your lifetime risk of developing ovarian cancer is 5%. This is higher than the average risk for women, which is 2%.
Your risk of ovarian cancer is higher than average because you have been found to have at least one lifestyle factor and several common genetic variants which are known to put women at increased risk of developing ovarian cancer.

OR

Your personal ovarian cancer risk assessment: results [Group 2 only]

Your result indicates that your lifetime risk of developing ovarian cancer is 10%. This is higher than the average risk for women, which is 2%.
Your risk of ovarian cancer is higher than average because you have been found to have at least one lifestyle factor and several common genetic variants which are known to put women at increased risk of developing ovarian cancer.

OR

Your personal ovarian cancer risk assessment: results [Group 3 only]

Your result indicates that your lifetime risk of developing ovarian cancer is 10%. This is higher than the average risk for women, which is 2%.
Your risk of ovarian cancer is higher than average because you have been found to have a rare genetic variant which is known to put women at increased risk of developing ovarian cancer.

AND

[All groups]

There are several options for women who are at higher than average risk of ovarian cancer.
Risk-reducing surgery involves removing the ovaries and fallopian tubes to prevent ovarian cancer from developing. However, removing the ovaries has downsides. For example, it causes a woman who has not yet been through her menopause to start her menopause (a natural process that usually happens in a woman's early 50 s).
Surveillance includes having a regular (e.g., annual) ultrasound of your ovaries to see if a tumour is present. This ultrasound is usually an internal (transvaginal) ultrasound. Effective screening has not been established.
Lifestyle changes include maintaining a healthy weight and quitting smoking. These types of lifestyle changes may reduce a woman's risk of developing ovarian cancer.

Appendix C

Questionnaire

Please carefully imagine what you would think and how you would feel if you had received this personal result from the ovarian cancer risk assessment. Now please answer the following questions.

Intention for Genetic Screening

Q1. If your GP offered you this ovarian cancer risk assessment on the NHS, would you take up the offer?

- No definitely not
- No probably not
- Yes probably
- Yes definitely

Q2. How likely do you think you are to develop ovarian cancer in your lifetime?

(a) ... Not at all likely
(b) ... Not very likely
(c) ... Quite likely
(d) ... Extremely likely

Behavioural outcome

Q3. If I had just received this personal ovarian cancer risk result, I would choose to ...

(a) ... have risk-reducing surgery to remove my ovaries.
(b) ... have surveillance such as regular ultrasound scans.
(c) ... make lifestyle changes.
(d) ... do nothing.
(e) ... I am not sure what I would choose.

(Please select one option only)

Perceived risk

Q4. If I had just received this personal ovarian cancer risk result, I would feel that my risk of developing ovarian cancer was ...

(a) ... much lower than other women of my age
(b) ... lower than other women of my age
(c) ... the same as other women of my age
(d) ... higher than other women of my age
(e) ... much higher than other women of my age

Perceived Response efficacy

How much do you agree or disagree with the following statement based on how you would feel if you had received this personal ovarian cancer risk result from the ovarian cancer risk assessment.

Q7. There is little that can be done to prevent ovarian cancer.

(a) ... Strongly agree
(b) ... Agree
(c) ... Neither agree or disagree
(d) ... Disagree
(e) ... Strongly disagree

Q8. Having surgery to remove your ovaries and fallopian tubes is an effective way to lower your risk of ovarian cancer.

(a) ... Strongly agree
(b) ... Agree
(c) ... Neither agree or disagree
(d) ... Disagree
(e) ... Strongly disagree

Perceived Response efficacy

Q9. Regular screening through transvaginal ultrasound is an effective way to lower your risk of ovarian cancer.

(a) ... Strongly agree
(b) ... Agree
(c) ... Neither agree or disagree
(d) ... Disagree
(e) ... Strongly disagree

Perceived severity

Q10. Developing ovarian cancer would have major consequences on my life

(a) ... Strongly agree
(b) ... Agree
(c) ... Neither agree or disagree
(d) ... Disagree
(e) ... Strongly disagree

Perceived severity

Q11. Ovarian cancer is a serious condition.

(a) ... Strongly agree
(b) ... Agree
(c) ... Neither agree or disagree
(d) ... Disagree
(e) ... Strongly disagree

Self-efficacy

Q12. How confident are you that you could go through with having risk-reducing surgery if you were motivated to do so?

(a) ... not at all confident
(b) ... somewhat confident
(c) ... fairly confident
(d) ... very confident
(e) ... extremely confident

Q13. Have you ever been diagnosed with cancer? (Please select one)

Yes
No
Not sure

Q14. If yes, what type of cancer is it/was it?

... ...

Q15. Do you have a family history of cancer?

Have anyfirst-degree family member(parents, brothers, sisters, children) orsecond-degree(aunts, uncles, nieces, nephews, grandparents, grandchildren) been diagnosed with cancer.

Yes

No
Not sure

Q15a. If yes, what type(s) of cancer?

… … … … … … … … … … … … … … … … … … ..

Q16. What is your current menstrual status? (Please select one)

Premenopausal (before menopause; having regular periods)
Perimenopause (menopause transition—changes in periods, but have not gone 12 months in a row without a period)
Postmenopausal (After menopause; periods have stopped for at least 12 months)
Don't know

Q17. If you have indicated that you have not had a period in the previous 12 months, what age were you at your last period?

Q18. If you are still having periods, how often do they occur? (Please respond in days)

Q19. Is there a recent change in how often you have periods?

Yes/No

Q20. Was your menopause:

Spontaneous ("natural")
Surgical (removal of both ovaries)
Due to chemotherapy or radiation therapy
Other
n/a—haven't yet reached menopause
(If indicated they are still having periods don't ask this question)

Q21. Women aged 25–49 years are invited for cervical screening (also called a smear or Pap test) every 3 years, and women aged 50–64 are invited every 5 years. Which of these statements best describes you?

I'm up to date with cervical screening
I'm overdue for cervical screening
I've never been for cervical screening
I'm 65 or over so I'm not invited any more

Q22. Women aged 50–70 years are invited for breast screening (also called a mammogram or mammography) every 3 years. Which of these statements best describes you?

I'm up to date with breast screening
I'm overdue for breast screening
I've never been for breast screening
I'm under 50 or over 70 so I'm not eligible for breast screening.

Q23. How old are you?

____

Q24. How would you describe your ethnic background? (Please select one)

White British
White non-British

Black
Asian
Mixed
Other
Do not wish to answer

Q25. What is the highest level of education you have achieved? (Please select one)

No formal qualifications
GCSEs/O levels or equivalent
A-Levels or equivalent
Undergraduate degree or equivalent
Postgraduate degree or equivalent
Other (please state)

Q26. What is your relationship status? (Please select one)

Single
In a relationship
Living with a partner
Married
Separated/divorced/widowed

Q27. How many children do you have? (Please select one)

0
1
2
3
4
5 or more

Q28. Do you plan to have any (more) children in the future? (Please select one)

Yes
No
Not sure

END OF SURVEY

References

1. Cancer Research UK, Ovarian Cancer Statistics. 2016. Available online: https://www.cancerresearchuk.org/health-professional/cancer-statistics/statistics-by-cancer-type/ovarian-cancer (accessed on 25 June 2017).
2. Hunn, J.; Rodriguez, G.C. Ovarian Cancer: Etiology, risk factors, and epidemiology. *Clin. Obstet. Gynecol.* **2012**, *55*, 3–23. [CrossRef] [PubMed]
3. Levy-Lahad, E.; Gabai-Kapara, E.; Kaufman, B.; Catane, R.; Segev, S.; Renbaum, P.; Beller, U.; King, M.; Lahad, A. Identification of BRCA1/BRCA2 carriers by screening in the healthy population and its implications. *J. Clin. Oncol.* **2011**, *29*, 1513. [CrossRef]
4. King, M.-C.; Levy-Lahad, E.; Lahad, A. Population-Based Screening for BRCA1 and BRCA2. *JAMA* **2014**, *312*, 1091–1092. [CrossRef] [PubMed]
5. Kuchenbaecker, K.B.; Hopper, J.L.; Barnes, D.R.; Phillips, K.-A.; Mooij, T.M.; Roos-Blom, M.-J.; Jervis, S.E.; Van Leeuwen, F.; Milne, R.L.; Andrieu, N.; et al. Risks of Breast, Ovarian, and Contralateral Breast Cancer for BRCA1 and BRCA2 Mutation Carriers. *JAMA* **2017**, *317*, 2402–2416. [CrossRef] [PubMed]

6. Manchanda, R.; Burnell, M.; Gaba, F.; Desai, R.; Wardle, J.; Gessler, S.; Side, L.; Sanderson, S.; Loggenberg, K.; Brady, A.F.; et al. Randomised trial of population-based BRCA testing in Ashkenazi Jews: Long-term outcomes. *BJOG: Int. J. Obstet. Gynaecol.* **2019**, *127*, 364–375. [CrossRef] [PubMed]
7. Manchanda, R.; Loggenberg, K.; Sanderson, S.; Burnell, M.; Wardle, J.; Gessler, S.; Side, L.; Balogun, N.; Desai, R.; Kumar, A.; et al. Population testing for cancer predisposing BRCA1/BRCA2 mutations in the Ashkenazi-Jewish community: A randomized controlled trial. *J. Natl. Cancer Inst.* **2014**, *107*, 379. [CrossRef]
8. Manchanda, R.; Blyuss, O.; Gaba, F.; Gordeev, V.S.; Jacobs, C.; Burnell, M.; Gan, C.; Taylor, R.; Turnbull, C.; Legood, R.; et al. Current detection rates and time-to-detection of all identifiable BRCA carriers in the Greater London population. *J. Med. Genet.* **2018**, *55*, 538–545. [CrossRef]
9. Jervis, S.; Song, H.; Lee, A.; Dicks, E.; Harrington, P.; Baynes, C.; Manchanda, R.; Easton, D.F.; Jacobs, I.; Pharoah, P.P.D.; et al. A risk prediction algorithm for ovarian cancer incorporating BRCA1, BRCA2, common alleles and other familial effects. *J. Med. Genet.* **2015**, *52*, 465–475. [CrossRef]
10. Manchanda, R.; Gaba, F. Population Based Testing for Primary Prevention: A Systematic Review. *Cancers* **2018**, *10*, 424. [CrossRef]
11. Evans, O.; Gaba, F.; Manchanda, R. Population-based genetic testing for Women's cancer prevention. *Best Pr. Res. Clin. Obstet. Gynaecol.* **2020**, *65*, 139–153. [CrossRef]
12. Gaba, F.; Blyuss, O.; Liu, X.; Goyal, S.; Lahoti, N.; Chandrasekaran, D.; Kurzer, M.; Kalsi, J.K.; Sanderson, S.C.; Lanceley, A.; et al. Population Study of Ovarian Cancer Risk Prediction for Targeted Screening and Prevention. *Cancers* **2020**, *12*, 1241. [CrossRef] [PubMed]
13. Rahman, B.; Side, L.; Gibbon, S.; Meisel, S.F.; Fraser, L.; Gessler, S.; Wardle, J.; Lanceley, A. Moving towards population-based genetic risk prediction for ovarian cancer. *BJOG: Int. J. Obstet. Gynaecol.* **2017**, *124*, 855–858. [CrossRef]
14. Manchanda, R.; Legood, R.; Antoniou, A.; Pearce, L.; Menon, U. Commentary on changing the risk threshold for surgical prevention of ovarian cancer. *BJOG: Int. J. Obstet. Gynaecol.* **2017**, *125*, 541–544. [CrossRef] [PubMed]
15. Manchanda, R.; Menon, U. Setting the Threshold for Surgical Prevention in Women at Increased Risk of Ovarian Cancer. *Int. J. Gynecol. Cancer* **2018**, *28*, 34–42. [CrossRef] [PubMed]
16. Manchanda, R.; Legood, R.; Antoniou, A.C.; Gordeev, V.S.; Menon, U. Specifying the ovarian cancer risk threshold of 'premenopausal risk-reducing salpingo-oophorectomy' for ovarian cancer prevention: A cost-effectiveness analysis. *J. Med. Genet.* **2016**, *53*, 591–599. [CrossRef] [PubMed]
17. Manchanda, R.; Legood, R.; Pearce, L.; Menon, U. Defining the risk threshold for risk reducing salpingo-oophorectomy for ovarian cancer prevention in low risk postmenopausal women. *Gynecol. Oncol.* **2015**, *139*, 487–494. [CrossRef] [PubMed]
18. Manchanda, R.; Patel, S.; Gordeev, V.S.; Antoniou, A.C.; Smith, S.; Lee, A.; Hopper, J.L.; MacInnis, R.J.; Turnbull, C.G.N.; Ramus, S.J.; et al. Cost-effectiveness of Population-Based BRCA1, BRCA2, RAD51C, RAD51D, BRIP1, PALB2 Mutation Testing in Unselected General Population Women. *J. Natl. Cancer Inst.* **2018**, *110*, 714–725. [CrossRef]
19. Chandrasekaran, D.; Manchanda, R. Germline and somatic genetic testing in ovarian cancer patients. *BJOG: Int. J. Obstet. Gynaecol.* **2018**, *125*, 1460. [CrossRef]
20. Meisel, S.F.; for the PROMISE-2016 Study Team; Rahman, B.; Side, L.; Fraser, L.; Gessler, S.; Lanceley, A.; Wardle, J. Genetic testing and personalized ovarian cancer screening: A survey of public attitudes. *BMC Women's Health* **2016**, *16*, 46. [CrossRef]
21. Manchanda, R.; Burnell, M.; Loggenberg, K.; Desai, R.; Wardle, J.; Sanderson, S.C.; Gessler, S.; Side, L.; Balogun, N.; Kumar, A.; et al. Cluster-randomised non-inferiority trial comparing DVD-assisted and traditional genetic counselling in systematic population testing for BRCA1/2 mutations. *J. Med. Genet.* **2016**, *53*, 472–480. [CrossRef]
22. Manchanda, R.; Legood, R.; Burnell, M.; McGuire, A.; Raikou, M.; Loggenberg, K.; Wardle, J.; Sanderson, S.; Gessler, S.; Side, L.; et al. Cost-effectiveness of Population Screening for BRCA Mutations in Ashkenazi Jewish Women Compared with Family History-Based Testing. *J. Natl. Cancer Inst.* **2015**, *107*, 380. [CrossRef] [PubMed]
23. Manchanda, R.; Patel, S.; Antoniou, A.C.; Levy-Lahad, E.; Turnbull, C.; Evans, D.G.; Hopper, J.L.; MacInnis, R.J.; Menon, U.; Jacobs, I.; et al. Cost-effectiveness of population based BRCA testing with varying Ashkenazi Jewish ancestry. *Am. J. Obstet. Gynecol.* **2017**, *217*, 578.e1–578.e12. [CrossRef] [PubMed]

24. Rebbeck, T.R.; Lynch, H.T.; Neuhausen, S.L.; Narod, S.A.; Veer, L.V.; Garber, J.E.; Evans, G.; Isaacs, C.; Daly, M.B.; Matloff, E.; et al. Prophylactic Oophorectomy in Carriers of BRCA1 or BRCA2 Mutations. *N. Engl. J. Med.* **2002**, *346*, 1616–1622. [CrossRef] [PubMed]
25. Manchanda, R.; Burnell, M.; Abdelraheim, A.; Johnson, M.; Sharma, A.; Benjamin, E.; Brunell, C.; Saridogan, E.; Gessler, S.; Oram, D.; et al. Factors influencing uptake and timing of risk reducing salpingo-oophorectomy in women at risk of familial ovarian cancer: A competing risk time to event analysis. *BJOG: Int. J. Obstet. Gynaecol.* **2012**, *119*, 527–536. [CrossRef]
26. Manchanda, R.; Abdelraheim, A.; Johnson, M.; Rosenthal, A.N.; Benjamin, E.; Brunell, C.; Burnell, M.; Side, L.; Gessler, S.; Saridogan, E.; et al. Outcome of risk-reducing salpingo-oophorectomy in BRCA carriers and women of unknown mutation status. *BJOG: Int. J. Obstet. Gynaecol.* **2011**, *118*, 814–824. [CrossRef]
27. Yang, X.; Song, H.; Leslie, G.; Engel, C.; Hahnen, E.; Auber, B.; Horváth, J.; Kast, K.; Niederacher, D.; Turnbull, C.; et al. Ovarian and Breast Cancer Risks Associated with Pathogenic Variants in RAD51C and RAD51D. *J. Natl. Cancer Inst.* **2020**. [CrossRef]
28. Yang, X.; Leslie, G.; Doroszuk, A.; Schneider, S.; Allen, J.; Decker, B.; Dunning, A.M.; Redman, J.; Scarth, J.; Plaskocinska, I.; et al. Cancer Risks Associated with Germline PALB2 Pathogenic Variants: An International Study of 524 Families. *J. Clin. Oncol.* **2020**, *38*, 674–685. [CrossRef]
29. Ramus, S.J.; Song, H.; Dicks, E.; Tyrer, J.P.; Rosenthal, A.N.; Intermaggio, M.P.; Fraser, L.; Gentry-Maharaj, A.; Hayward, J.; Philpott, S.; et al. Germline Mutations in the BRIP1, BARD1, PALB2, and NBN Genes in Women with Ovarian Cancer. *J. Natl. Cancer Inst.* **2015**, *107*. [CrossRef]
30. Jacobs, I.; Menon, U.; Ryan, A.; Gentry-Maharaj, A.; Burnell, M.; Kalsi, J.K.; Amso, N.N.; Apostolidou, S.; Benjamin, E.; Cruickshank, D.; et al. Ovarian cancer screening and mortality in the UK Collaborative Trial of Ovarian Cancer Screening (UKCTOCS): A randomised controlled trial. *Lancet* **2016**, *387*, 945–956. [CrossRef]
31. Rosenthal, A.N.; Fraser, L.S.; Philpott, S.; Manchanda, R.; Burnell, M.; Badman, P.; Hadwin, R.; Rizzuto, I.; Benjamin, E.C.; Singh, N.; et al. Evidence of Stage Shift in Women Diagnosed with Ovarian Cancer during Phase II of the United Kingdom Familial Ovarian Cancer Screening Study. *J. Clin. Oncol.* **2017**, *35*, 1411–1420. [CrossRef]
32. Kauff, N.D.; Domchek, S.M.; Friebel, T.M.; Robson, M.E.; Lee, J.; Garber, J.E.; Isaacs, C.; Evans, D.G.; Lynch, H.; Eeles, R.A.; et al. Risk-Reducing Salpingo-Oophorectomy for the Prevention of BRCA1- and BRCA2-Associated Breast and Gynecologic Cancer: A Multicenter, Prospective Study. *J. Clin. Oncol.* **2008**, *26*, 1331–1337. [CrossRef] [PubMed]
33. Hollands, G.J.; French, D.P.; Griffin, S.J.; Prevost, A.T.; Sutton, S.; King, S.; Marteau, T.M. The impact of communicating genetic risks of disease on risk-reducing health behaviour: Systematic review with meta-analysis. *BMJ* **2016**, *352*, i1102. [CrossRef] [PubMed]
34. Hallowell, N.; kConFab Psychosocial Group on Behalf of the kConFab Investigators; Baylock, B.; Heiniger, L.; Butow, P.N.; Patel, D.; Meiser, B.; Saunders, C.M.; Price, M.A. Looking different, feeling different: Women's reactions to risk-reducing breast and ovarian surgery. *Fam. Cancer* **2011**, *11*, 215–224. [CrossRef] [PubMed]
35. Meiser, B.; Butow, P.; Friedlander, M.; Barratt, A.; Schnieden, V.; Watson, M.; Brown, J.; Tucker, K. Psychological impact of genetic testing in women from high-risk breast cancer families. *Eur. J. Cancer* **2002**, *38*, 2025–2031. [CrossRef]
36. Pruthi, S.; Gostout, B.S.; Lindor, N.M. Identification and Management of Women with BRCA Mutations or Hereditary Predisposition for Breast and Ovarian Cancer. *Mayo Clinic Proc.* **2010**, *85*, 1111–1120. [CrossRef]
37. Rebbeck, T.R.; Kauff, N.D.; Domchek, S.M. Meta-analysis of Risk Reduction Estimates Associated with Risk-Reducing Salpingo-oophorectomy in BRCA1 or BRCA2 Mutation Carriers. *J. Natl. Cancer Inst.* **2009**, *101*, 80–87. [CrossRef]
38. Marteau, T.M.; French, D.P.; Griffin, S.J.; Prevost, T.; Sutton, S.; Watkinson, C.; Attwood, S.; Hollands, G.J. Effects of communicating DNA-based disease risk estimates on risk-reducing behaviours. *Cochrane Database Syst. Rev.* **2010**, CD007275. [CrossRef]
39. Cameron, L.D.; Sherman, K.; Marteau, T.M.; Brown, P.M. Impact of genetic risk information and type of disease on perceived risk, anticipated affect, and expected consequences of genetic tests. *Health Psychol.* **2009**, *28*, 307–316. [CrossRef]

40. French, D.P.; Southworth, J.; Howell, A.; Harvie, M.; Stavrinos, P.; Watterson, D.; Sampson, S.; Evans, D.G.; Donnelly, L.S. Psychological impact of providing women with personalised 10-year breast cancer risk estimates. *Br. J. Cancer* **2018**, *118*, 1648–1657. [CrossRef]
41. Hart, M.R.; Biesecker, B.B.; Blout, C.L.; Christensen, K.D.; Amendola, L.M.; Bergstrom, K.L.; Biswas, S.; Bowling, K.M.; Brothers, K.B.; Conlin, L.K.; et al. Secondary findings from clinical genomic sequencing: Prevalence, patient perspectives, family history assessment, and health-care costs from a multisite study. *Genet. Med.* **2019**, *21*, 1100–1110. [CrossRef]
42. Witte, K.; Allen, M. A Meta-Analysis of Fear Appeals: Implications for Effective Public Health Campaigns. *Heal. Educ. Behav.* **2000**, *27*, 591–615. [CrossRef] [PubMed]
43. Meisel, S.F.; Side, L.; Fraser, L.; Gessler, S.; Wardle, J.; Lanceley, A. Population-Based, Risk-Stratified Genetic Testing for Ovarian Cancer Risk: A Focus Group Study. *Public Health Genom.* **2013**, *16*, 184–191. [CrossRef] [PubMed]
44. Waller, J.L.; Osborne, K.; Wardle, J.F.C. Enthusiasm for cancer screening in Great Britain: A general population survey. *Br. J. Cancer* **2015**, *112*, 562–566. [CrossRef] [PubMed]
45. Mai, P.L.; Piedmonte, M.; Han, P.K.J.; Moser, R.P.; Walker, J.L.; Rodriguez, G.C.; Boggess, J.; Rutherford, T.J.; Zivanovic, O.; Cohn, D.E.; et al. Factors associated with deciding between risk-reducing salpingo-oophorectomy and ovarian cancer screening among high-risk women enrolled in GOG-0199: An NRG Oncology/Gynecologic Oncology Group study. *Gynecol. Oncol.* **2017**, *145*, 122–129. [CrossRef] [PubMed]
46. Witte, K. Putting the fear back into fear appeals: The extended parallel process model. *Commun. Monogr.* **1992**, *59*, 329–349. [CrossRef]
47. Claassen, L.; Henneman, L.; De Vet, R.; Knol, D.; Marteau, T.M.; Timmermans, D. Fatalistic responses to different types of genetic risk information: Exploring the role of Self-Malleability. *Psychol. Health* **2010**, *25*, 183–196. [CrossRef] [PubMed]
48. Marteau, T.M. Genetic risk and behavioural change. *BMJ* **2001**, *322*, 1056–1059. [CrossRef]
49. Marteau, T.M.; Weinman, J. Self-regulation and the behavioural response to DNA risk information: A theoretical analysis and framework for future research. *Soc. Sci. Med.* **2006**, *62*, 1360–1368. [CrossRef]
50. Evans, R.E.; Beeken, R.J.; Steptoe, A.; Wardle, J. Cancer information and anxiety: Applying the Extended Parallel Process Model. *J. Health Psychol.* **2012**, *17*, 579–589. [CrossRef]
51. Meisel, S.F.; Freeman, M.; Waller, J.; Fraser, L.; Gessler, S.; Jacobs, I.; Kalsi, J.K.; Manchanda, R.; Rahman, B.; Side, L.; et al. Impact of a decision aid about stratified ovarian cancer risk-management on women's knowledge and intentions: A randomised online experimental survey study. *BMC Public Health* **2017**, *17*, 882. [CrossRef]
52. Evans, O.; Manchanda, R. Population-based Genetic Testing for Precision Prevention. *Cancer Prev. Res.* **2020**, *13*, 643–648. [CrossRef] [PubMed]
53. Manchanda, R.; Lieberman, S.; Gaba, F.; Lahad, A.; Levy-Lahad, E. Population Screening for Inherited Predisposition to Breast and Ovarian Cancer. *Annu. Rev. Genom. Hum. Genet.* **2020**, *21*, 373–412. [CrossRef] [PubMed]
54. Gurmankin, A.D.; Shea, J.; Williams, S.V.; Quistberg, D.A.; Armstrong, K. Measuring Perceptions of Breast Cancer Risk. *Cancer Epidemiol. Biomarkers Prev.* **2006**, *15*, 1893–1898. [CrossRef] [PubMed]
55. Peipins, L.A.; Mccarty, F.; Hawkins, N.A.; Rodriguez, J.L.; Scholl, L.E.; Leadbetter, S. Cognitive and affective influences on perceived risk of ovarian cancer. *Psycho-Oncology* **2015**, *24*, 279–286. [CrossRef] [PubMed]
56. Rawl, S.; Champion, V.; Menon, U.; Loehrer, P.J.; Vance, G.H.; Skinner, C.S. Validation of Scales to Measure Benefits of and Barriers to Colorectal Cancer Screening. *J. Psychosoc. Oncol.* **2001**, *19*, 47–63. [CrossRef]

6

High Galectin-7 and Low Galectin-8 Expression and the Combination of both are Negative Prognosticators for Breast Cancer Patients

Anna Trebo [1,†], Nina Ditsch [1,2,†], Christina Kuhn [1], Helene Hildegard Heidegger [1], Christine Zeder-Goess [1], Thomas Kolben [1], Bastian Czogalla [1], Elisa Schmoeckel [3], Sven Mahner [1], Udo Jeschke [1,2,*] and Anna Hester [1]

1 Department of Obstetrics and Gynecology, University Hospital, Ludwig-Maximilians-Universität (LMU) Munich, 81377 Munich, Germany; Anna.trebo@campus.lmu.de (A.T.); nina.ditsch@uk-augsburg.de (N.D.); christina.kuhn@med.uni-muenchen.de (C.K.); helene.heidegger@med.uni-muenchen.de (H.H.H.); christine.goess@med.uni-muenchen.de (C.Z.-G.); thomas.kolben@med.uni-muenchen.de (T.K.); bastian.czogalla@med.uni-muenchen.de (B.C.); sven.mahner@med.uni-muenchen.de (S.M.); anna.hester@med.uni-muenchen.de (A.H.)

2 Department of Obstetrics and Gynecology, University Hospital Augsburg, 86156 Augsburg, Germany

3 Institute of Pathology, LMU Munich, 81377 Munich, Germany; elisa.schmoeckel@med.uni-muenchen.de

* Correspondence: udo.jeschke@med.uni-muenchen.de

† These authors contributed equally to this work.

Abstract: Galectins are commonly overexpressed in cancer cells and their expression pattern is often associated with the aggressiveness and metastatic phenotype of the tumor. This study investigates the prognostic influence of the expression of galectin-7 (Gal-7) and galectin-8 (Gal-8) in tumor cell cytoplasm, nucleus and on surrounding immune cells. Primary breast cancer tissue of 235 patients was analyzed for the expression of Gal-7 and Gal-8 and correlated with clinical and pathological data and the outcome. To identify immune cell subpopulations, immunofluorescence double staining was performed. Significant correlations of Gal-7 expression in the cytoplasm with HER2-status, PR status, patient age and grading, and of Gal-8 expression in the cytoplasm with HER2-status and patient age and of both galectins between each other were found. A high Gal-7 expression in the cytoplasm was a significant independent prognosticator for an impaired progression free survival (PFS) ($p = 0.017$) and distant disease-free survival (DDFS) ($p = 0.030$). Gal-7 was also expressed by tumor-infiltrating macrophages. High Gal-8 expression in the cytoplasm was associated with a significantly improved overall survival (OS) ($p = 0.032$). Clinical outcome in patients showing both high Gal-7 and with low Gal-8 expression was very poor. Further understanding of the role of galectins in the regulation and interaction of tumor cells and macrophages is essential for finding new therapeutic targets.

Keywords: breast cancer; galectins; galectin-7; galectin-8; prognostic markers; tumor infiltrating macrophages

---

1. Introduction

Breast cancer is one of the three most prevalent cancers worldwide and the most frequent malignant tumor in women [1]. In 2018, about 2.1 million female patients were diagnosed with breast cancer and it represented the leading cause of tumor-related deaths in over 100 countries [2].

Based on gene profiling studies, breast cancer can be classified into different intrinsic subtypes [3]. In daily clinical practice, a surrogate system based on immunohistochemical and molecular characteristics is generally used: luminal A-like tumors show a strong expression of estrogen (ER) and progesterone (PR) receptors, low proliferation rates and a good prognosis. Luminal B-like human epidermal growth factor receptor 2 (HER2), and negative tumors show a lower hormone receptor expression and higher grading than Luminal A-like tumors and have an intermediate prognosis. Tumors that show an amplification of HER2 can be further classified based on hormone receptor expression in Luminal B-like HER2+ and in HER2+ non-luminal tumors. Triple negative breast cancers (TNBC) lack the expression of both hormone receptors and HER2, and show the worst prognosis of all breast cancer subtypes [3,4]. Even though therapy has improved in recent years, [1] new therapeutic strategies aiming at specific targets are needed [5–7]. This is especially important for TNBC, because patients still have a poor outcome and cannot be treated with endocrine therapy or targeted therapies like anti-HER2-therapy [8].

The discovery of galectins in 1994 [9,10] led to investigations on their impact on tumor development, progression and metastasis [11]. Galectins are a group of proteins able to bind to β-galactoside-binding sugars, either by N-linked or O-linked glycosylation, and they share primary structural homology in their carbohydrate-recognition domains (CRDs) [10]. A total of 12 different human galectin coding genes were found, including two for galectin-9 [12]. Galectins are divided into the subgroups of dimeric galectins (galectin-1,-2,-7,-10,-13,-14) with two identical CRD subunits, tandem galectins (galectin-4,-8,-9,-12) with two distinct CRD subunits, and chimeric galectins (galectin-3) with one or even multiple subunits of the same type [10,12]. Galectins are commonly overexpressed in cancer cells and cancer-associated stromal cells [13]. This altered galectin expression often correlates with the aggressiveness of the tumor and the metastatic phenotype [14]. In breast cancer, a connection between diverse galectin expression patterns and different cancer characteristics—like a correlation of galectin-1 (Gal-1) expression with tumor grading—was found [11,15]. Recently, the role of Gal-1 and galectin-3 (Gal-3) was thoroughly investigated [14]. Silencing Gal-1 led to both impaired tumor growth and reduced metastasis in a breast cancer mouse model [16]. Furthermore, it was found that Gal-1 interacts with E-selectin and influences adhesion [17]. However, targeting Gal-1 still has not come to clinical practice because no strategy of a fully specific Gal-1 blocking has been established yet. Gal-3 was identified as a molecular signature of breast cancer [18] and also as a potential therapeutic target [19]. Galectin-9, however, was described as anti-tumorigenic with possible antimetastatic potential in breast cancer [20]. Galectin-7 (Gal-7), like Gal-1 and Gal-3, seems to have tumor-promoting effects: in a Gal-7 deficient mouse model, a delayed development of HER2+ breast cancer was observed. Further investigations showed a positive correlation of Gal-7 expression with the frequency of HER2+ breast cancer. Furthermore, an association of Gal-7 expression with increased lymph node axillary metastasis in HER2+ tumors was seen [21,22]. Another study revealed an augmented Gal-7 expression in aggressive molecular subtypes, notably in estrogen receptor negative breast cancer and in cell lines with a basal-like phenotype. High expression of Gal-7 caused a higher metastatic risk, rendering cancer cells more resistant to apoptosis in a mouse model. Gal-7 might be part of the p53-promoted cancer progression pathway [23]. It is not known if these effects are specific to Gal-7, as most of the studies focused on one galectin and did not compare all individual galectins with each other. There is no detailed analysis of all galectins and their specific effects in breast cancer and most galectins, like galectin-8 (Gal-8), have not been studied in detail. There are only limited data suggesting that silencing a Gal-8-dependent pathway might lead to impaired tumor growth, especially in TNBC [24].

In this study, the specific role of Gal-7 and Gal-8 in a bigger cohort of human primary non-metastatic breast cancer was evaluated. The analysis included the specific location of galectin expression in the nucleus or cytoplasm and the expression in tumor-surrounding immune cells.

2. Results

2.1. Gal-7 and Gal-8 Expression in Breast Cancer and Correlation to Different Clinical and Pathological Characteristics

2.1.1. Gal-7 and Gal-8 Expression in Breast Cancer Cytoplasm and Nucleus

Expression of both galectins was observed in the cytoplasm as well as in the nucleus, being more pronounced for Gal-7. Gal-7 expression could not be evaluated in 19 sections (due to technical issues). Seven cases showed no Gal-7 expression in the cytoplasm and 35 no staining in the nucleus. For Gal-8, 20 tissue sections could not be analyzed (due to technical issues), and 15 and 63 samples revealed no staining in the cytoplasm and in the nucleus, respectively. The distribution of the immunoreactivity score (IRS) for the staining in the cytoplasm and in the nucleus is shown in Table 1; Table 2. The mean IRS for staining in the cytoplasm was 4.88 for Gal-7 and 4.37 for Gal-8, while it was 2.51 for staining in the nucleus for Gal-7 and 2.56 for Gal-8.

Table 1. Staining results of Gal-7 in the cytoplasm and the nucleus. Gal = galectin; NA = not applicable; IRS = immunoreactivity score.

Gal-7 Cytoplasm			**Gal-7 Nucleus**		
IRS	n	%	**IRS**	n	%
0	7	3.0	0	35	14.9
1	2	0.9	1	17	7.2
2	43	18.3	2	64	27.2
3	21	8.9	3	51	21.7
4	40	17.0	4	25	10.6
6	60	25.5	6	24	10.2
8	27	11.5	NA	19	8.1
9	8	3.4	total	235	100.0
12	8	3.4			
NA	19	8.1			
total	235	100.0			

Table 2. Staining results of Gal-8 in the cytoplasm and the nucleus. Gal = galectin; NA = not applicable; IRS = immunoreactivity score.

Gal-8 Cytoplasm			**Gal-8 Nucleus**		
IRS	n	%	**IRS**	n	%
0	15	6.4	0	63	26.8
1	12	5.1	1	14	6.0
2	50	21.3	2	55	23.4
3	27	11.5	3	7	3.0
4	18	7.7	4	43	18.3
6	54	23.0	6	22	9.4
8	16	6.8	8	1	0.4
9	18	7.7	9	9	3.8
12	5	2.1	12	1	0.4
NA	20	8.5	NA	20	8.5
total	235	100.0	total	235	100.0

2.1.2. Gal-7 and Gal-8 Expression and Correlation with Clinical Characteristics, Histopathological Breast Cancer Subtypes and Grading

Both Gal-7 and Gal-8 expression in the cytoplasm and in the nucleus did not correlate with the clinical parameters: tumor size and lymph node status. Gal-7 and Gal-8 expression in the cytoplasm correlated negatively with patient age (see Spearman correlation analyses in Supplementary Data: Tables S1 and S2).

The Gal-7 expression correlated negatively with the histopathological subtype. Kruskal–Wallis test and boxplots analysis showed that Gal-7 expression in the cytoplasm was significantly higher in no special type (NST) tumors compared to non-NST tumors (median IRS 6 in NST vs. 4 in non-NST, $p < 0.001$) (Figure 1a). Similarly, Gal-7 expression in the nucleus was significantly higher in NST tumors ($p = 0.042$). The Gal-8 expression did not differ concerning the histological subtype.

Regarding tumor grading, a positive correlation with the cytoplasmic Gal-7 expression was found (Spearman correlation analysis in Table S1). Kruskal–Wallis test showed that Gal-7 expression in the cytoplasm was higher in higher tumor grading (Gal-7 in G1 median IRS 3 and in G2/3 median IRS 6, $p = 0.003$, Figure 1b). The Gal-7 expression in the nucleus and the Gal-8 expression in the cytoplasm were not associated with tumor grading. The Gal-8 expression in the nucleus correlated negatively with the tumor grading and showed a trend towards a lower IRS in higher tumor grading ($p = 0.089$). Exemplary immunohistochemical Gal-7 and Gal-8 staining in tumors with different gradings are shown in Figure 2.

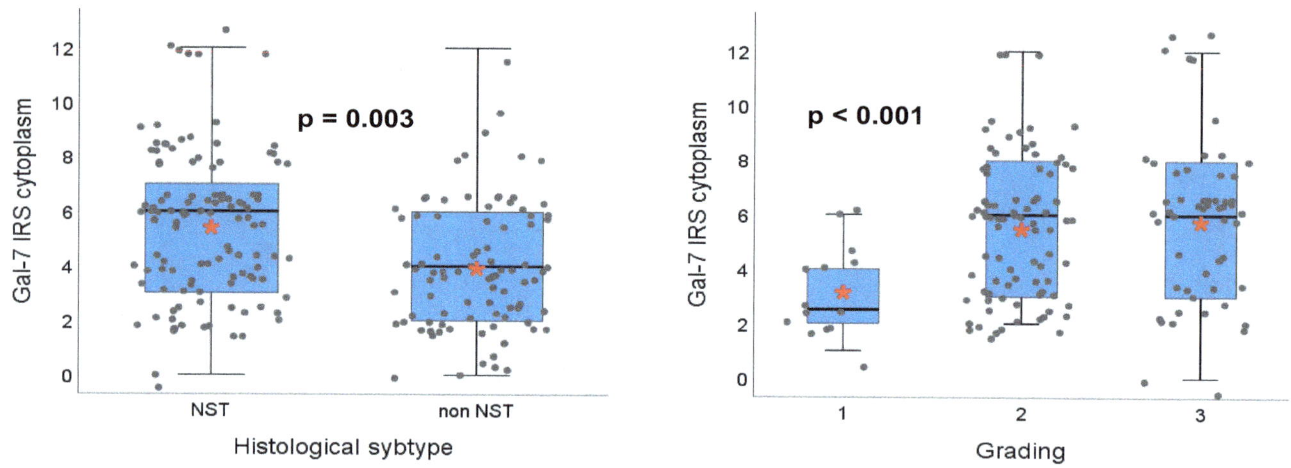

(a) (b)

Figure 1. Association of Gal-7 expression with histological subtype and tumor grading. Boxplots of the median IRS of Gal-7 staining in the cytoplasm dependent on histological subtype (**a**) and tumor grading (**b**) of the tumor are shown. (**a**) In non-NST tumors, Gal-7 expression in the cytoplasm is significantly lower than in NST tumors. (**b**) Tumors with G2/3 grading show a significantly higher Gal-7 expression in the cytoplasm compared to G1 tumors. Red asterisks indicate means. Please note that individual datapoints have been jittered to avoid overlap.

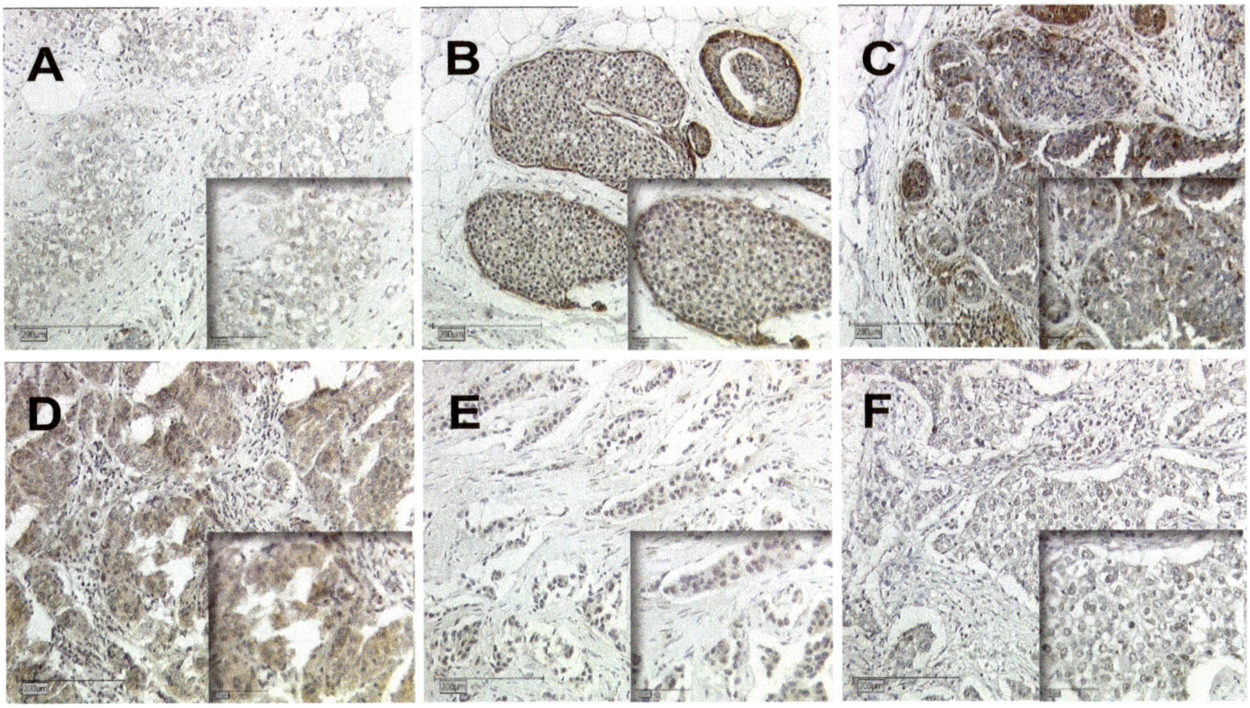

Figure 2. Gal-7 and Gal-8 expression dependent on tumor grading. Exemplary immunohistochemical staining of Gal-7 in grade 1 (**A**), 2 (**B**), and 3 (**C**) tumors and of Gal-8 in grade 1 (**D**), 2 (**E**), 3 (**F**) tumors are shown. Magnification: main images x10, image sections x25.

2.1.3. Gal-7 and Gal-8 Expression and Correlation with Hormone Receptor Status, HER2 Amplification and Surrogate Intrinsic Subtypes

Spearman analysis revealed that Gal-7 expression in the cytoplasm did correlate to PR-status and Gal-8 expression in the nucleus to ER-status (Spearman analysis in Tables S1 and S2). In the Kruskal–Wallis analysis, the Gal-7 staining in the cytoplasm was significantly higher in PR-negative compared to PR-positive tumors (median IRS in PR-positive: 4 vs. in PR-negative: 6, $p = 0.038$, Figure 3b), but was not significantly different concerning ER-status ($p = 0.159$, Figure 3a). The Gal-8 expression in the nucleus was significantly higher in ER-positive tumors ($p = 0.026$, Figure 3c) and a trend towards a higher Gal-8 expression in PR-positive compared to PR-negative tumors was observed ($p = 0.098$, Figure 3d). Both Gal-7 expression in the nucleus and Gal-8 in the cytoplasm did not correlate with the ER- or PR-status.

Both Gal-7 and Gal-8 staining in the cytoplasm correlated significantly with the HER2-status (Spearman analysis in Tables S1 and S2). HER2-positive breast cancer samples showed a distinctly higher Gal-7 expression in the cytoplasm compared to HER2-negative tumor sections (median IRS in HER2+: 8 vs. in HER2-: 4, $p < 0.001$, Figure 3e). Gal-8 expression in the cytoplasm in HER2-positive tissue sections was significantly higher than in HER2-negative samples (median IRS in HER2+: 6 vs. in HER2-: 3, $p = 0.004$, Figure 3f). Gal-7 and Gal-8 staining in the nucleus were not significantly associated with HER2-status (Figure S1).

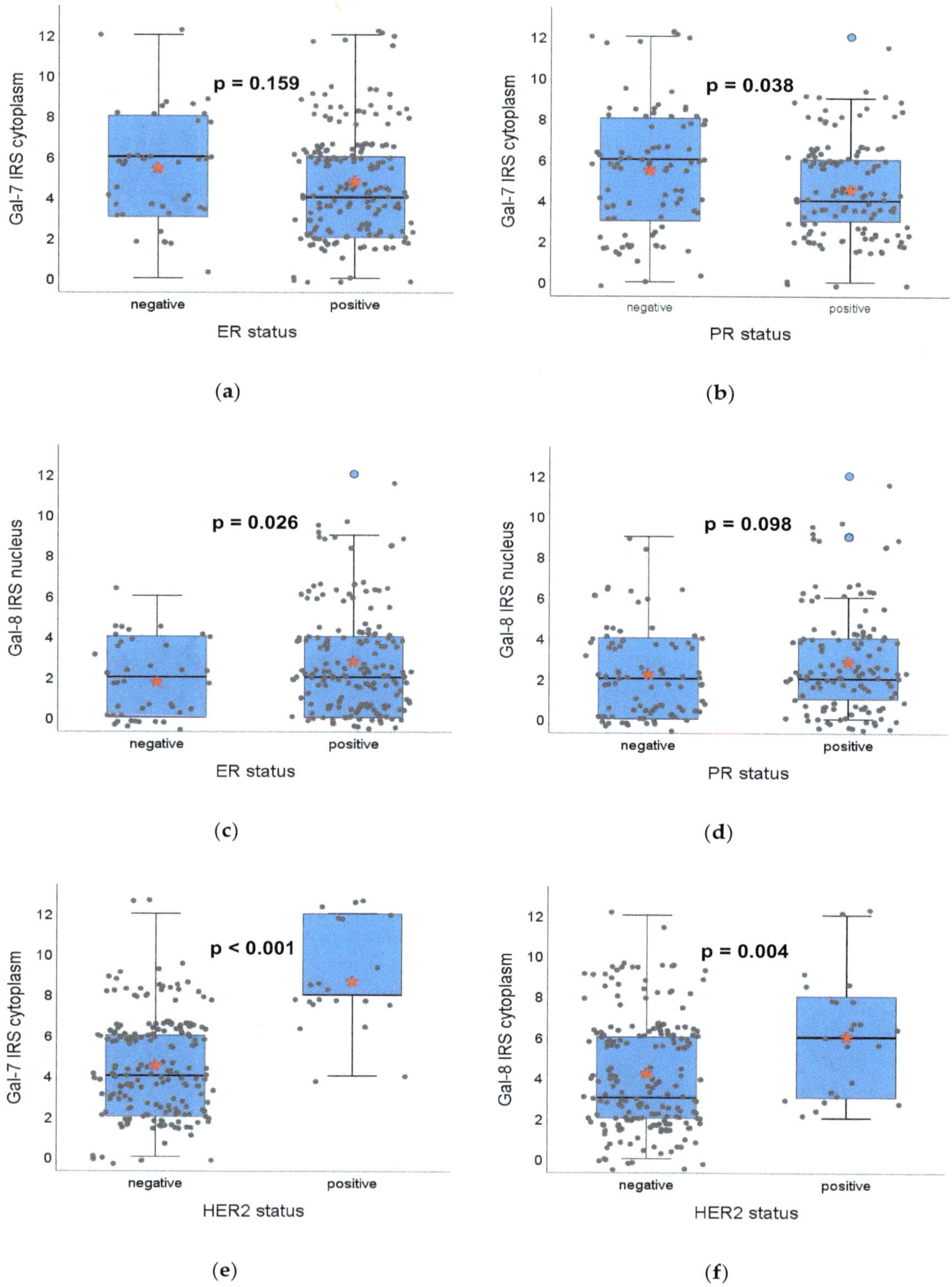

Figure 3. Association of Gal-7 and Gal-8 expression with the ER-, PR- and HER2-status. Boxplots of the median IRS of Gal-7 staining in the cytoplasm dependent on ER-status (**a**), PR-status (**b**) and HER2-status (**e**) and of Gal-8 staining in the nucleus dependent on ER-status (**c**) and PR-status (**d**) as well as Gal-8 staining in the cytoplasm dependent on HER2-status (**f**) are shown. ER-positive tumors do not differ concerning Gal-7 staining but show a higher Gal-8 staining. PR-positive tumors show lower Gal-7 staining and a trend towards higher Gal-8 staining. HER2-positive tumors show a significantly higher Gal-7 and Gal 8 expression in the cytoplasm compared to HER2-negative tumors. Staining in the nucleus does not show significant differences. Red asterisks indicate means. Please note that individual data points have been jittered to avoid overlap.

The Gal-7 expression in the cytoplasm differed significantly regarding the different surrogate intrinsic subtypes ($p < 0.001$) (Figure 4): HER2-positive tumors (both luminal B-like and non-luminal) clearly showed the highest Gal-7 expression in the cytoplasm compared to all other subtypes (Luminal A-like and B-like and TNBC). The distribution of Gal-8 staining, neither in the cytoplasm (Figure S2) nor in the nucleus, and Gal-7 expression in the nucleus in the different surrogate intrinsic subtypes showed no significant differences.

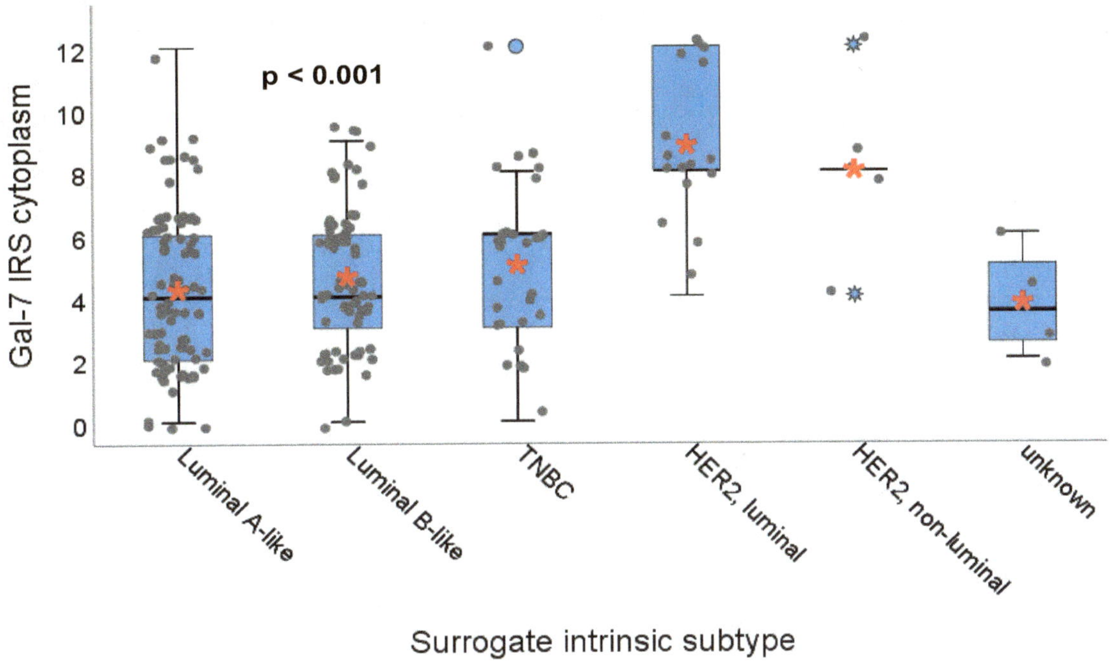

Figure 4. Association of Gal-7 expression with different surrogate intrinsic subtype. Boxplot of the median IRS of Gal-7 staining in the cytoplasm dependent on the surrogate intrinsic subtype of the tumor is shown. HER2-positive, both luminal and non-luminal tumors show a significantly higher Gal-7 expression in the cytoplasm compared to the other subtypes. Red asterisks indicate means. Please note that individual datapoints have been jittered to avoid overlap.

2.1.4. Correlation of Gal-7 and Gal-8 Expression

Gal-7 expression in the nucleus and cytoplasm correlated to each other as well as Gal-8 expression in the nucleus and cytoplasm (Table 3). Gal-7 and Gal-8 expressions in the nucleus and cytoplasm also correlated with each other.

2.2. *Correlation of Gal-7 and Gal-8 Expression with Survival in Breast Cancer Patients*

Median overall survival (OS), progression-free survival (PFS) and distant disease-free survival (DDFS) in the whole cohort was not reached (NR). The prognostic relevance of Gal-7 and -8 was analyzed concerning PFS, DDFS and OS and tumors were categorized in "high" and "low" expressing tumors using ROC-curve analysis.

2.2.1. High Gal-7 Expression in the Cytoplasm is a Negative Prognosticator for Survival in Breast Cancer Patients

High Gal-7 expression in the cytoplasm (IRS > 6) was associated with a worse outcome: tumors with high Gal-7 expression in the cytoplasm showed a significantly impaired PFS ($p = 0.017$, median PFS in Gal-7 high: 9.7 years, median PFS in Gal-7 low: NR) (Figure 5a) and DDFS ($p = 0.030$, median DDFS in both subgroups NR) (Figure 5b). Concerning OS, no significant difference was detected ($p = 0.927$, median OS in both subgroups NR) (Figure 5c).

Table 3. Spearman correlation analysis of Gal-7 and Gal-8 expression in the nucleus and cytoplasm. Significant correlations are displayed in bold. ** indicates a significance level of $p < 0.01$.

		Gal-7 IRS Cytoplasm	Gal-7 IRS Nucleus	Gal-8 IRS Cytoplasm	Gal-8 IRS Nucleus
Gal-7 IRS cytoplasm	Correlation Coefficient	1.000	**0.467** **	**0.332** **	**0.188** **
	Sig. (2-tailed)		<0.001	<0.001	0.007
	N	216	216	206	206
Gal-7 IRS nucleus	Correlation Coefficient	**0.467** **	1.000	**0.185** **	**0.301** **
	Sig. (2-tailed)	<0.001		0.008	<0.001
	N	216	216	206	206
Gal-8 IRS cytoplasm	Correlation Coefficient	**0.332** **	**0.185** **	1.000	**0.594** **
	Sig. (2-tailed)	<0.001	0.008		0.000
	N	206	206	215	215
Gal-8 IRS nucleus	Correlation Coefficient	**0.188** **	**0.301** **	**0.594** **	1.000
	Sig. (2-tailed)	0.007	<0.001	<0.001	
	N	206	206	215	215

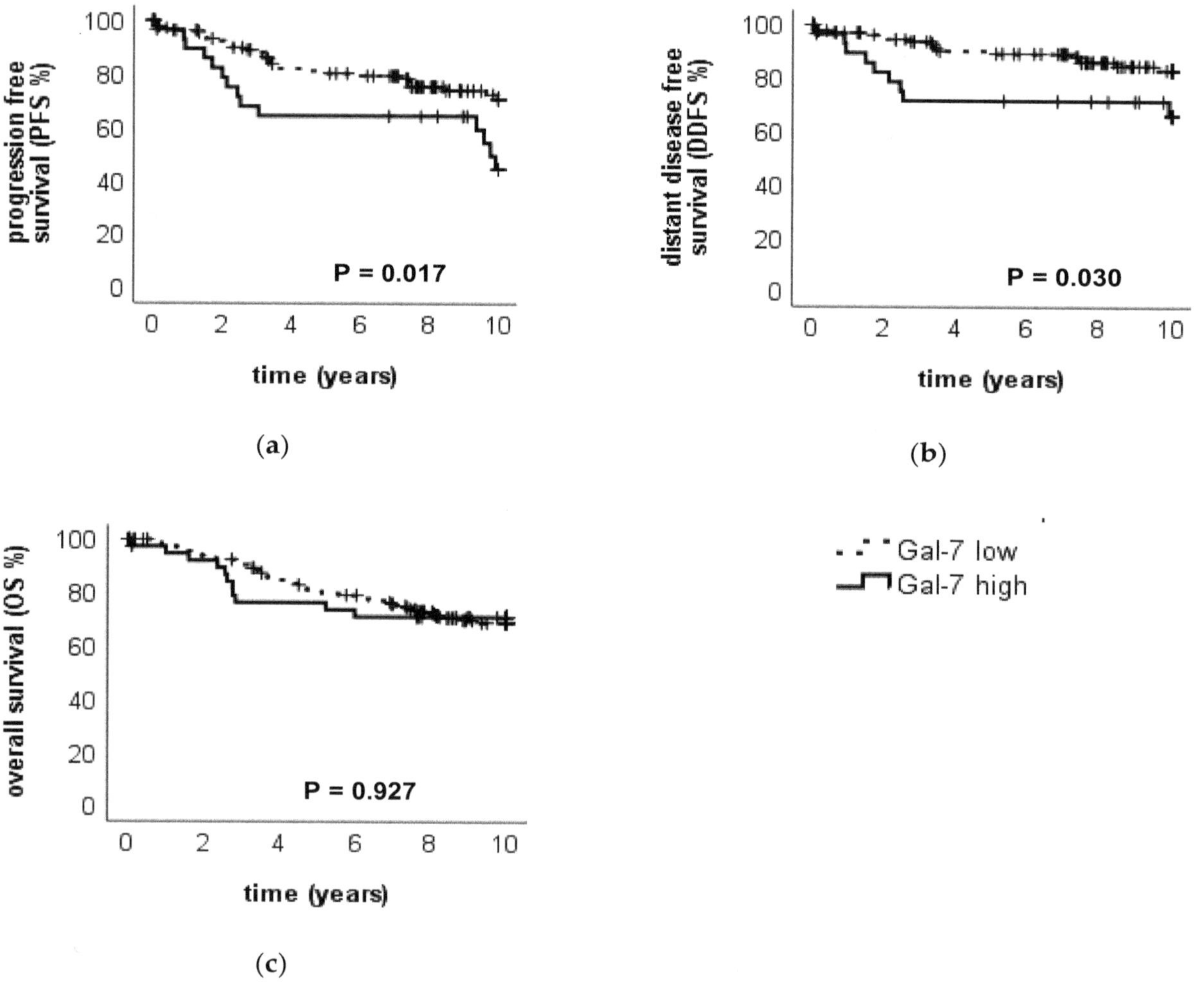

Figure 5. Association of Gal-7 expression in the cytoplasm to the clinical outcome. Kaplan–Meier analysis of PFS (**a**), DDFS (**b**) and OS (**c**) in Gal-7 high- and low-expressing tumors (in the cytoplasm) is shown. Tumors with high Gal-7 expression in the cytoplasm showed a significantly impaired PFS and DDFS.

Multivariate COX regression analysis revealed Gal-7 expression as an independent prognostic factor for PFS (Table 4) but not for DDFS (Table S3). Concerning OS, where Gal-7 was not significant in the univariate analysis, COX regression analysis revealed ER-status, nodal status and age as independent prognosticators (Table S4).

Table 4. Multivariate analysis of PFS concerning Gal 7 expression in the cytoplasm. Significant factors are highlighted in bold.

Prognostic Factor	B	SE	Wald	df	Sig.	Exp(B)	95,0% CI for Exp(B)	
							Lower	Upper
Histological subtype (NST vs. non-NST)	0.245	0.459	0.286	1	0.593	1.278	0.520	3.140
Grading (G1 vs. G2-3)	0.312	0.817	0.146	1	0.702	1.367	0.276	6.773
Tumor size (pT1 vs. pT2-4)	0.284	0.377	0.564	1	0.453	1.328	0.634	2.783
Nodal status (pN0 vs. pN1-3)	0.553	0.397	1.935	1	0.164	1.738	0.798	3.788
HER2 status (positive vs. negative)	−0.161	0.538	0.090	1	0.764	0.851	0.297	2.443
ER (positive vs. negative)	−0.823	0.459	3.219	1	0.073	0.439	0.179	1.079
PR (positive vs. negative)	−0.345	0.460	0.565	1	0.452	0.708	0.288	1.743
Patient age (continuous)	0.010	0.017	0.329	1	0.566	1.010	0.977	1.043
Gal-7 expression in the cytoplasm (high vs. low)	0.806	0.410	3.860	1	**0.049**	2.239	1.002	5.003

Subgroup analysis revealed that Gal-7 expression in the cytoplasm had prognostic relevance for an impaired PFS in the ER-negative (but not in ER-positive) ($p = 0.036$, median PFS in Gal-7 high 2.52 years, Figure S3), in the pT1 (but not in pT > 1) ($p = 0.014$) and in the pN0 (but not in pN > 0) ($p = 0.043$) subgroups. A trend towards an impaired PFS could be observed in PR positive (but not PR negative) ($p = 0.098$) and in HER2 positive (but not in HER2 negative) tumors ($p = 0.084$, Figure S4).

Gal-7 expression in the nucleus did not show prognostic relevance for PFS, DDFS or for the OS (Figure S5). Subgroup analysis did also not show any new prognostic relevance of nuclear Gal-7 expression concerning the subgroups of PR-positive vs. -negative, HER2-positive vs. -negative tumors, grading, tumor size and lymph node status. However, in ER-negative tumors, a high nuclear Gal-7 expression showed an impaired OS while nuclear Gal-7 expression was not relevant in ER-positive tumors even if statistical significance was not reached ($p = 0.082$. Similarly, a worse outcome regarding PFS could be seen in lower grading (G1, $p = 0.058$) (but not in G2-3) when nuclear Gal-7 expression was high.

2.2.2. High Gal-8 Expression in the Cytoplasm is a Positive Prognosticator for Overall Survival in Breast Cancer Patients

High Gal-8 expression in the cytoplasm (IRS > 5) was associated with an improved outcome: Tumors with a high Gal-8 expression in the cytoplasm showed a significantly improved OS compared to tumors with low Gal-8 expression in the cytoplasm ($p = 0.032$, median OS in both subgroups NR) (Figure 6a). No significance in the outcome regarding PFS ($p = 0.974$, median PFS in both subgroups NS, Figure 6b) and DDFS ($p = 0.138$, median DDFS in both subgroups NR, Figure 6c) was found.

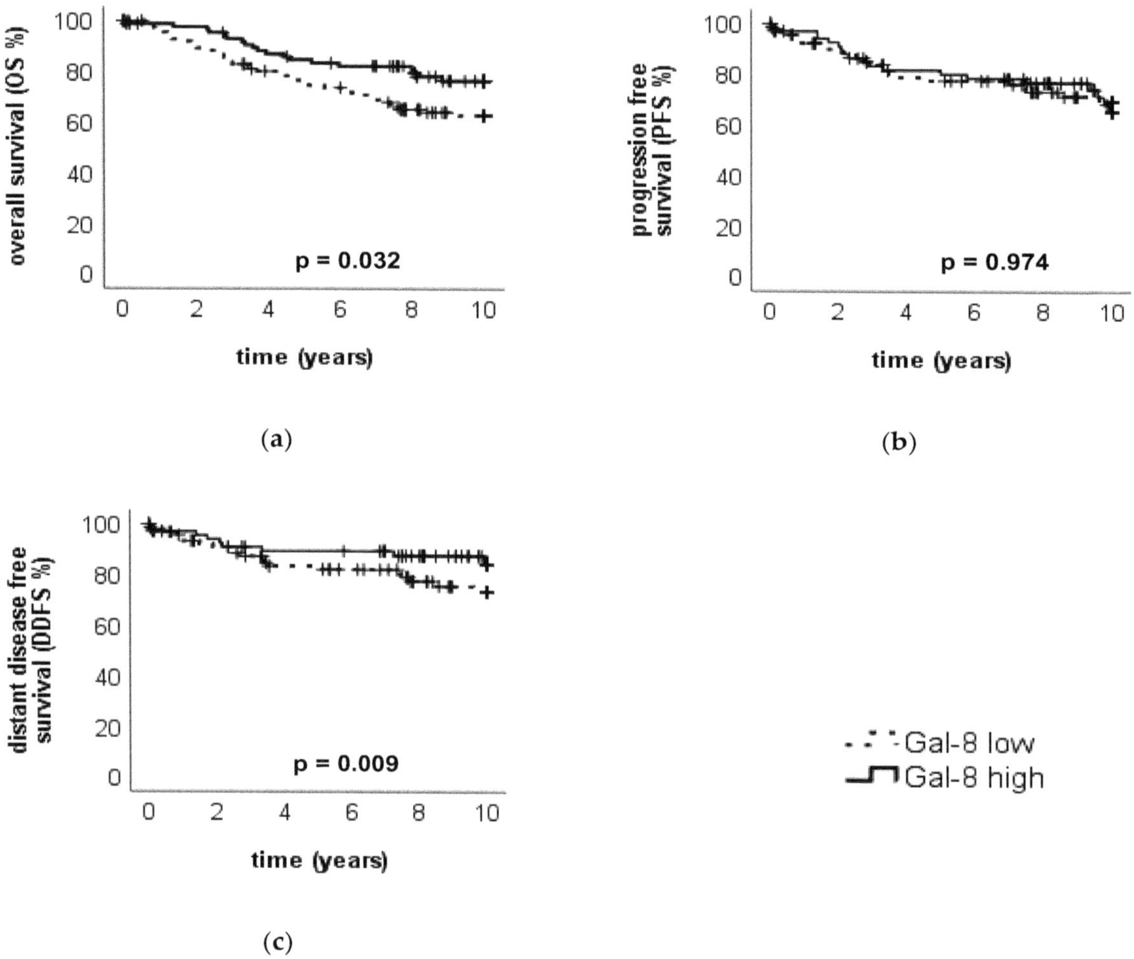

Figure 6. Association of Gal-8 expression in the cytoplasm to the clinical outcome. Kaplan–Meier analysis of OS (**a**), PFS (**b**) and DDFS (**c**) in Gal-8 high- and low-expressing tumors (in the cytoplasm) is shown. Tumors with high Gal-8 expression in the cytoplasm showed a significantly improved OS.

The multivariate COX regression analysis could not confirm Gal-8 expression in the cytoplasm as an independent prognostic factor (Table 5) for OS. In contrast, age at the surgery, ER status and lymph-node status (pN) were detected as independent prognosticators for the OS. Gal-8 was also not prognostically relevant in COX regression for PFS or DDFS.

Table 5. Cox regression analysis of prognostic factors for OS in breast cancer patients. Significant factors are highlighted in bold.

Prognostic Factor	B	SE	Wald	df	Sig.	Exp(B)	95,0% CI for Exp(B)	
							Lower	Upper
Histological subtype (NST vs. non-NST)	0.199	0.456	0.190	1	0.663	1.220	0.499	2.983
Grading (G1 vs. G2-3)	−0.321	0.591	0.295	1	0.587	0.725	0.228	2.311
Tumor size (pT1 vs. pT2-4)	0.237	0.385	0.378	1	0.539	1.267	0.596	2.693
Nodal status (pN0 vs. pN1-3)	1.144	0.406	7.927	1	**0.005**	3.140	1.416	6.964
HER2 status (positive vs. negative)	0.429	0.617	0.483	1	0.487	1.535	0.458	5.143
ER (positive vs. negative)	−1.178	0.504	5.466	1	**0.019**	0.308	0.115	0.827
PR (positive vs. negative)	0.568	0.483	1.381	1	0.240	1.765	0.684	4.551
Patient age (continuous)	0.051	0.017	9.367	1	**0.002**	1.053	1.019	1.088
Gal-8 expression in the cytoplasm (high vs. low)	−0.258	0.372	0.479	1	0.489	0.773	0.372	1.603

Subgroup analysis revealed that Gal-8 expression in the cytoplasm had prognostic relevance with a better outcome for the OS in NST (but not non-NST) tumors ($p = 0.049$), in HER2-negative (but not HER2-positive) ($p = 0.029$, Figure S6) in ER-positive (but not ER-negative) ($p = 0.055$, Figure S7) and in pT1 (but not in pT2-4) ($p = 0.038$). Concerning PFS and DDFS, no significant prognostic impact could be found for Gal-8 in the different subgroups.

Similar to Gal-7 staining in the nucleus, Gal-8 staining in the nucleus did not show prognostic relevance for neither PFS, DDFS or OS (Figure S8). However, subgroup analysis revealed that high Gal-8 staining in the nucleus was associated with improved PFS in ER-positive patients ($p = 0.041$) but not in ER negative patients and to tendentially ($p = 0.081$) better OS in pT2-4 (but not in pT1) tumors. Regarding the other subgroups (PR-positive vs. -negative, HER2-positive vs. -negative, nodal status, histological subtype), nuclear Gal-8 staining did not show significant prognostic influence, similar to the overall cohort.

2.2.3. Survival Analysis Using Combined Gal-7 and Gal-8 Staining

Survival analysis was also performed in subgroups with high or low Gal-7 expression in the cytoplasm in combination with low or high Gal-8 expression in the cytoplasm, respectively. A high Gal-7 combined with a low Gal-8 expression in the cytoplasm was associated with an impaired OS compared to all other patients ($p = 0.201$, median OS in all subgroups NR, Figure 7a). When Gal-7 expression was high and Gal-8 was low, DDFS was significantly impaired ($p = 0.009$, median DDFS in all subgroups NR, Figure 7b) compared to the rest of the patients, as well as PFS with a borderline significance ($p = 0.067$, median PFS in all subgroups NR, Figure 7c). In summary, two different groups regarding the outcome could be defined: The first group, representing 6.8% of the patients, consisted of tumors expressing Gal-7 high (IRS > 6) and Gal-8 low (IRS ≤ 5) in the cytoplasm. This subgroup showed a poor OS. The second group, formed by 13.6% of the patients with high Gal-8 (IRS > 5) and low Gal-7 (IRS ≤ 6) expression in the cytoplasm, showed good OS (Figure 7a). Comparing the three subgroups concerning PFS and DDFS, the "advantageous" subgroup (high Gal-8, low Gal-7) seems to be less relevant (survival curves similar to the "others" subgroup, Figure S9).

2.2.4. Immune Cell Infiltration Stained with Gal-7

Gal-7 had an interesting expression pattern in the tumor tissue, with staining on only the outer layer of cancer cells and expression in the immune cells next to the tumor cells as well (Figure 8a–d). Gal-7 staining in the immune cells was not included as part of the IRS-scoring for the cancer specimen in the analyses described above. The immune cell staining of Gal-7 correlated significantly with the tumor grading: in tissue sections defined as grade 1 no stained immune cell infiltration was observed, whereas in grade 2 and 3, stained immune cells were detected ($p = 0.008$, Figure S10a). Gal-7-expressing immune cells were furthermore found significantly more often in NST compared to non-NST tumors ($p = 0.001$, Figure S10b) and in tumors with lymph node metastasis ($p = 0.038$, Figure S10c). A double immunofluorescence staining with Gal-7 and CD68 (a macrophage marker) showed that the Gal-7 stained immune cells were macrophages (Figure 8e–g).

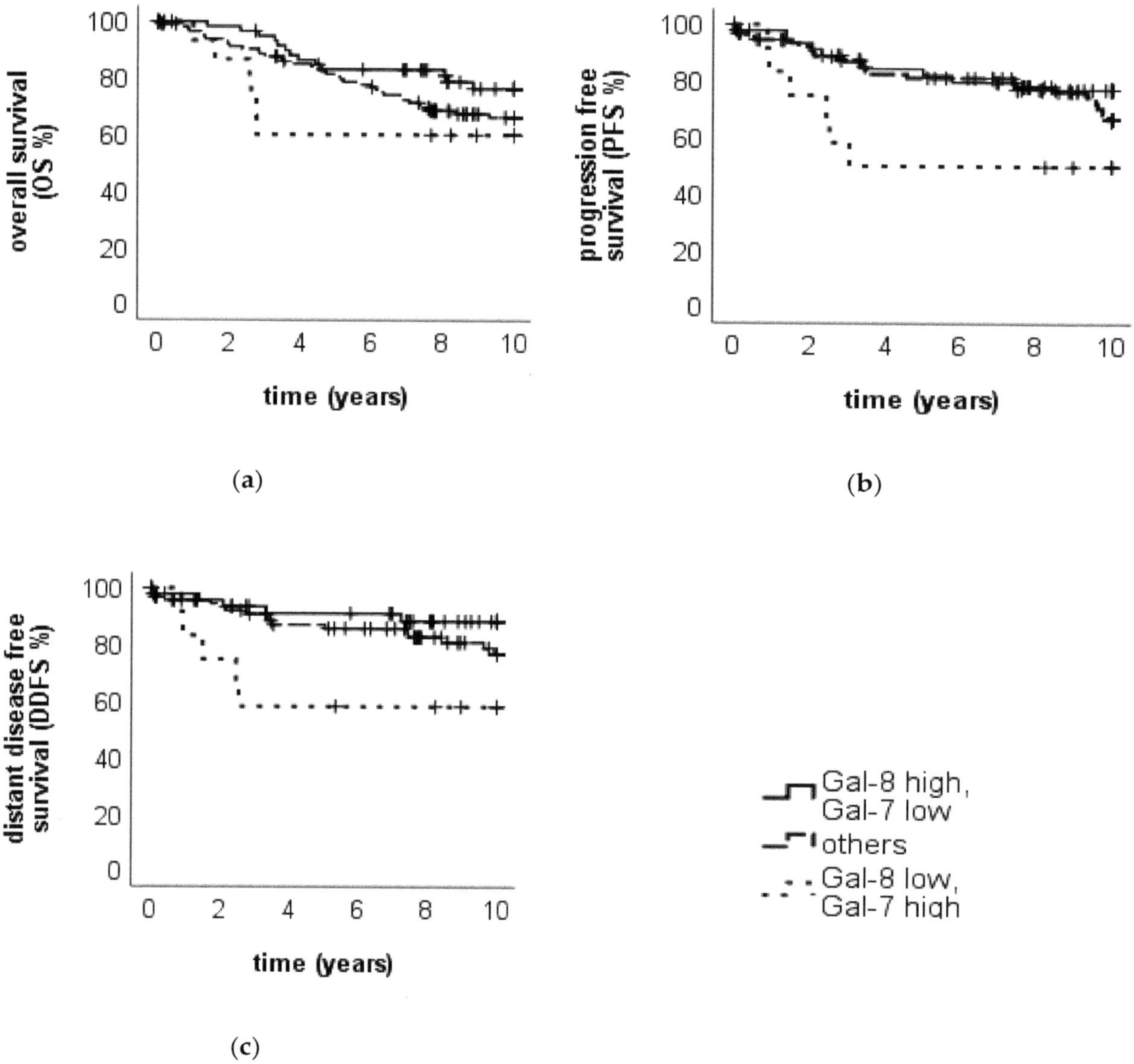

Figure 7. OS, PFS and DDFS for the two groups. Kaplan–Meier analysis of OS (**a**), PFS (**b**) and DDFS (**c**) in tumors with combined high or low Gal-7 expression with low or high Gal-8 expression (in the cytoplasm), respectively, are shown. Tumors with high Gal-7 and low Gal-8 expression in the cytoplasm show the trend of an impaired OS, while tumors with high Gal-8 and low Gal 7 expression show the trend of an improved OS. Tumors with high Gal-7 and low Gal-8 expression in the cytoplasm show the trend of an impaired PFS and a significantly reduced DDFS, while tumors with high Gal-8 and low Gal-7 expression show the trend of an improved PFS and a DDFS.

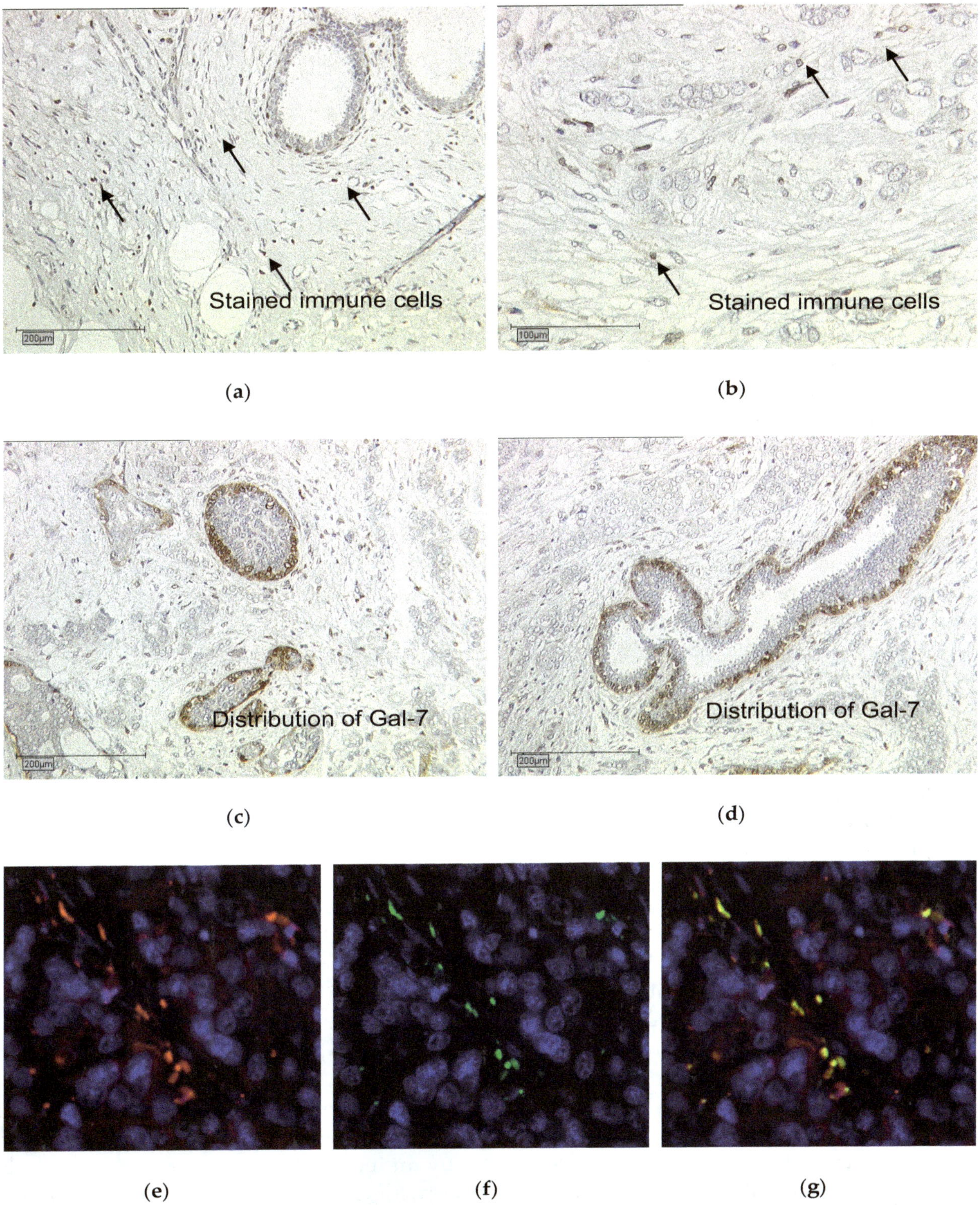

Figure 8. Gal-7-staining results (**a**–**d**) and double immunofluorescence staining with Gal 7 and CD68 (**e**–**g**). Exemplary pictures of Gal 7-staining results are shown, revealing the distribution of Gal 7-staining in tumor cells (**a**,**b**). Stained immune cells in Gal 7-expressing tumors are shown in (**c**) and (**d**). Immunofluorescence results: Gal-7 is shown in red (**e**), CD68 in green (**f**) and the nucleus is stained with DAPI in blue. Picture (**g**) shows that Gal 7- and CD8-staining is overlapping in some cells, which appear yellow, showing that these are macrophages. Magnification: Images 8a, 8c and 8d x10, and images 8b, 8e, 8f and 8g x25.

3. Discussion

Galectins have been shown to be a pivotal factor in carcinogenesis. However, data on their relevance in breast cancer are still sparse. As recently proposed [22,25], we could show in our cohort of primary breast cancer patients that Gal-7 was a negative prognosticator for the clinical outcome. Gal-7 expression in the cytoplasm had a negative prognostic impact on PFS and DDFS, a negative trend on OS and was even an independent negative prognosticator for PFS in the multivariate analysis. A strong association between a high Gal-7 expression in the cytoplasm and HER2 amplification was observed, suggesting that HER2-positive tumors might be especially interesting for potentially targeting Gal-7. In HER2-positive tumors—like in the overall cohort—high Gal-7 expression was associated with an impaired prognosis. Gal-8 expression in the cytoplasm, however, was associated with an improved OS.

Our data are in line with Grosset et al., [21,25] who found high Gal-7 expression only in HER2-positive tumors and in TNBC. Recent studies showed Gal-3 as a modifier of the epidermal growth factor receptor (EGFR), which is a regulator of cell growth and survival in normal and cancerous tissues [26–28]. EGFR and HER2 are both known as members of the ErbB receptor family and, when activated, they stimulate the activation of many signaling pathways [29]. Apart from Gal-3, no functional associations between galectins and ErbB receptors have been reported to date. However, these data suggest a functional connection between these two families which might also exist between Gal-7 and HER2.

Other groups showed in an in silico mRNA survival analysis that Gal-7 and Gal-8 did not have a prognostic impact in breast cancer patients. However, regarding protein level—similarly to our data—high Gal-7 expression was associated with an impaired PFS (although not statistically significant), whereas no effect could be shown for Gal-8 (both in the overall cohort) [25].

Our results suggest that combining Gal-7 and Gal-8 expression might further improve prognostic accuracy. Two different groups could be defined: a small group (high Gal-8, low Gal-7) with a very good outcome (6.8% of the patients), compared to a second group (high Gal-7, low Gal-8) with a worse outcome, consisting of 13.6% of the patients. This is especially interesting, as Gal-7 and Gal-8 expressions are strongly correlated. Similar effects have been shown for galectin ligands: in BC patients, high levels of- Gal-1 ligands and low levels of Gal-8 ligands have been observed, making their ratio a strong marker for BC [30]. A similar ratio could be established using the Gal-7/Gal-8 expression for prognostic considerations.

Galectin expression was also associated with tumor cell differentiation: Gal-7 expression was significantly higher in less differentiated cells (reflected by higher grading), whereas Gal-8 expression was highest in highly differentiated cells (reflected by lower grading). This is similar to other data where high Gal-4 (which belongs to the same family as Gal-8) expression in highly differentiated, and low Gal-1 (which belongs to the same family as Gal-7) expression in poorly differentiated, tumors have been shown [31]. Furthermore, in our study, poor tumor cell differentiation was also associated with high Gal-7 expression in tumor-surrounding macrophages, who are known to correlate with poor breast cancer survival rates.

Regarding mechanisms of the regulation of galectin expression and distribution between nucleus and cytoplasm, it is important to consider that Gal-7 is also provided extracellularly: The extracellular Gal-7 controls the intracellular pool of Gal-7, firstly by an increase in the gene transcription, and secondly by a re-entry pathway into the cells [32]. Similarly, for Gal-1 (which belongs to the same group as Gal-7) an extracellular to nucleus transfer has been shown and nuclear Gal-1 accumulation drove epithelial invasiveness. Extracellular glycans that bear N-acetyllactosamins (LacNAc) epitopes bind Gal-1 and trap it extracellularly. An α-2,6-sialylation of these LacNAc epitopes inhibits Gal-1-binding and drives the nuclear transfer of Gal-1 [33]. We could observe in our study that Gal-7 was also present in macrophages next to the tumor cells. Therefore, these macrophages might also provide a source of extracellular Gal-7 for tumor cells and might regulate the intracellular Gal-7 pool. Tumor-associated macrophages are correlated with poor survival rates of breast cancer [34], rendering Gal-7 even more interesting as a therapeutic target. Functional effects that have been described for Gal-8 include the activation of the activated leukocyte cell adhesion molecule (ALCAM) [23,35,36] and the activation of the endothelial nitric oxide synthase (eNOS) pathway on endothelial cells [37]. However, these pathways all describe a tumorigenic potential of Gal-8, while Gal-8 was a positive prognosticator in our study. Therefore, other tumor-suppressing pathways that need further investigation might exist.

First attempts in targeting galectins in breast cancer have already been made: Grosset et al. demonstrated that targeting CRD-independent cytosolic Gal-7 in breast cancer cells, and therefore impairing p53-functions, might be a valuable strategy for the treatment of breast cancer [35]. Targeting Gal-8 has not been performed to date. Gal-3 knockdown enhanced the sensitivity of tumor cells to the apoptotic agent arsenic trioxide (ATO, which is already approved by the US Food and Drug Administration for the treatment of acute myeloid leukemia) [19], making Gal-3 an interesting therapeutic target. An orally applied Gal-3 antagonist was already studied in a mouse model, leading to less lung adenocarcinoma growth [36]. Furthermore, a Gal-1 inhibitor that showed synergistic activity with the chemotherapeutic paclitaxel in BC has been discovered [37]. As Gal-7 belongs to the same family as Gal-1, similar therapeutic potential could exist for Gal-7.

4. Materials and Methods

4.1. Patients

Formalin-fixed, paraffin-embedded (FFPE) primary breast cancer samples of 235 patients were examined in this study (Table 6).

We included in our study all patients that were diagnosed with primary non-metastatic breast cancer and underwent surgery at the Department of Gynaecology and Obstetrics, Ludwig-Maximilians-University Munich, Germany, from the period 1998 to 2000.

Therefore, there was no pre-selection and a complete group of patients attending the clinic was analysed. Only women with benign tumors of the breast were excluded from the study.

Clinical, pathological and follow-up data (up to ten years) were retrieved from patients' charts and from the Munich Cancer Registry. Patient characteristics are displayed in Table 6. In terms of clinical and pathological characteristics and tumor biology, the collective represents the reality of the wide BC spectrum.

Histopathological subtype (no specific type (NST) vs. non-NST), tumor grading (G1-3) according to the Elston and Ellis criteria (1993) [4,38,39], and staging using the TNM-System [40] (T for tumor size, N for the lymph node status and M for metastasis) were determined by a gynecological pathologist. As tumor grading could only be obtained in about 70% of all patients, the results have to be regarded with limited reliability. HER2-positivity is defined by the DAKO Scoring system (DAKO, HER2 FISH pharmDx™ Kit, Agilent Technologies, Waldbronn, Germany). As HER2 status was not determined routinely in Germany before 2001, it was retrospectively assessed. HER2 status was determined as recommended in the national guidelines, i.e., by DAKO Score and FISH analysis in cases of DAKO 2+.

Endpoints regarding the survival data were defined as follows: OS = overall survival, period of time from the date of surgery until the date of death or date of last follow-up; PFS = progression free survival, period of time until local recurrence or metastasis were diagnosed and DDFS = distant disease free survival: period of time until metastasis was diagnosed.

Table 6. Patients' characteristics.

Patients' Characteristics	Median	SD
Age	58.2	13.3
	N	**%**
Histological subtype		
NST	126	53.6
Non-NST	96	40.9
NA	13	5.5
Intrinsic surrogate subtype		
Luminal A-like	103	43.8
Luminal B-like	73	31.1
HER2-positive, luminal	17	7.2
HER2-positive, non-luminal	7	3.0
TNBC	31	13.2
NA	4	1.7
Grading		
Grade 1	17	7.2
Grade 2	90	38.3
Grade 3	55	23.4
NA	73	31.1
Lymph node involvement (pN)		
pN0	128	54.5
pN1	87	37.0
pN2	10	4.3
NA	10	4.3
Tumor size (pT)		
pT1 (≤2 cm)	160	68.1
pT2 (2–5 cm)	68	28.9
pT3 (>5 cm)	1	0.4
pT4 (with infiltration in the epidermis or the thoracic wall)	5	2.1
NA	1	0.4
HER2 status		
Positive	24	10.2
Negative	208	88.5
NA	3	1.3
ER status		
Positive	192	81.7
Negative	43	18.3
PR status		
Positive	141	60.0
Negative	94	40.0

NST = no special type, NA = not available, ER = estrogen receptor, PR = progesterone receptor, HER2 = human epidermal growth factor receptor 2, TNBC = triple negative breast cancer.

4.2. Immunohistochemistry

Paraffine-embedded breast cancer tissue samples were analyzed by immunohistochemistry. The samples were fixed in neutral buffered formalin and embedded in paraffin after surgery. For histopathological investigations, tissue sections (3 μm) were deparaffinized in Roticlear (Carl Roth GmbH + Co. KG) for 20 min and then the endogenous peroxidase was inactivated with 3% hydrogen peroxide (VWR International GmbH) in methanol. The slides were rehydrated in a descending gradient of ethanol (100%, 75% and 50%) and prepared for epitope retrieval in a pressure cooker for 5 min in sodium citrate buffer (0.1 mol/L citric acid, 0.1 mol/L sodium citrate, pH 6.0). After washing in distilled water and phosphate-buffered saline (PBS), all tissue slides were blocked using a blocking solution (Reagent 1; ZytoChem Plus HRP Polymer System (Mouse/Rabbit); Zytomed Systems GmbH, Berlin,

Germany) for 5 min at room temperature (RT) in order to block non-specific binding of the primary antibodies. Then, a specific procedure followed for each Galectin: the slides were incubated with Gal-7 primary antibody (rabbit, polyclonal; Abcam, ab10482) at a final concentration of 2.5 µg/mL in PBS Dulbecco (Biochrom GmbH) for 16 h at 4 °C. Gal-8 primary antibody (rabbit, monoclonal, Abcam, ab109519) was used for incubation at a final concentration of 3.3 µg/mL in PBS for 1 h at RT. Afterwards, the staining specimens were incubated in post block reagent (Reagent 2) and HRP-polymer (Reagent 3) containing secondary antibodies (anti-mouse/-rabbit) and peroxidase according to the manufacturer's protocol. These antibodies are part of the provided Reagent 3, exact concentrations are not specified by the manufacturer. (Reagent 2 and 3, ZytoChem Plus HRP Polymer System, Mouse/Rabbit). All slides were washed in PBS after every incubation step. The slides were then stained with 3,3′-diaminobenzidine chromogen (DAB; Dako, Glostrup, Denmark) for visualization and counterstained in Mayer acidic hematoxylin. After dehydrating in an ascending ethanol gradient and Roticlear they were cover slipped with Roti-Mount (Carl Roth GmbH + Co. KG). Appropriate tissue slides were used as positive controls (sigma tissue for Gal-7 and placenta for Gal-8). To obtain expression results, the semiquantitative immunoreactive score (IRS, Remmele and Stegner 1987 [41] was performed using a Leitz Diaplan microscope (Leitz, Wetzlar, Germany). The score was optically obtained by multiplying the predominant staining intensity (0: none; 1: low; 2: moderate; 3: strong) and the percentage of positively stained cancer cells (0 = 0%, 1= 1–10%, 2 = 11–50%, 3 = 51%–80%, and 4 = 81%–100% stained cells). The IRS was determined separately in the cytoplasm and the nucleus of the cancer cells. The staining of other cells, like immune cells, was not included in the IRS. Images were taken with a CCD color camera (JVC, Victor Company of Japan, Japan).

Furthermore, immune cells stained with Gal-7 were analyzed independently of the tumor IRS for Gal-7 and evaluated using following scoring system: 0 = no immune cells were stained, 1 = <50% and 2 = >50% of the immune cells were stained.

4.3. *Immunofluorescence*

Paraffine-embedded breast cancer tissue samples were also used for immunofluorescence-analyses. The samples were fixed in neutral buffered formalin and embedded in paraffin after surgery. After deparaffinization in Roticlear (Carl Roth GmbH + Co. KG) for 20 min, the slides were rehydrated in a descending gradient of ethanol (100%, 75% and 50%) and prepared for epitope retrieval in a pressure cooker for 5 min in sodium citrate buffer (0.1 mol/L citric acid, 0.1 mol/L sodium citrate, pH 6.0). After washing in distilled water and PBS, all tissue slides were blocked with Ultra V Block (Thermo scientific) for 15 min. The primary antibodies were diluted in Dako Antibody Diluent (Dako North America) incubated with the slides for 16 h at 4 degrees. Gal-7 (rabbit, polyclonal; Abcam, ab10482) was diluted at a final concentration of 2,5 µg/mL and CD68 (mouse, monoclonal, Sigma AldrichAMAb90874) at a concentration of 0.1 µg/mL. Next, the light in the room was dimmed and an incubation with the secondary antibodies for 30 min at RT followed. Secondary antibodies: Goat-Anti Rabbit IgG Cy3 (Dianova/Jackson, 111-165-144) diluted at a concentration of 3 µg/mL and Goat-Anti-Mouse-AlexaFluor488-IgG (Dianova/Jackson, 115-546-062) at a concentration of 15 µg/mL. After the slices were dried in the dark, they were cover slipped with mounting medium for fluorescence with DAPI (Vectashield H-1200). The samples were then analyzed using a Zeiss AxioPhot microscope with an Axiocam MRm within one day.

4.4. *Statistical Analysis*

Data analyses were performed with SPSS Statistics 25 (Armonk, NY: IBM Corp.). *p*-values lower than 0.05 were considered as statistically significant. Correlations between staining results and ordinal variables were tested with Spearman's rank correlation coefficient. Group comparisons regarding the IRS of galectins between different clinical and pathological subgroups were tested with Kruskal–Wallis test and displayed as boxplot graphs. Survival times between different groups were compared by Kaplan–Meier analysis, and differences were tested for significance by Log-Rank (Mantel-Cox),

Breslow- and Tarone-Ware-tests. Censored cases are cases for which the second event is not recorded (for example, people still alive at the end of the study). The Kaplan–Meier procedure is a method of estimating time-to-event models in the presence of censored cases. The Kaplan–Meier model is based on estimating conditional probabilities at each time point when an event occurs and taking the product limit of those probabilities to estimate the survival rate at each point in time. Cox-regression analysis was used to determine the independence of prognostic factors.

Concerning survival analysis dependent on Gal-7 and Gal-8 expression, patients were grouped into high and low expression. Cut-off points were selected considering the distribution pattern of IR-scores in the collective. Therefore, the receiver operator curve (ROC curve) was drawn using SPSS software, which is considered as one of the most reliable methods for cut-off point selection. In this context, the ROC curve is a plot representing sensitivity on the y-axis and (1-specificity) the x-axis. Consecutively Youden index, defined as the maximum (sensitivity + specificity−1), was used to find the optimal cut-off maximizing the sum of sensitivity and specificity (exemplary results of the ROC curve analysis in Table S5). Furthermore, the medians of Kruskal–Wallis tests were observed and evaluated in order to find the ideal cutoff. The cytoplasmatic Gal-7 expression was regarded as low with an IRS 0–6 and as high with an IRS > 6. The cytoplasmatic Gal-8 expression was regarded as low with an IRS 0–5 and as high with an IRS > 5.

4.5. Ethics Approval and Consent to Participate

This study has been approved by the Ethics Committee of the Ludwig-Maximilian-University Munich (approval number 048–08). The breast cancer specimens were obtained in clinically indicated surgeries. When the current study was performed, all diagnostic procedures were completed, and the patients' data were anonymized. The ethical principles adopted in the Declaration of Helsinki 1975 have been respected. As per the declaration of our ethics committee, no written informed consent of the participants or permission to publish is needed given the circumstances described above. Researchers were blinded from patient data during experimental and statistical analysis.

5. Conclusions

In summary, our results suggest that Gal-7 might be an independent negative prognostic factor in breast cancer and therapeutic target, especially in HER2-positive breast cancer. Furthermore, Gal-8 was observed to be a positive predictor for overall survival and upregulation should be further investigated. The role of Gal-7 and Gal-8 should be validated in a BC collective treated with today's standard of therapy—even if this might be outdated at the time point of the analysis. Additional studies are required to detect the signaling pathways in which both Gal-7 and Gal-8 are involved, as the combination of both markers showed strong prognostic impact. Gal-7 and Gal-8, as well as the whole group of galectins, seem to be interesting therapeutic and prognostic targets that might help to improve therapies and outcome for breast cancer patients in the future.

Supplementary Materials:
Figure S1: Association of Gal 7 and Gal¬ 8 expression in the nucleus with HER2 status. Figure S2: Association of Gal-8 expression in the cytoplasm to the different surrogate intrinsic subtypes. Figure S3: Association of Gal-7 expression in the cytoplasm in ER negative tumors to the clinical outcome. Figure S4: Association of Gal-7 expression in the cytoplasm in HER2 positive tumors to the clinical outcome. Figure S5: Association of Gal-7 expression in the nucleus to the clinical outcome. Figure S6: Association of Gal-8 expression in the cytoplasm in HER2 negative tumors to the clinical outcome. Figure S7: Association of Gal-8 expression in the cytoplasm in ER positive tumors to the clinical outcome. Figure S8: Association of Gal-8 expression in the nucleus to the clinical outcome. Figure S9: OS, PFS and DDFS comparing high Gal 7 and low Gal 8 expressing tumors to the rest of the patients. Figure S10: Association of Gal 7 expression in immune cells with tumor grading, histological subtype and lymph node status. Table S1: Correlations of Gal 7 expression with clinical and histological parameters. Table S2: Correlations of Gal 8 expression with clinical and histological parameters. Table S3: Multivariate analysis of DDFS concerning Gal 7 expression in the cytoplasm. Table S4: Multivariate analysis of OS concerning Gal 7 expression in the cytoplasm. Table S5: Coordinates of ROC Curve exemplary for Gal-7 expression in the cytoplasm.

Author Contributions: A.T.: Participated in design and coordination of the study, participated in immunohistochemistry assays and analysis and performed the statistical analysis. C.K. performed technical assistance in immunohistochemistry assays and analysis. A.T. and A.H. wrote the manuscript. N.D.: participated in the design of the study and carefully read the manuscript for important intellectual content. E.S.: supervised immunohistochemistry as a gynecologic pathologist and participated in immunohistochemistry analysis as well as in the design and coordination of the study. C.Z.-G., T.K., B.C., and H.H.H. and S.M. revised the manuscript for important intellectual content. U.J. and A.H.: conceived of the study and participated in its design and coordination, approved the final version of the manuscript. All authors analyzed and interpreted the data and read and approved the final manuscript.

Acknowledgments: The authors thank Christina Kuhn for her excellent technical assistance. Furthermore, Kerstin Hermelink helped us with the revisions with statistical advice and imaging our data. Thank you very much. We also thank Michael Semmlinger for proofreading of the manuscript.

References

1. Harbeck, N.; Gnant, M. Breast cancer. *Lancet* **2017**, *389*, 1134–1150. [CrossRef]
2. Bray, F.; Ferlay, J.; Soerjomataram, I.; Siegel, R.L.; Torre, L.A.; Jemal, A. Global cancer statistics 2018: GLOBOCAN estimates of incidence and mortality worldwide for 36 cancers in 185 countries. *CA A Cancer J. Clin.* **2018**, *68*, 394–424. [CrossRef] [PubMed]
3. Sorlie, T.; Tibshirani, R.; Parker, J.; Hastie, T.; Marron, J.S.; Nobel, A.; Deng, S.; Johnsen, H.; Pesich, R.; Geisler, S.; et al. Repeated observation of breast tumor subtypes in independent gene expression data sets. *Proc. Natl. Acad. Sci. USA* **2003**, *100*, 8418–8423. [CrossRef] [PubMed]
4. Perou, C.M.; Sorlie, T.; Eisen, M.B.; van de Rijn, M.; Jeffrey, S.S.; Rees, C.A.; Pollack, J.R.; Ross, D.T.; Johnsen, H.; Akslen, L.A.; et al. Molecular portraits of human breast tumours. *Nature* **2000**, *406*, 747–752. [CrossRef]
5. Cho, S.H.; Jeon, J.; Kim, S.I. Personalized medicine in breast cancer: A systematic review. *J. Breast Cancer* **2012**, *15*, 265–272. [CrossRef]
6. Harris, E.E.R. Precision medicine for breast cancer: The paths to truly individualized diagnosis and treatment. *Int. J. Breast Cancer* **2018**, *2018*, 4809183. [CrossRef]
7. Gaudet, M.M.; Gierach, G.L.; Carter, B.D.; Luo, J.; Milne, R.L.; Weiderpass, E.; Giles, G.G.; Tamimi, R.M.; Eliassen, A.H.; Rosner, B.; et al. Pooled analysis of nine cohorts reveals breast cancer risk factors by tumor molecular subtype. *Cancer Res.* **2018**, *78*, 6011–6021. [CrossRef]
8. Foulkes, W.D.; Smith, I.E.; Reis-Filho, J.S. Triple-negative breast cancer. *N. Engl. J. Med.* **2010**, *363*, 1938–1948. [CrossRef]
9. Barondes, S.H.; Castronovo, V.; Cooper, D.N.W.; Cummings, R.D.; Drickamer, K.; Felzi, T.; Gitt, M.A.; Hirabayashi, J.; Hughes, C.; Kasai, K.-I.; et al. Galectins: A family of animal β-galactoside-binding lectins. *Cell* **1994**, *76*, 597–598. [CrossRef]
10. Barondes, S.H.; Cooper, D.N.; Gitt, M.A.; Leffler, H. Galectins. Structure and function of a large family of animal lectins. *J. Biol. Chem.* **1994**, *269*, 20807–20810.
11. Ebrahim, A.H.; Alalawi, Z.; Mirandola, L.; Rakhshanda, R.; Dahlbeck, S.; Nguyen, D.; Jenkins, M.; Grizzi, F.; Cobos, E.; Figueroa, J.A.; et al. Galectins in cancer: Carcinogenesis, diagnosis and therapy. *Ann. Transl. Med.* **2014**, *2*, 88. [CrossRef] [PubMed]
12. Cummings, R.D.; Liu, F.T. Galectins. In *Essentials of Glycobiology*, 2nd ed.; Varki, A., Cummings, R.D., Esko, J.D., Freeze, H.H., Stanley, P., Bertozzi, C.R., Hart, G.W., Etzler, M.E., Eds.; Cold Spring Harbor Laboratory Press: Cold Spring Harbor, NY, USA; The Consortium of Glycobiology Editors: La Jolla, CA, USA, 2009.
13. Thijssen, V.L.; Heusschen, R.; Caers, J.; Griffioen, A.W. Galectin expression in cancer diagnosis and prognosis: A systematic review. *Biochim. Biophys. Acta* **2015**, *1855*, 235–247. [CrossRef] [PubMed]
14. Liu, F.T.; Rabinovich, G.A. Galectins as modulators of tumour progression. *Nat. Rev. Cancer* **2005**, *5*, 29–41. [CrossRef] [PubMed]

15. Kolbl, A.C.; Andergassen, U.; Jeschke, U. The role of glycosylation in breast cancer metastasis and cancer control. *Front. Oncol.* **2015**, *5*, 219. [CrossRef] [PubMed]
16. Dalotto-Moreno, T.; Croci, D.O.; Cerliani, J.P.; Martinez-Allo, V.C.; Dergan-Dylon, S.; Mendez-Huergo, S.P.; Stupirski, J.C.; Mazal, D.; Osinaga, E.; Toscano, M.A.; et al. Targeting galectin-1 overcomes breast cancer-associated immunosuppression and prevents metastatic disease. *Cancer Res.* **2013**, *73*, 1107–1117. [CrossRef] [PubMed]
17. Reynolds, N.M.; Mohammadalipour, A.; Hall, C.R.; Asghari Adib, A.; Farnoud, A.M.; Burdick, M.M. Galectin-1 influences breast cancer cell adhesion to e-selectin via ligand intermediaries. *Cell Mol. Bioeng.* **2018**, *11*, 37–52. [CrossRef]
18. Simone, G.; Malara, N.; Trunzo, V.; Renne, M.; Perozziello, G.; Di Fabrizio, E.; Manz, A. Galectin-3 coats the membrane of breast cells and makes a signature of tumours. *Mol. Biosyst.* **2014**, *10*, 258–265. [CrossRef]
19. Zhang, H.; Luo, M.; Liang, X.; Wang, D.; Gu, X.; Duan, C.; Gu, H.; Chen, G.; Zhao, X.; Zhao, Z.; et al. Galectin-3 as a marker and potential therapeutic target in breast cancer. *PLoS ONE* **2014**, *9*, e103482. [CrossRef]
20. Irie, A.; Yamauchi, A.; Kontani, K.; Kihara, M.; Liu, D.; Shirato, Y.; Seki, M.; Nishi, N.; Nakamura, T.; Yokomise, H.; et al. Galectin-9 as a prognostic factor with antimetastatic potential in breast cancer. *Clin. Cancer Res.* **2005**, *11*, 2962–2968. [CrossRef]
21. Grosset, A.A.; Poirier, F.; Gaboury, L.; St-Pierre, Y. Galectin-7 expression potentiates her-2-positive phenotype in breast cancer. *PLoS ONE* **2016**, *11*, e0166731. [CrossRef]
22. Demers, M.; Rose, A.A.; Grosset, A.A.; Biron-Pain, K.; Gaboury, L.; Siegel, P.M.; St-Pierre, Y. Overexpression of galectin-7, a myoepithelial cell marker, enhances spontaneous metastasis of breast cancer cells. *Am. J. Pathol.* **2010**, *176*, 3023–3031. [CrossRef] [PubMed]
23. Campion, C.G.; Labrie, M.; Lavoie, G.; St-Pierre, Y. Expression of galectin-7 is induced in breast cancer cells by mutant p53. *PLoS ONE* **2013**, *8*, e72468. [CrossRef] [PubMed]
24. Ferragut, F.; Cagnoni, A.J.; Colombo, L.L.; Sanchez Terrero, C.; Wolfenstein-Todel, C.; Troncoso, M.F.; Vanzulli, S.I.; Rabinovich, G.A.; Marino, K.V.; Elola, M.T. Dual knockdown of Galectin-8 and its glycosylated ligand, the activated leukocyte cell adhesion molecule (ALCAM/CD166), synergistically delays in vivo breast cancer growth. *Biochim. Biophys. Acta Mol. Cell Res.* **2019**, *1866*, 1338–1352. [CrossRef] [PubMed]
25. Grosset, A.A.; Labrie, M.; Vladoiu, M.C.; Yousef, E.M.; Gaboury, L.; St-Pierre, Y. Galectin signatures contribute to the heterogeneity of breast cancer and provide new prognostic information and therapeutic targets. *Oncotarget* **2016**, *7*, 18183–18203. [CrossRef]
26. Piyush, T.; Chacko, A.R.; Sindrewicz, P.; Hilkens, J.; Rhodes, J.M.; Yu, L.G. Interaction of galectin-3 with MUC1 on cell surface promotes EGFR dimerization and activation in human epithelial cancer cells. *Cell Death Differ.* **2017**, *24*, 1937–1947. [CrossRef]
27. Kuo, H.Y.; Hsu, H.T.; Chen, Y.C.; Chang, Y.W.; Liu, F.T.; Wu, C.W. Galectin-3 modulates the EGFR signalling-mediated regulation of Sox2 expression via c-Myc in lung cancer. *Glycobiology* **2016**, *26*, 155–165. [CrossRef]
28. Wu, K.L.; Kuo, C.M.; Huang, E.Y.; Pan, H.M.; Huang, C.C.; Chen, Y.F.; Hsiao, C.C.; Yang, K.D. Extracellular galectin-3 facilitates colon cancer cell migration and is related to the epidermal growth factor receptor. *Am. J. Transl. Res.* **2018**, *10*, 2402–2412.
29. Wang, Z. ErbB receptors and cancer. *Methods Mol. Biol.* **2017**, *1652*, 3–35. [CrossRef]
30. Carlsson, M.C.; Balog, C.I.; Kilsgard, O.; Hellmark, T.; Bakoush, O.; Segelmark, M.; Ferno, M.; Olsson, H.; Malmstrom, J.; Wuhrer, M.; et al. Different fractions of human serum glycoproteins bind galectin-1 or galectin-8, and their ratio may provide a refined biomarker for pathophysiological conditions in cancer and inflammatory disease. *Biochim. Biophys. Acta* **2012**, *1820*, 1366–1372. [CrossRef]
31. Huflejt, M.E.; Leffler, H. Galectin-4 in normal tissues and cancer. *Glycoconj. J.* **2004**, *20*, 247–255. [CrossRef]
32. Bibens-Laulan, N.; St-Pierre, Y. Intracellular galectin-7 expression in cancer cells results from an autocrine transcriptional mechanism and endocytosis of extracellular galectin-7. *PLoS ONE* **2017**, *12*, e0187194. [CrossRef] [PubMed]
33. Bhat, R.; Belardi, B.; Mori, H.; Kuo, P.; Tam, A.; Hines, W.C.; Le, Q.T.; Bertozzi, C.R.; Bissell, M.J. Nuclear repartitioning of galectin-1 by an extracellular glycan switch regulates mammary morphogenesis. *Proc. Natl. Acad. Sci. USA* **2016**, *113*, E4820–E4827. [CrossRef] [PubMed]

34. Zhao, X.; Qu, J.; Sun, Y.; Wang, J.; Liu, X.; Wang, F.; Zhang, H.; Wang, W.; Ma, X.; Gao, X.; et al. Prognostic significance of tumor-associated macrophages in breast cancer: A meta-analysis of the literature. *Oncotarget* **2017**, *8*, 30576–30586. [CrossRef] [PubMed]
35. Grosset, A.A.; Labrie, M.; Gagne, D.; Vladoiu, M.C.; Gaboury, L.; Doucet, N.; St-Pierre, Y. Cytosolic galectin-7 impairs p53 functions and induces chemoresistance in breast cancer cells. *BMC Cancer* **2014**, *14*, 801. [CrossRef]
36. Vuong, L.; Kouverianou, E.; Rooney, C.M.; McHugh, B.J.; Howie, S.E.M.; Gregory, C.D.; Forbes, S.J.; Henderson, N.C.; Zetterberg, F.R.; Nilsson, U.J.; et al. An orally active galectin-3 antagonist inhibits lung adenocarcinoma growth and augments response to pd-l1 blockade. *Cancer Res.* **2019**, *79*, 1480–1492. [CrossRef]
37. Shih, T.C.; Liu, R.; Fung, G.; Bhardwaj, G.; Ghosh, P.M.; Lam, K.S. A novel galectin-1 inhibitor discovered through one-bead two-compound library potentiates the antitumor effects of paclitaxel in vivo. *Mol. Cancer Ther.* **2017**, *16*, 1212–1223. [CrossRef]
38. Elston, C.W.; Ellis, I.O. Pathological prognostic factors in breast cancer. I. The value of histological grade in breast cancer: Experience from a large study with long-term follow-up. *Histopathology* **1991**, *19*, 403–410. [CrossRef]
39. Makki, J. Diversity of breast carcinoma: Histological subtypes and clinical relevance. *Clin. Med. Insights Pathol.* **2015**, *8*, 23–31. [CrossRef]
40. Cserni, G.; Chmielik, E.; Cserni, B.; Tot, T. The new TNM-based staging of breast cancer. *Virchows Arch.* **2018**, *472*, 697–703. [CrossRef]
41. Remmele, W.; Stegner, H.E. Recommendation for uniform definition of an immunoreactive score (IRS) for immunohistochemical estrogen receptor detection (ER-ICA) in breast cancer tissue. *Pathologe* **1987**, *8*, 138–140.

7

Population Study of Ovarian Cancer Risk Prediction for Targeted Screening and Prevention

Faiza Gaba [1,2], Oleg Blyuss [3,4,5], Xinting Liu [1], Shivam Goyal [1], Nishant Lahoti [1], Dhivya Chandrasekaran [1,2], Margarida Kurzer [2], Jatinderpal Kalsi [6], Saskia Sanderson [7], Anne Lanceley [6], Munaza Ahmed [8], Lucy Side [9], Aleksandra Gentry-Maharaj [10], Yvonne Wallis [11], Andrew Wallace [12], Jo Waller [13], Craig Luccarini [14], Xin Yang [14], Joe Dennis [14], Alison Dunning [14], Andrew Lee [14], Antonis C. Antoniou [14], Rosa Legood [15], Usha Menon [10], Ian Jacobs [16] and Ranjit Manchanda [1,2,10,*]

1 Wolfson Institute of Preventative Medicine, Barts CRUK Cancer Centre, Queen Mary University of London, Charterhouse Square, London EC1M 6BQ, UK; f.gaba@qmul.ac.uk (F.G.); xintingliu@yahoo.co.uk (X.L.); s.goyal@smd15.qmul.ac.uk (S.G.); n.lahoti@smd15.qmul.ac.uk (N.L.); d.chandrasekaran@qmul.ac.uk (D.C.)

2 Department of Gynaecological Oncology, St Bartholomew's Hospital, Barts Health NHS Trust, London EC1A 7BE, UK; m.kurzer@nhs.net

3 School of Physics, Astronomy and Mathematics, University of Hertfordshire, College Lane, Hatfield AL10 9AB, UK; o.blyuss@qmul.ac.uk

4 Department of Paediatrics and Paediatric Infectious Diseases, Sechenov First Moscow State Medical University, Moscow 119146, Russia

5 Department of Applied Mathematics, Lobachevsky State University of Nizhny Novgorod, Nizhny Novgorod 603098, Russia

6 Department of Women's Cancer, Elizabeth Garrett Anderson Institute for Women's Health, University College London, London WC1E 6AU, UK; j.k.kalsi@ucl.ac.uk (J.K.); a.lanceley@ucl.ac.uk (A.L.)

7 Department of Behavioural Science and Health, University College London, 1-19 Torrington Place, London WC1E 6BT, UK; saskia.sanderson@ucl.ac.uk

8 Department Clinical Genetics, North East Thames Regional Genetics Unit, Great Ormond Street Hospital, London WC1N 3JH, UK; munaza.ahmed@gosh.nhs.uk

9 Department of Clinical Genetics, University Hospital Southampton NHS Foundation Trust, Southampton SO16 6YD, UK; Lucy.Side@uhs.nhs.uk

10 Medical Research Council Clinical Trials Unit at UCL, Institute of Clinical Trials and Methodology, University College London, 90 High Holborn, London WC1V 6LJ, UK; a.gentry-maharaj@ucl.ac.uk (A.G.-M.); u.menon@ucl.ac.uk (U.M.)

11 West Midlands Regional Genetics Laboratory, Birmingham Women's NHS Foundation Trust, Birmingham B15 2TG, UK; y.wallis@nhs.net

12 Manchester Centre for Genomic Medicine, 6th Floor Saint Marys Hospital, Oxford Rd, Manchester M13 9WL, UK; Andrew.Wallace@mft.nhs.uk

13 Cancer Prevention Group, King's College London, Great Maze Pond, London SE1 9RT, UK; jo.waller@kcl.ac.uk

14 Centre for Cancer Genetic Epidemiology, Department of Public Health and Primary Care, University of Cambridge, Strangeways Laboratory, Worts Causeway, Cambridge CB1 8RN, UK; craig@srl.cam.ac.uk (C.L.); xy249@medschl.cam.ac.uk (X.Y.); jgd29@cam.ac.uk (J.D.); amd24@medschl.cam.ac.uk (A.D.); ajl65@medschl.cam.ac.uk (A.L.); aca20@medschl.cam.ac.uk (A.C.A.)

15 Department of Health Services Research and Policy, London School of Hygiene and Tropical Medicine, London WC1E 7HT, UK; Rosa.Legood@lshtm.ac.uk

16 Department of Women's Health, University of New South Wales, Australia, Level 1, Chancellery Building, Sydney 2052, Australia; i.jacobs@unsw.edu.au

* Correspondence: r.manchanda@qmul.ac.uk

Abstract: Unselected population-based personalised ovarian cancer (OC) risk assessment combining genetic/epidemiology/hormonal data has not previously been undertaken. We aimed to perform a feasibility study of OC risk stratification of general population women using a personalised OC risk tool followed by risk management. Volunteers were recruited through London primary care networks. Inclusion criteria: women ≥18 years. Exclusion criteria: prior ovarian/tubal/peritoneal cancer, previous genetic testing for OC genes. Participants accessed an online/web-based decision aid along with optional telephone helpline use. Consenting individuals completed risk assessment and underwent genetic testing (*BRCA1/BRCA2/RAD51C/RAD51D/BRIP1*, OC susceptibility single-nucleotide polymorphisms). A validated OC risk prediction algorithm provided a personalised OC risk estimate using genetic/lifestyle/hormonal OC risk factors. Population genetic testing (PGT)/OC risk stratification uptake/acceptability, satisfaction, decision aid/telephone helpline use, psychological health and quality of life were assessed using validated/customised questionnaires over six months. Linear-mixed models/contrast tests analysed impact on study outcomes. Main outcomes: feasibility/acceptability, uptake, decision aid/telephone helpline use, satisfaction/regret, and impact on psychological health/quality of life. In total, 123 volunteers (mean age = 48.5 (SD = 15.4) years) used the decision aid, 105 (85%) consented. None fulfilled NHS genetic testing clinical criteria. OC risk stratification revealed 1/103 at ≥10% (high), 0/103 at ≥5%–<10% (intermediate), and 100/103 at <5% (low) lifetime OC risk. Decision aid satisfaction was 92.2%. The telephone helpline use rate was 13% and the questionnaire response rate at six months was 75%. Contrast tests indicated that overall depression ($p = 0.30$), anxiety ($p = 0.10$), quality-of-life ($p = 0.99$), and distress ($p = 0.25$) levels did not jointly change, while OC worry ($p = 0.021$) and general cancer risk perception ($p = 0.015$) decreased over six months. In total, 85.5–98.7% were satisfied with their decision. Findings suggest population-based personalised OC risk stratification is feasible and acceptable, has high satisfaction, reduces cancer worry/risk perception, and does not negatively impact psychological health/quality of life.

Keywords: population genetic testing; ovarian cancer risk; risk stratification; *BRCA1*; BRCA2; RAD51C; RAD51D; BRIP1; SNP; risk modelling

---

1. Introduction

BRCA1/BRCA2 pathogenic variants have a 17–44% ovarian cancer (OC) risk until age 80 years [1]. Testing for OC susceptibility genes (CSGs)—*RAD51C* (lifetime OC risk = 11%) [2], *RAD51D* (lifetime OC risk = 13%) [2] and *BRIP1* (lifetime OC risk = 5.8%) [3]—is now part of clinical practice. Genome-wide association studies (GWAS) have discovered ~30 validated single-nucleotide polymorphisms (SNPs) which modify OC risk [4,5]. Newer risk prediction models incorporating validated SNPs as a polygenic risk score with epidemiologic/family history(FH)/hormonal data and moderate–high-penetrance CSGs can be used to predict lifetime OC risk, improving the precision of risk estimation and allowing population division into risk strata, enabling targeted downstream risk-stratified prevention/screening for those at increased risk [4,6].

The current practice of identifying high-risk women uses clinical criteria/FH-based testing for CSGs, misses >50% CSG carriers who do not fulfil genetic testing criteria and requires people to get cancer before identifying unaffected family members who can benefit from prevention [7–10]. Given the effective cancer risk management/prevention options available, the adequacy of current practice, representing massive missed opportunities for risk-stratified prevention, is questionable. Unselected population genetic testing (PGT) overcomes these limitations and identifies many more individuals at increased OC risk. PGT can be cost effective and prevent thousands of more OC/BC cases than clinical criteria/FH-based genetic testing [11].

Most PGT evidence comes from UK/Israeli/Canadian studies in Ashkenazi Jewish (AJ) populations [9,10,12]. These show that AJ population-based *BRCA* testing is acceptable, feasible, can be community based, doubles the *BRCA* pathogenic variant individuals identified, does not harm psychological health/quality of life (QoL), reduces long-term anxiety, has high satisfaction rates (90–95%) [9,10,13], and is extremely cost effective (potentially cost saving) for the UK/US health systems [14]. However, prospective/unbiased PGT data and model-based OC risk stratification for a general (non-Jewish) low-risk population are lacking.

We describe results from a feasibility study in order to stratify a general population using predicted lifetime OC risk and offer risk management options of screening and prevention, within the Predicting Risk of Ovarian Malignancy Improved Screening and Early detection programme (PROMISE-FS, ISRCTN54246466). This article reports on (1) the acceptability, feasibility, and uptake of PGT/OC risk stratification; (2) perceived risks/limitations; (3) decision aid (DA)/telephone helpline use; (4) satisfaction; (5) cancer worry/risk perception; (6) impact on psychological health/QoL.

2. Results

Between June 2017 and August 2017, 218 women registered and 123 viewed the online DA. In total, 105/123 (85%) DA users consented to genetic testing/risk assessment, and two withdrew. In total, 103 were eligible for analysis (Figure 1). In total, 2/103 were excluded from RPA assessment (Figure 1). Women who chose not to participate declined providing information on factors affecting decision making. The follow-up questionnaire response rate was 94%, 84%, and 75% at seven days, three months and six months post results, respectively.

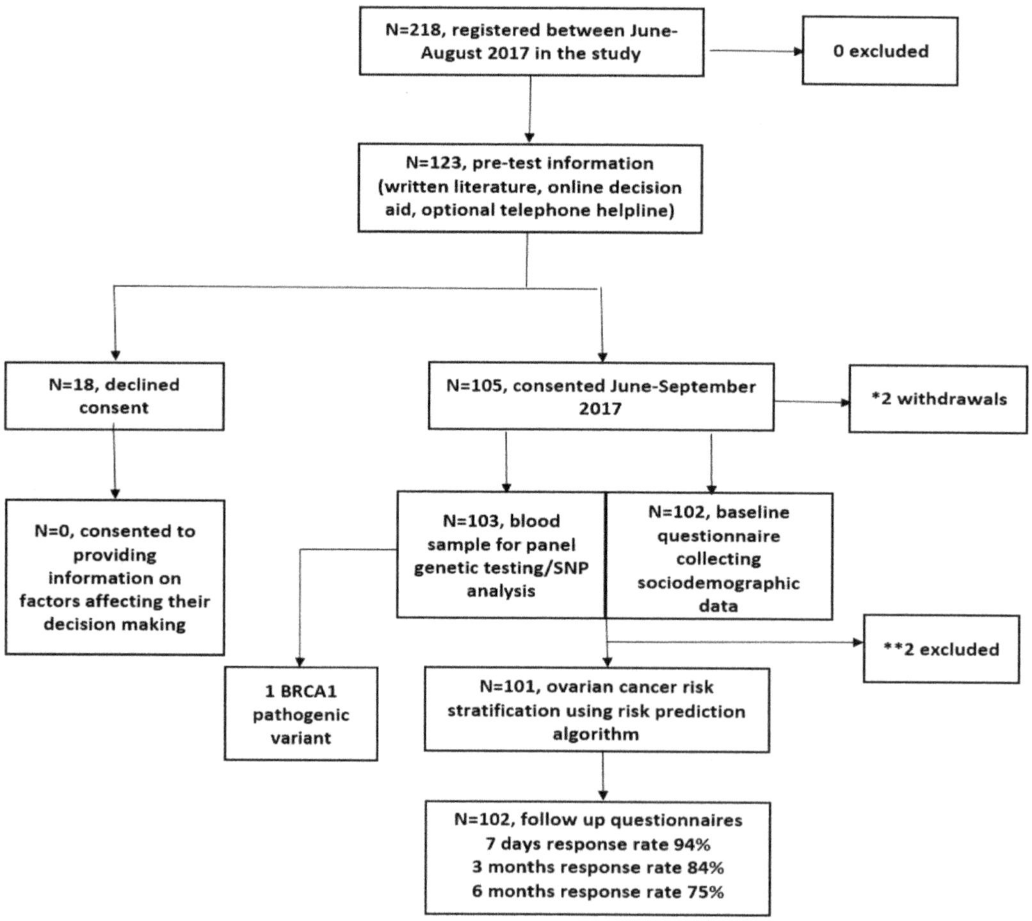

Figure 1. Study flow chart. * Reasons for withdrawal: miscarriage ($n = 1$) and inability to use public transport to attend an outpatient blood test appointment for genetic testing ($n = 1$). ** Reasons for exclusion: one participant was excluded because she entered this study at age 84 and the model predicts risks to age 80; the second participant did not provide the baseline demographic information required to run the algorithm.

Table 1 summarises cohort baseline characteristics. The mean age of participants was 48.5 (SD = 15.4; range = 18–85) years; 44.6% (n = 45) had university level education; 55.7% (n = 54) had a household income >£40,000; 74.5% (n = 76) were Caucasian; 7% (n = 7) were smokers; 64% (n = 63) ate >5 portions of fruit/vegetables daily; 78% (n = 80) were physically active over the last month. None had a clinically significant FH of cancer (fulfilling NHS genetic testing criteria). RPA revealed 1/103 at ≥10%, 0/103 at ≥5%–<10% and 100/103 at <5% lifetime OC risk. As expected using the algorithm, the epidemiological risk factors alone provide a greater level of OC risk stratification among the participants compared to the polygenic risk score (PRS) alone (Figure S1). However, risk stratification is further improved when the full model incorporating both epidemiological risk factors and PRS is considered. One high-risk participant, aged 35 years, had a lifetime OC risk of 42%. She had a pathogenic duplication of exon-13 in BRCA1. History included one second-degree relative with OC—parity = 1, 10 years oral contraceptive pill (OCP) use, endometriosis, BMI = 30.4, and no tubal ligation/hormone-replacement therapy (HRT) use. Following results, the participant opted for Risk of Ovarian Cancer Algorithm (ROCA)-based screening (24) within a research study (ALDO, https://www.uclh.nhs.uk/OurServices/ServiceA-Z/Cancer/NCV/Pages/TheALDOproject.aspx) and for risk-reducing early salpingectomy within a clinical trial (PROTECTOR, ISRCTN25173360, http://www.protector.org.uk/). She underwent MRI screening for BC risk. Four Class-3 variants of uncertain significance (VUS) were detected (BRCA1:c.3328_3330delAAG, c.2998_3003del; BRCA2:c.1438T>G; RAD51D:c.482T>C).

Table 1. Baseline characteristics of cohort.

Characteristic	%	N
Mean age, years (SD, range)		48.54 (15.42, 18–85)
Marital status		
Single	20	20/100
Married	52	52/100
Cohabiting/living with partner	15	15/100
Divorced/separated	11	11/100
Widowed	2	2/100
Children		
Have children	65.69	67/102
Mean number of children (SD, range)		1.34 (1.23, 0–5)
Education		
No formal qualification	5.94	6/101
GCSE/O-level/CSE	17.82	18/101
NVQ1/NVQ2	0.99	1/101
A-level/NVQ3	26.73	27/101
NVQ4	3.96	4/101
Bachelors	26.73	27/101
Masters	13.86	14/101
PhD	3.96	4/101
Income (£)		
<10,000	13.4	13/97
10,000–19,000	7.22	7/97
20,000–29,000	13.4	13/97
30,000–39,900	10.31	10/97
40,000–49,900	11.34	11/97
>50,000	44.33	43/97

Table 1. *Cont.*

Characteristic	%	N
Ethnicity		
White	74.51	76/102
Asian	13.73	14/102
Black/Afro-Caribbean	2.94	3/102
Mixed	6.86	7/102
Other	1.96	2/102
Religion		
Christian	59.41	60/101
Muslim	6.93	7/101
Jewish	4.95	5/101
Buddhist	0.99	1/101
Hindu	1.98	2/101
Sikh	1.98	2/101
No religion	22.77	23/101
Other	0.99	1/101
FH/clinical criteria positive	0	0/102
FH of cancer		
Total number of participants with any FH of ovarian cancer	11.76	12/102
Number of participants with a FDR with ovarian cancer	5.88	6/102
Number of participants with a SDR with ovarian cancer	5.88	6/102
Number of participants with a TDR with ovarian cancer	0	0/102
Total number of participants with any FH of breast cancer	44.12	45/102
Number of participants with a FDR with breast cancer	14.71	15/102
Number of participants with a SDR with breast cancer	23.53	24/102
Number of participants with a TDR with breast cancer	5.88	6/102
Total number of participants with a FH of breast and ovarian cancer	0.98	1/102
Total number of participants with any FH of prostate cancer	17.65	18/102
Number of participants with a FDR with prostate cancer	7.84	8/102
Number of participants with a SDR with prostate cancer	7.84	8/102
Number of participants with a TDR with prostate cancer	1.96	2/102
Total number of participants with any FH of pancreatic cancer	4.9	5/102
Number of participants with a FDR with pancreatic cancer	0.00	0/102
Number of participants with a SDR with pancreatic cancer	3.92	4/102
Number of participants with a TDR with pancreatic cancer	0.98	1/102
Psychiatric history		
Depression	9	9/100
Other psychiatric condition	5	5/100
Current medication for psychiatric condition	5	5/100
Personal history of non-ovarian cancer		
Breast cancer	0	0/102
Other cancers	3.92	4/102
Previous genetic testing unrelated to HBOC	1.98	2/101
Breast self-examination in the last 12 months		
Never	29.41	30/102
<once a month	48.04	49/102
once a month	14.71	15/102
>once a month	7.84	8/102
Clinical screening for breast cancer		
Ever had a clinical breast exam	56.57	56/99
Ever had a MRI	4	4/100
Ever had a mammogram	54.46	55/101

Table 1. *Cont.*

Characteristic	%	N
Ovarian cancer screening		
Currently undergoing screening	1.96	2/102
Have previously undergone screening	11.11	11/99
Previous surgical prevention to prevent ovarian cancer	0	0/102
Health behaviour and lifestyle		
Smoking		
Ever smokers	25.49	26/102
Current smokers	7.07	7/99
Alcohol consumption in the past 12 months		
Every week	48.04	49/102
Every month	14.71	15/102
Less frequently than once a month	21.57	22/102
Not at all	15.69	16/102
Median alcohol consumption on a typical day in units (IQR)		2 (1–2)
≥5 portions of fruit and vegetables	63.64	63/99
Number of participants who consume red meat	81.37	83/102
Number of participants currently using vitamin supplements	51.51	51/99
Physical exercise (past month)	78.43	80/102
Risk prediction algorithm results		
High lifetime ovarian cancer risk	0.97	1/103
Intermediate ovarian cancer risk	0	0/103
Low lifetime ovarian cancer risk	97.09	100/103
Excluded *	1.94	2/103
Mean lifetime risk prediction score (excluding the high-risk participant (SD, range))		1.39 (0.69, 0.56–4.38)
Mean lifetime risk prediction score (including the high-risk participant (SD, range))		1.80 (4.10, 0.56–41.98)

FH: family history; FDR: first-degree relative; SDR: second-degree relative; TDR: third-degree relative; HBOC: hereditary breast and ovarian cancer; SD: standard deviation. * One participant was excluded because she entered this study at age 84 and the model predicts risks to age 80. A second participant was excluded because she did not provide any baseline demographic information. Both participants were provided with their high-penetrance gene results, but personalised risk scores were not provided.

Key perceived benefits/risks of PGT/OC risk assessment are shown in Table S1. Need for reassurance, reduction in uncertainty, enhancing cancer prevention, benefiting research, knowledge about enhanced screening/prevention and children's risks were rated somewhat/very important by ~70–98% women. Important risks/limitations of PGT/OC risk assessment rated somewhat/very important included concern about effect on family (56.4%) and being unable to handle it emotionally (38.6%). A minority felt stigmatization (9%) or targeting of an ethnic group (11%) was a somewhat/very important risk. Insurance and confidentiality were highlighted as somewhat/very important by 28% and 24.7% respectively.

Participant responses to the ten DA items are shown in Table S2. The mean number of times DA was viewed was non-significantly higher in consenters versus decliners (1.61 vs. 1.05; $p = 0.06$). The mean DA score was not significantly different between consenters and decliners (8.1 vs. 7.4; $p = 0.14$). Consenters were older than decliners (48.5 vs. 40, $p = 0.016$). The mean age of volunteers who registered but did not view the DA was 45.5 years and not significantly different from consenters ($p = 0.16$) or decliners ($p = 0.24$). There was no statistically significant difference in 9/10 DA item responses between consenters and decliners. (Table S2). In total, 88.3% of consenters versus 75% of decliners ($p = 0.036$) would regret not participating if they developed OC in the future. In total, 23/123 viewed the DA on multiple occasions, and DA scores increased on repeat attempts (Tables S3 and S4). For 122/123 participants, there was concordance between participant decision making and

DA outcome category. One participant (85 years, Caucasian, no OC-FH) consented to PGT/OC risk stratification despite DA advice to the contrary (DA score = −1). Table 2 summarises responses to the DA evaluation questionnaire. In total, 92.2% (94/102) were very satisfied/satisfied and 82.2% (83/101) would recommend the DA. The amount of information provided, length of time taken to view and level of detail available was deemed just right by 98% (100/102), 97.1% (99/102), and 97% (98/101), respectively. No part of the DA needed omitting.

Table 2. Decision aid evaluation questionnaire responses.

Satisfaction	%	N
Very satisfied	47.06	48/102
Satisfied	45.1	46/102
Neither satisfied nor dissatisfied	5.88	6/102
Dissatisfied	0.98	1/102
Very dissatisfied	0.98	1/102
Amount of information provided		
Too little	1.96	2/102
About right	98.04	100/102
Too much	0	0/102
Length of time taken to view DA		
Too short	0	0/102
About right	97.06	99/102
Too long	2.94	3/102
Do any parts of the DA require more detail?		
Yes	2.97	3/101
No	97.03	98/101
Are there any parts of the DA that should be left out?		
Yes	0	0/99
No	100	99/99
Would you recommend DA use?		
Yes	82.18	83/101
No	0.99	1/101
Not sure	16.83	17/101

How much the DA improved understanding of:	**Not at all**		**Not very much**		**Somewhat**		**Quite a bit**		**A lot**	
	%	N	%	N	%	N	%	N	%	N
OC	7.92	8/101	12.87	13/101	34.65	35/101	28.71	29/101	15.84	16/101
Disadvantages of discovering OC risk (%)	3.96	4/101	6.93	7/101	40.59	41/101	28.71	29/101	19.8	20/101
Advantages of discovering OC risk	2.97	3/101	7.92	8/101	26.73	27/101	36.63	37/101	25.74	26/101
Genetic testing for OC genes	1.98	2/101	8.91	9/101	29.7	30/101	33.66	34/101	25.74	26/101
Implications of carrying OC gene alteration	3.96	4/101	5.94	6/101	36.63	37/101	28.71	29/101	24.75	25/101
Emotional response to DA										
Worried/concerned	56.44	57/101	27.72	28/101	13.86	14/101	1.98	2/101	0	0/101
Reassured	6.86	7/102	12.75	13/102	35.29	36/102	25.49	26/102	19.61	20/102
Upset	80.2	81/101	14.85	15/101	3.96	4/101	0	0/101	0.99	1/101

In total, 13% (13/103) of consenters used the optional telephone helpline (Table 3), and 8/13 filled in an evaluation questionnaire. No decliner used the telephone helpline. The mean number of calls to the telephone helpline was 1.38 (SD = 1.12; range = 1–5). In total, 12.5% (1/8) used the telephone helpline to aid decision making and 75% (6/8) had study specific queries—of which, DA technical assistance queries (4/8) were the most common. All helpline users were very satisfied/satisfied with their experience and 75% (6/8) would recommend the helpline. In total, 37.5% (3/8) felt that the helpline aided decision making. There was no difference in baseline characteristics between helpline users and non-users. When comparing how much the DA improved understanding of OC/gene testing/advantages and disadvantages of discovering personalised OC risk or DA satisfaction, there was no statistically significant difference between helpline users/non-users. Helpline users had a significantly greater degree of worry (2/13 vs. 0/89; $p = 0.02$) and upset (1/13 vs. 0/89; $p = 0.003$) when viewing the DA in comparison to non-users. Helpline users had a higher DA mean score than non-users (9.123 vs. 8.019; $p = 0.032$)

Table 3. Telephone helpline evaluation questionnaire responses.

Telephone Helpline Evaluation Questionnaire	%	N
Total number of women using the helpline	12.62	13/103
Number of participants using helpline who consented to this study	100	13/13
Mean number of times used (SD, range)		1.38 (1.12, 1–5)
Reason for helpline use		
To help decide whether to take part in this study	12.5	1/8
To ask a study specific question not related to decision making	75	6/8
Technical assistance with the decision aid	50	4/8
Pregnancy related query	25	2/8
Results query	12.5	1/8
Satisfaction with helpline		
Very satisfied	75	6/8
Satisfied	25	2/8
Neither satisfied nor dissatisfied	0	0/8
Dissatisfied	0	0/8
Very dissatisfied	0	0/8
Did the helpline help with decision making?		
Yes	37.5	3/8
No	50	4/8
Not sure	12.5	1/8
Would you recommend helpline use?		
Yes	75	6/8
No	0	0/8
Not sure	25	2/8

SD: standard deviation; 8/13 participants who used the telephone helpline completed the telephone helpline questionnaire. Data are presented for these eight participants.

Mean Hospital Anxiety and Depression Scale (HADS)/EuroQol-5D-5L (EQ-5D-5L)/Impact of Events Scale (IES)/Cancer Risk Perception questionnaire (CRP)/Cancer Worry Scale questionnaire (CWS)/Decision Regret Satisfaction questionnaire (DRS) questionnaire scores at baseline and at seven days/three months/six months follow up are shown in Table 4.

Table 4. Mean questionnaire scores at baseline and at seven days, three months and six months follow up.

Validated Questionnaire	Baseline	7 Days Post Results	3 Months Post Results	6 Months Post Results
HADS				
Total	9.06 (SD = 6.11, range 0–23)	10.43 (SD = 6.26, range 0–30)	9.78 (SD = 7.1, range 0–31)	9.64 (SD = 7.06, range 0–28)
Anxiety	6.11 (SD = 4.05, range 0–17)	7.02 (SD = 4.02, range 0–18)	6.35 (SD = 3.97, range 0–16)	6.1 (SD = 4.06, range 0–15)
Depression	2.92 (SD = 2.9, range 0–11)	3.41 (SD = 3.07, range 0–14)	3.36 (SD = 3.71, range 0–16)	3.55 (SD = 3.62, range 0–14)

Table 4. *Cont.*

Validated Questionnaire	Baseline	7 Days Post Results	3 Months Post Results	6 Months Post Results
EQ-5D-5L				
Total	0.86 (SD = 0.14, range 0.382–1)	0.84 (SD = 0.17, range 0.259–1)	0.83 (SD = 0.21, range 0.051–1)	0.84 (SD = 0.17, range −0.035–1)
VAS	81.27 (SD = 13.9, range 35–100)	80.61 (SD = 16.11, range 4–100)	80.45 (SD = 18.81, range 15–100)	80.76 (SD = 15.3, range 20–100)
Mobility	1.25 (SD = 0.57, range 1–3)	1.26 (SD = 0.55, range 1–3)	1.35 (SD = 0.8, range 1–5)	1.47 (SD = 0.92, range 1–5)
Self-care	1.08 (SD = 0.39, range 1–4)	1.04 (SD = 0.2, range 1–2)	1.12 (SD = 0.57, range 1–5)	1.21 (SD = 0.82, range 1–5)
Usual activities	1.25 (SD = 0.57, range 1–4)	1.24 (SD = 0.52, range 1–3)	1.38 (SD = 0.77, range 1–5)	1.42 (SD = 0.94, range 1–5)
Pain/discomfort	1.55 (SD = 0.71, range 1–4)	1.65 (SD = 0.8, range 1–4)	1.68 (SD = 0.95, range 1–5)	1.71 (SD = 0.82, range 1–5)
Anxiety/depression	1.43 (SD = 0.69, range 1–4)	1.58 (SD = 0.88, range 1–5)	1.58 (SD = 0.88, range 1–5)	1.53 (SD = 0.71, range 1–3)
IES		7.93 (SD = 15.06, range 0–67)	7.57 (SD = 17.07, range 0–73)	4.95 (SD = 10.61, range 0–48)
CWS	5.8 (SD = 1.96, range 4–14)	5.13 (SD = 1.61, range 4–12)	5.04 (SD = 1.51, range 4–11)	5.17 (SD = 1.61, range 4–11)
CRP				
CRP Likert scale	2.93 (SD = 0.78, range 1–5)	2.72 (SD = 0.83, range 1–5)	2.86 (SD = 0.66, range 1–5)	2.93 (SD = 0.74, range 1–5)
CRP VAS	46.05 (SD = 22.1, range 0–90)	44.51 (SD = 24.61, range 2–90)	47.43 (SD = 21.81, range 0–90)	49.67 (SD = 22.84, 1–90)
DRS				
DRS scale			27 (SD = 52.11, range 0–250)	
DRS Madalinska			1.16 (SD = 0.4, range 1–3)	

HADS: Hospital Anxiety and Depression Scale questionnaire; IES: Impact of Events Scale questionnaire; CRP: Cancer Risk Perception questionnaire; CWS: Cancer Worry Scale questionnaire; DRS: Decision Regret Satisfaction questionnaire; VAS: Visual Analogue Scale. HADS: 14 item questionnaire, with 7 items pertaining to anxiety and 7 to depression. Each item is scored on a 4-point Likert scale, from 0 to 3, with total scores ranging from 0 to 42. Higher scores indicate higher levels of anxiety/depression. EQ-5D-5L: EuroQol-5D-5L 5 item questionnaire. Each item (mobility, self-care, usual activities, pain/discomfort, and anxiety/depression) is scored on a 5-point Likert scale, from 1 to 5. Higher scores indicate poorer health. Total scores are then converted into a utility value using published reference values for the UK by the EuroQol Research Foundation. Utility values range from 0 to 1, with 0 indicating the worst health and 1 the best health. In addition, participants are asked to state "how good or bad your health is today" using a Visual Analogue Scale ranging from 0 (worst health) to 100 (best health). IES: 15 item questionnaire. Each item is scored on a 4-point Likert scale, from 0 to 5, with total scores ranging from 0 to 75. Higher scores indicate higher distress levels. CWS: 4 item questionnaire. Each item is scored on a 4-point Likert scale, from 1 to 4, with total scores ranging from 4 to 16. Higher scores indicate greater worry of developing ovarian cancer. CRP: 1 item questionnaire. The item is scored on a 5-point Likert scale, from 1 to 5. A higher score indicates that the individual perceives that they are at greater risk of developing cancer of any type at some point in their life compared to other women of the same age. In addition, participants are asked to state "on a scale from 0 to 100, where 0 is no chance at all, and 100 is absolutely certain, what do you think are the chances that you will get cancer (of any type) sometime during your lifetime?" DRS: First part consists of a 5 item questionnaire (Decision Satisfaction Regret Scale. Each item is scored on a 5-point Likert scale, from 0 to 100, with total scores ranging from 0 to 500. Higher scores indicate less satisfaction/more regret. Second part consists of a 1 item questionnaire (Madalinska). The item is scored on a 5-point Likert scale, from 0 to 100. Higher scores indicate less satisfaction/more regret.

Linear random-effects mixed-model outputs showing the association of covariates with different outcomes are shown in Table 5. There was a transient increase in HADS anxiety at seven days ($p = 0.048$), returning to baseline by three months ($p = 0.318$). Compared to baseline, there was a small increase in HADS depression scores at individual time points of 3 months ($p = 0.027$) and

6 months ($p \leq 0.001$), while QoL scores were marginally lower at three ($p = 0.025$) and six months ($p = 0.036$). However, the absolute level of change from baseline in all these scores was extremely small (HADS depression = 2.92 to 3.55; HADS anxiety = 6.11 to 7.02; EQ-5D-5L = 0.86 to 0.84) and not clinically meaningful. Additionally, contrast tests evaluating whether overall mean values at seven days, three months and six months were jointly different from the baseline suggested that anxiety, depression and QoL at these time points were not jointly different from the baseline value for the cohort (Table 5). Distress scores decreased with time and were significantly lower at six months versus 7 days ($p = 0.042$). Compared to baseline, OC worry was significantly lower at 7 days ($p \leq 0.001$), 3 months ($p \leq 0.001$) and 6 months ($p \leq 0.001$). Contrast tests evaluating the overall time effect showed a significant decrease in OC worry scores ($p = 0.02$) but not distress scores ($p = 0.25$) over time (Table 5). General cancer risk perception showed a decrease at 7 days ($p = 0.012$), returning to baseline by 6 months ($p = 0.45$).

Table 5. Linear random-effects mixed models and overall contrast tests for study outcomes.

Model and Variable	Coef.	Std. Err	$p > \|z\|$	95% CI
HADS Total				
FH Breast Cancer	1.66	1.334	0.217	−0.782 to 4.3
FH Ovarian Cancer	0.426	2.146	0.843	−3.766 to 4.616
* 7 Days	1.068	0.513	0.039	0.159 to 2.071
3 Months	0.986	0.537	0.068	−0.094 to 2.148
* 6 Months	1.268	0.557	0.024	0.215 to 2.385
Age	−0.015	0.046	0.742	−0.101 to 0.078
Income	−0.633	0.411	0.127	−1.452 to 0.178
Marital Status	1.321	1.424	0.356	−1.608 to 4.675
Ethnicity	3.349	1.899	0.081	−0.716 to 7.141
Religion: Jewish	−1.715	3.116	0.584	−7.559 to 4.456
Religion: Muslim	−6.223	3.228	0.057	−12.655 to 0.751
Religion: Atheist	−0.736	1.582	0.643	−3.893 to 2.478
Religion: Other	−3.759	2.848	0.19	−9.587 to 2.509
HADS Total	**df**	**Chi-sq**	***p*-value**	
# BL vs. Overall (joint)	3	5.2	0.158	
HADS Anxiety				
FH Breast Cancer	0.933	0.801	0.248	−0.63 to 2.625
FH Ovarian Cancer	−0.142	1.285	0.912	−2.552 to 2.373
* 7 Days	0.649	0.326	0.048	0.006 to 1.278
3 Months	0.339	0.339	0.318	−0.377 to 1.022
6 Months	0.172	0.353	0.628	−0.498 to 0.88
Age	−0.026	0.028	0.346	−0.083 to 0.028
Income	−0.216	0.247	0.383	−0.66 to 0.255
Marital Status	0.505	0.856	0.557	−1.285 to 2.123
Ethnicity	1.688	1.143	0.143	−0.433 to 3.799
Religion: Jewish	0.039	1.871	0.984	−3.838 to 3.558
* Religion: Muslim	−4.136	1.941	0.036	−7.79 to −0.387
Religion: Atheist	−0.89	0.951	0.352	−2.71 to 1.051
Religion: Other	−1.975	1.707	0.251	−5.541 to 1.271
HADS Anxiety	**df**	**Chi-sq**	***p*-value**	
# BL vs. Overall (joint)	3	6.22	0.102	
HADS Depression				
FH Breast Cancer	0.778	0.655	0.238	−0.55 to 2.141
FH Ovarian Cancer	0.942	1.086	0.387	−1.201 to 3.16
7 Days	0.481	0.292	0.101	−0.03 to 1.048
* 3 Months	0.68	0.304	0.027	0.062 to 1.257
* 6 Months	1.155	0.317	<0.001	0.54 to 1.772
Age	0.012	0.022	0.586	−0.033 to 0.054

Table 5. *Cont.*

* Income	−0.403	0.2	0.047	−0.805 to −0.031
Marital Status	0.8	0.702	0.258	−0.579 to 2.132
Ethnicity	1.642	0.925	0.079	−0.249 to 3.377
Religion: Jewish	−1.782	1.53	0.248	−5.021 to 1.214
Religion: Muslim	−1.996	1.562	0.205	−5.08 to 1.209
Religion: Atheist	0.148	0.776	0.85	−1.312 to 1.787
Religion: Other	−1.769	1.388	0.206	−4.607 to 1.095
HADS Depression	**df**	**Chi-sq**	***p*-value**	
# BL vs. Overall (joint)	3	3.7	0.296	
EQ-5D-5L Total				
FH Breast Cancer	−0.068	0.031	0.034	−0.135 to −0.008
FH Ovarian Cancer	−0.066	0.052	0.204	−0.171 to 0.028
7 Days	−0.026	0.015	0.082	−0.056 to 0.003
* 3 Months	−0.034	0.015	0.025	−0.062 to −0.004
6 Months	−0.033	0.016	0.036	−0.069 to −0.005
Age	−0.002	0.001	0.138	−0.004 to 0.001
Income	0.013	0.01	0.19	−0.007 to 0.032
Marital Status	−0.01	0.034	0.756	−0.076 to 0.061
Ethnicity	−0.05	0.044	0.262	−0.136 to 0.038
Religion: Jewish	−0.011	0.073	0.885	−0.155 to 0.136
Religion: Muslim	0.059	0.075	0.435	−0.106 to 0.209
Religion: Atheist	0.058	0.037	0.12	−0.012 to 0.136
Religion: Other	0.078	0.066	0.242	−0.058 to 0.202
EQ-5D-5L Total	**df**	**Chi-sq**	***p*-value**	
# BL vs. Overall (joint)	3	0.14	0.987	
EQ-5D-5L VAS				
FH Breast Cancer	−4.74	2.792	0.093	−10.024 to 0.915
FH Ovarian Cancer	−6.613	4.908	0.18	−16.246 to 3.636
7 Days	−1.537	1.68	0.361	−5.063 to 2.159
3 Months	−3.244	1.749	0.065	−6.533 to 0.491
6 Months	−2.492	1.798	0.167	−6.161 to 1.046
Age	0.048	0.097	0.621	−0.143 to 0.243
* Income	1.819	0.859	0.037	0.267 to 3.524
Marital Status	−0.386	2.997	0.898	−6.607 to 5.465
Ethnicity	−7.129	4.004	0.078	−15.297 to −0.015
Religion: Jewish	−1.73	6.474	0.79	−14.671 to 10.225
Religion: Muslim	10.205	6.774	0.136	−3.622 to 25.287
Religion: Atheist	0.921	3.322	0.782	−6.351 to 7.29
Religion: Other	2.139	5.9	0.718	−9.416 to 14.159
EQ-5D-5L VAS	**df**	**Chi-sq**	***p*-value**	
# BL vs. Overall (joint)	3	1.63	0.654	
IES				
FH Breast	−2.691	2.783	0.337	−8.768 to 2.934
FH Ovarian	−2.838	4.625	0.541	−11.282 to 6.296
3 Months	0.541	1.688	0.749	−2.841 to 3.86
* 6 Months	−3.533	1.724	0.042	−6.764 to −0.456
Age	−0.009	0.1	0.93	−0.183 to 0.178
Income	−1.53	0.895	0.091	−3.193 to 0.129
Marital Status	−1.252	3.005	0.678	−7.493 to 4.494
Ethnicity	1.551	4.379	0.724	−6.956 to 10.635
Religion: Jewish	7.084	6.242	0.26	−5.696 to 18.636
Religion: Muslim	−12.871	7.211	0.078	−25.685 to 2.043
* Religion: Atheist	−8.159	3.377	0.018	−15.396 to −1.292
Religion: Other	−3.833	6.028	0.527	−16.369 to 8.471

Table 5. *Cont.*

IES	df	Chi-sq	*p*-value	
# BL vs. Overall (joint)	2	2.78	0.249	
CWS				
FH Breast Cancer	0.019	0.306	0.952	−0.616 to 0.639
FH Ovarian Cancer	−0.138	0.535	0.797	−1.316 to 1.001
* 7 Days	−0.73	0.182	<0.001	−1.096 to −0.399
* 3 Months	−0.802	0.189	<0.001	−1.173 to −0.448
* 6 Months	−0.775	0.195	<0.001	−1.16 to −0.358
Age	−0.013	0.011	0.215	−0.035 to 0.009
Income	−0.126	0.094	0.186	−0.325 to 0.065
Marital Status	0.335	0.329	0.311	−0.374 to 0.973
Ethnicity	0.585	0.44	0.187	−0.264 to 1.439
Religion: Jewish	1.375	0.71	0.056	−0.091 to 2.772
Religion: Muslim	−1.073	0.737	0.149	−2.593 to 0.455
Religion: Atheist	−0.491	0.365	0.182	−1.224 to 0.247
Religion: Other	1.157	0.647	0.078	−0.035 to 2.428
CWS	**df**	**Chi-sq**	***p*-value**	
# BL vs. Overall (joint)	3	9.7	0.021	
CRP Likert Scale				
FH Breast Cancer	0.436	0.138	0.002	0.135 to 0.696
FH Ovarian Cancer	0.248	0.238	0.299	−0.207 to 0.748
* 7 Days	−0.195	0.077	0.012	−0.349 to −0.041
3 Months	−0.093	0.079	0.241	−0.251 to 0.068
6 Months	−0.062	0.083	0.454	−0.237 to 0.111
Age	−0.007	0.005	0.131	−0.017 to 0.002
Income	0.024	0.042	0.58	−0.071 to 0.107
Marital Status	−0.032	0.148	0.83	−0.308 to 0.269
Ethnicity	−0.089	0.197	0.654	−0.475 to 0.309
Religion: Jewish	0.173	0.321	0.592	−0.475 to 0.73
Religion: Muslim	−0.179	0.332	0.59	−0.89 to 0.524
Religion: Atheist	−0.115	0.164	0.486	−0.44 to 0.196
Religion: Other	0.127	0.292	0.665	−0.459 to 0.714
CRP Likert Scale	**df**	**Chi-sq**	***p*-value**	
# BL vs. Overall (joint)	3	10.44	0.015	
CRP VAS				
FH Breast Cancer	6.455	4.416	0.148	−2.004 to 15.098
FH Ovarian Cancer	−4.31	7.495	0.566	−19.607 to 9.766
7 Days	−2.985	2.441	0.223	−7.692 to 2.013
3 Months	0.579	2.675	0.829	−4.12 to 5.918
6 Months	−0.093	2.77	0.973	−5.488 to 5.632
Age	−0.194	0.153	0.207	−0.487 to 0.084
Income	1.471	1.353	0.28	−1.386 to 4.059
Marital Status	0.794	4.727	0.867	−9.788 to 9.475
Ethnicity	−9.792	6.261	0.121	−22.644 to 3.523
Religion: Jewish	3.429	10.238	0.739	−15.525 to 24.542
Religion: Muslim	−0.805	10.561	0.939	−22.586 to 20.999
Religion: Atheist	−6.437	5.263	0.225	−16.92 to 3.543
Religion: Other	1.36	9.434	0.886	−17.183 to 21.316
CRP VAS	**df**	**Chi-sq**	***p*-value**	
# BL vs. Overall (joint)	3	2.51	0.474	
DRS scale				
FH Breast Cancer	1.741	12.287	0.888	−22.846 to 26.328
FH Ovarian Cancer	11.808	17.974	0.514	−24.157 to 47.773

Table 5. *Cont.*

Age	0.208	0.437	0.636	−0.667 to 1.083
Income	−0.001	<0.001	0.216	−0.001 to 0
Marital Status	24.362	14.121	0.09	−3.894 to 52.617
* Ethnicity	47.091	20.396	0.024	6.28 to 87.902
Religion: Jewish	24.538	25.272	0.336	−26.031 to 75.108
Religion: Muslim	−11.145	32.366	0.732	−75.909 to 53.62
Religion: Atheist	10.411	16.022	0.518	−21.65 to 42.471
* Religion: Other	62.958	25.021	0.015	12.891 to 113.024
DRS Madalinska				
FH Breast Cancer	0.118	0.093	0.21	−0.068 to 0.303
FH Ovarian Cancer	0.022	0.136	0.871	−0.25 to 0.294
Age	0.001	0.003	0.849	−0.006 to 0.007
* Income	<0.001	<0.001	0.045	0 to 0
* Marital Status	0.247	0.107	0.025	0.033 to 0.46
Ethnicity	0.18	0.154	0.248	−0.129 to 0.488
Religion: Jewish	0.145	0.191	0.451	−0.238 to 0.528
Religion: Muslim	−0.151	0.245	0.541	−0.641 to 0.34
Religion: Atheist	0.068	0.121	0.573	−0.173 to 0.31
* Religion: Other	0.642	0.189	0.001	0.263 to 1.021

HADS: Hospital Anxiety and Depression Scale questionnaire; IES: Impact of Events Scale questionnaire; CRP: Cancer Risk Perception questionnaire; CWS: Cancer Worry Scale questionnaire; DRS: Decision Regret Satisfaction questionnaire; VAS: Visual Analogue Scale; FH: family history; Coef: coefficient; Std. Err: standard error. FH of breast cancer: positive versus negative (reference category); FH of ovarian cancer: positive versus negative (reference category); 7 days: questionnaire scores at 7 days versus baseline (reference category); 3 months: questionnaire scores at 3 months versus baseline (reference category); 6 months: questionnaire scores at 6 months versus baseline (reference category); age: age in years (continuous variable); income: as a continuous variable, but measured in £10,000 increments; marital status: cohabiting/living with partner/married (reference category) versus divorced/separated/single/widowed; ethnicity: Caucasian (reference category) versus non-Caucasian; religion Jewish: Christian (reference category) versus Jewish; religion Muslim: Christian (reference category) versus Muslim; Atheist: Christian (reference category) versus atheist; religion other (Hindu, Buddhist, Sikh): Christian (reference category) versus other. # BL vs. Overall (joint): Overall contrast test reflecting whether the mean outcome scale values at each time point (7 days, 3 months, or 6 months) were jointly different from the baseline for the whole group. This showed a significant decrease for CWS and CRP (Likert), but no significant change for HADS, HADS anxiety, HADS depression, EQ-5D-5L, IES and CRP (VAS) outcomes jointly over time. * Variables of statistical significance ($p < 0.05$).

In total, 85.5% strongly agreed and 13.2% agreed that their decision to undergo PGT/OC risk stratification was the right decision and that they were satisfied with it. In total, 95% would make the same choice again. Only 1.3% regretted their decision. Table 6 summarises responses to the DRS questionnaire.

Table 6. Decision Regret Satisfaction questionnaire responses according to individual questionnaire items.

Questionnaire Items	Questionnaire Responses									
	Strongly Disagree		Disagree		Neither Agree nor Disagree		Agree		Strongly Agree	
	%	N	%	N	%	N	%	N	%	N
It was the right decision	0	0/76	0	0/76	1.32	1/76	13.16	10/76	85.53	65/76
I regret the choice that was made	80.26	61/76	14.47	11/76	2.63	2/76	1.32	1/76	1.32	1/76
I would go for the same choice if I had to do it over again	0	0/76	1.32	1/76	3.95	3/76	13.16	10/76	81.58	62/76
The choice did me a lot of harm	89.33	67/75	8	6/75	2.67	2/75	0	0/75	0	0/75
The decision was a wise one	1.32	1/76	0	0/76	2.63	2/76	13.16	10/76	82.89	63/76
I am satisfied with the decision I have made	0	0/76	0	0/76	1.32	1/76	13.16	10/76	85.53	65/76

A FH of BC ($p = 0.034$) but not OC ($p = 0.20$) was negatively associated with QOL. Having a FH of OC was not associated with an increase in OC worry or general cancer risk perception.

However, women with a FH of BC perceived themselves to be at higher cancer risk ($p = 0.002$) but did not have increased OC worry.

Results from contrast tests assessing the joint effect of between-group and within-group differences in various outcomes over six months compared to baseline are shown in Table 7. There was no statistically significant between-group difference for groups 'with' and 'without' a FH of OC for HADS total/HADS depression/HADS anxiety/QoL/distress/OC worry/general cancer risk perception over time. There was no statistically significant within-group difference for groups 'with' and 'without' a FH of OC for HADS total/HADS anxiety/QoL/general cancer risk perception over six months. However, there was a statistically significant within-group difference for individuals 'without' a FH of OC but not 'with' a FH of OC for HADS depression ($p = 0.003$, $p = 0.866$, respectively), distress ($p = 0.043$, $p = 0.524$ respectively) and OC worry ($p \leq 0.001$, $p = 0.582$, respectively) over six months. Viewing the contrast tests together in combination with the linear random-effects mixed-model outputs would suggest a small increase in HADS depression scores not of clinical significance and a decrease in distress and OC worry over six months for the 'without' a FH of OC group.

Table 7. Contrast tests for between-group and within-group analyses over time.

HADS total	**df**	**Chi-sq**	***p*-value**	**CRP Likert scale**	**df**	**Chi-sq**	***p*-value**
Event#Group				**Event#Group**			
BL vs. 7 Days (joint)	1	0.43	0.51	BL vs. 7 Days (joint)	1	1.16	0.281
BL vs. 3 Months (joint)	1	0.07	0.797	BL vs. 3 Months (joint)	1	2.7	0.101
BL vs. 6 Months (joint)	1	0.13	0.719	BL vs. 6 Months (joint)	1	0.78	0.378
BL vs. Overall (joint)	3	1.05	0.788	BL vs. Overall (joint)	3	2.8	0.423
Event|Group				**Event|Group**			
BL vs. Joint|OC FH−	3	7.08	0.07	BL vs. Joint|OC FH−	3	6.69	0.083
BL vs. Joint|OC FH+	3	2.57	0.463	BL vs. Joint|OC FH+	3	6.59	0.086
HADS anxiety	**df**	**Chi-sq**	***p*-value**	**CRP VAS**	**df**	**Chi-sq**	***p*-value**
Event#Group				**Event#Group**			
BL vs. 7 Days (joint)	1	0.62	0.431	BL vs. 7 Days (joint)	1	2.23	0.135
BL vs. 3 Months (joint)	1	<0.01	0.972	BL vs. 3 Months (joint)	1	0.51	0.477
BL vs. 6 Months (joint)	1	0.04	0.849	BL vs. 6 Months (joint)	1	1.1	0.294
BL vs. Overall (joint)	3	1.05	0.79	BL vs. Overall (joint)	3	5.63	0.131
Event|Group				**Event|Group**			
BL vs. Joint|OC FH−	3	4.39	0.222	BL vs. Joint|OC FH−	3	2.37	0.5
BL vs. Joint|OC FH+	3	3.51	0.319	BL vs. Joint|OC FH+	3	4.37	0.224
HADS depression	**df**	**Chi-sq**	***p*-value**	**EQ-5D-5L UK score**	**df**	**Chi-sq**	***p*-value**
Event#Group				**Event#Group**			
BL vs. 7 Days (joint)	1	0.03	0.869	BL vs. 7 Days (joint)	1	2.36	0.125
BL vs. 3 Months (joint)	1	<0.01	0.971	BL vs. 3 Months (joint)	1	2.44	0.118
BL vs. 6 Months (joint)	1	0.91	0.339	BL vs. 6 Months (joint)	1	2.25	0.133
BL vs. Overall (joint)	3	1.18	0.759	BL vs. Overall (joint)	3	3.66	0.3
Event|Group				**Event|Group**			
* BL vs. Joint|OC FH−	3	14.18	0.003	BL vs. Joint|OC FH−	3	7	0.072
BL vs. Joint|OC FH+	3	0.73	0.866	BL vs. Joint|OC FH+	3	1.11	0.774
IES Score	**df**	**Chi-sq**	***p*-value**	**EQ-5D-5L VAS**	**df**	**Chi-sq**	***p*-value**
Event#Group				**Event#Group**			
BL vs. 3 Months (joint)	1	1.09	0.297	BL vs. 7 Days (joint)	1	0.64	0.425
BL vs. 6 Months (joint)	1	0.01	0.93	* BL vs. 3 Months (joint)	1	6.47	0.011
BL vs. Overall (joint)	2	1.3	0.523	BL vs. 6 Months (joint)	1	1.4	0.237

Table 7. *Cont.*

Event|Group				BL vs. Overall (joint)	3	6.74	0.081
* BL vs. Joint|OC FH−	2	6.31	0.043	**Event|Group**			
BL vs. Joint|OC FH+	2	1.29	0.524	BL vs. Joint|OC FH−	3	3.89	0.273
CWS Score	**df**	**Chi-sq**	***p*-value**				
Event#Group							
BL vs. 7 Days (joint)	1	0.99	0.32				
BL vs. 3 Months (joint)	1	0.25	0.615				
BL vs. 6 Months (joint)	1	0.18	0.675				
BL vs. Overall (joint)	3	1	0.802				
Event|Group							
* BL vs. Joint|OC FH−	3	26.92	<0.001				
BL vs. Joint|OC FH+	3	1.95	0.582				

BL: baseline; FH: family history; HADS: Hospital Anxiety and Depression Scale questionnaire; IES: Impact of Events Scale questionnaire; CRP: Cancer Risk Perception questionnaire; CWS: Cancer Worry Scale questionnaire; VAS: Visual Analogue Scale. 'Group' refers to either participants with a family history of ovarian cancer (OC FH+ group) or no family history of ovarian cancer (OC FH− group). 'Event#Group' refers to the group–time interaction, which reflects the 'between-group' (OC FH+ vs. OC FH−) difference over time. BL vs. 7 days (joint), BL vs. 3 months (joint), and BL vs. 6 months (joint) reflect whether the mean between-group difference at each time point (7 days, 3 months, or 6 months) was different from baseline. BL vs. Overall (joint) reflects whether the mean between-group differences at each time point (7 days, 3 months, or 6 months) were jointly different from the baseline between-group difference. Event|Group refers to the group–time interaction, which reflects the 'within-group' difference over time. BL vs. Joint |OC FH− reflects whether the mean outcome scale value at each time point (7 days, 3 months, or 6 months) was jointly different from the baseline within the ovarian cancer family history negative group. BL vs. Joint |OC FH+ reflects whether the mean outcome scale value at each time point (7 days, 3 months, or 6 months) was jointly different from the baseline within the ovarian cancer family history positive group. * Statistical significance ($p < 0.05$).

3. Discussion

This is the first unselected population-based, prospective cohort study recruiting participants without cancer history in self/family, evaluating the feasibility of personalised lifetime OC risk stratification followed by offering risk management options. Data suggest that OC risk stratification using genetic/non-genetic (epidemiological/hormonal) factors in general population women is feasible and acceptable.

The 85% uptake of PGT and OC risk stratification suggests high acceptability, similar to previously published data indicating putative 85% uptake of PGT (n = 734/829 in a survey study assessing attitudes of a general population of women to unselected PGT and risk-stratified OC screening [15,16]. Findings are also similar to data showing the high acceptability of unselected *BRCA* testing in AJ populations (up to 88% uptake) [17]. The 85%–98% overall satisfaction we found with PGT is similar to rates reported with population-based *BRCA* testing in AJ populations [9,12].

Data from unselected *BRCA* testing in the AJ population [9,10,14,18,19] show acceptability/feasibility/effectiveness/cost effectiveness/lack of detrimental impact on psychological health/QoL, and support the concept of population-based *BRCA* testing in Jewish populations. However, these inferences cannot be directly generalized to a non-Jewish general population. Our findings of overall time effect contrast tests showing levels of anxiety/depression/QoL/distress not being jointly different from baseline values but a significant reduction in OC-specific worry/general cancer risk perception following OC risk stratification are reassuring. Small changes in scores observed in some outcomes at individual time points were not clinically meaningful. While larger studies are warranted, these initial findings concur with short-/long-term outcome data following unselected *BRCA* testing in AJ populations [9,13] and are similar to findings amongst high-risk individuals undergoing clinical criteria-based genetic testing [20–22]. In total, 25.5% of our cohort was non-Caucasian (13.7% Asian). We found no difference in psychological health/QoL outcomes amongst non-Caucasians versus Caucasians. More research is required for understanding the role of various risk factors in non-Europeans.

Our online DA was successfully completed by women from a wide range of ages (18–85), education levels, and ethnicities, with high levels (92.2%) of satisfaction. Women who used the optional telephone helpline reported higher levels of worry/upset when viewing the DA. In total, 75% of women using the telephone helpline did so for technical DA assistance. All went on to successfully view the online DA. The telephone helpline appears to have been used as a source of emotional/technical support, emphasising the importance/need for a telephone helpline as an adjunct to online web applications to facilitate access/decision making for PGT/OC risk stratification. That one volunteer consented despite her DA score (−1) indicating she was "leaning against taking part", highlights that whilst decision aids are adjuncts aiding decision making, individuals retain ultimate autonomy. While we showed the feasibility of using an online DA and helpline approach for PGT, this has not been compared in randomised trials to more standard/established methods (face-to-face/telephone-based/DVD-assisted counselling).

Our study strengths include population-based recruitment in a non-Jewish, ethnically diverse general population. We engaged and worked with primary care networks prior to study commencement. They helped increase awareness of this study, identify eligible women and facilitate recruitment. Engagement with primary care would be vital for the implementation of any national population-based model for PGT/OC risk stratification. Other advantages include a good questionnaire response rate, ranging from 99% (baseline) to 75% (six months follow up).

Limitations include the small sample size, lack of long-term follow up on QoL/psychological health/health behaviours. Additionally, this study was non-randomised and a control arm (without genetic testing) to compare any change in outcomes was lacking. However, the high-risk individual identified did opt for appropriate screening and preventive interventions to reduce OC/BC risk. Lack of intermediate-risk women identified probably reflects the small sample size.

In our cohort, 45% vs. 40% [23] of the UK general population had a university level education; 7% vs. 15% [23] were current smokers; 64% vs. 32% [23] ate the recommended ≥5 portions of fruit/vegetables daily; 78% vs. 64% [23] were physically active over the last month; median total household income was >£50,000 vs. £29,000 in the UK general population [23]. Higher income, education levels and healthy lifestyle behaviour in our study participants compared to the UK's general population may indicate a London bias. The income/education levels/lifestyle choices are similar to those of the UK Jewish population [9,17]. Significant associations of some study outcome variables seen with demographic variables of income/age are consistent with observations from population-based data reported in other population cohorts.

Precision prevention is a prevention strategy incorporating individual variation in genetic, epi-genetic and non-genetic (e.g., environment, hormonal, lifestyle, behavioural) risk factors. This comprises primary prevention to prevent occurrence of disease and, secondary prevention for screening/early detection of pre-symptomatic disease. Next-generation sequencing technologies, falling costs and advances in computational bioinformatics makes personalised risk-stratified prevention feasible. Improvements in the precision of risk estimation, genetic understanding of disease and increasing awareness offers an opportunity to apply this knowledge and technology at a broad population scale to make an important shift in health care towards disease prevention. Over 50% of OCs occur in 9% of the population, which is at >5% OC risk [4]. This provides a huge opportunity for population stratification for precision prevention. Identification of unaffected women at increased risk offers opportunities for risk-stratified prevention to reduce cancer burden. Women at increased OC risk can opt for risk-reducing salpingo-oophorectomy (RRSO) to prevent tubal cancer/OC [24], now advocated at >4–5% lifetime OC risk [25–27].

Access to and uptake of testing for CSGs remains restricted. Only a small proportion of at-risk *BRCA* carriers have been identified [7,8]. Our approach offers opportunities to maximise pathogenic variant identification and population stratification for OC prevention. While recent data suggest that population-based genetic testing for OC/BC gene pathogenic variants could be cost effective in general population women [11], additional research including general population implementation studies are needed to address knowledge gaps before considering this. Additional looked for findings have recently been offered and returned following post hoc sequencing and/or analysis of some large genomic study cohorts. These studies would enable evaluation of CSG pathogenic variant carriage rates. However, this would not address in a prospective unbiased fashion key questions around the (i) logistics of population testing; (ii) information giving, a priori informed consent, and uptake of testing; (iii) uptake of preventive options. This 'bolt-on' paradigm of returning additional 'secondary findings' cannot be equated to prospective uptake of testing CSGs in an unselected unaffected population.

A prospective, Canadian cohort study offering *BRCA1/BRCA2* testing to unselected men/women (The Screen Project) is ongoing. The study is evaluating the feasibility of a direct-to-consumer approach, satisfaction, OC worry, prevalence of *BRCA1/BRCA2* pathogenic variants and the number of OCs/BCs prevented. Results from our feasibility study would inform the development of a larger UK-wide study that implements PGT/OC risk-stratified prevention. An important challenge is identifying optimum implementation pathways. It is likely that different context-specific models are needed for various health care systems internationally. Risk assessment pathways could be established through a community/primary care-based approach outside the traditional hospital-based genetics clinic model. A key issue that needs resolving is a system for monitoring/managing VUS. Commissioning/funding of a system where laboratory reports can be reviewed and re-issued in light of new evidence is needed. A framework/structure for data management and legal and regulatory protections will also need to be established.

4. Materials and Methods

4.1. Design

A multicentre, prospective cohort, feasibility study (ISRCTN:54246466). Inclusion criteria: women ≥18 years. Exclusion criteria: history of ovarian/tubal/primary peritoneal cancer or previous genetic testing for OC CSGs.

4.2. Recruitment

Recruitment was by self-referral. Study information/leaflets were made available through North-East London primary care practices. Interested volunteers received a detailed participant information sheet and access to an online DA prior to consent to genetic testing/participation. All had access to use an 'optional' telephone helpline for support/advice/queries. The helpline was manned by a doctor/research nurse experienced in cancer genetic risk assessment/management. Individuals deciding to undergo PGT/OC risk assessment consented. Decliners were asked to provide information on factors affecting decision making.

4.3. Decision Aid (DA)

A bespoke web-based DA was developed, enabling potential participants to make an informed decision on whether they wish to determine their OC risk and undergo PGT/OC risk assessment [16,28]. The DA (Table S2) included information on OC, genetic testing and the PROMISE programme, followed by ten questions/items on potential advantages/disadvantages of learning about OC risk. Responses were rated according to two different 3-point Likert scales. Individual questions were scored according to responses ((a) 1 = in favour of taking part, −1 = against taking part, 0 = neither in-favour or against taking part; or (b) 1 = agree, −1 = disagree, 0 = unsure). Sum of all questions/items scores taken together ranged from −10 to 10. Women with total scores between −10 and −1 were considered "leaning against taking part", 0–5 "undecided", and 6–10 "leaning towards taking part".

4.4. Genetic Analysis

Genetic testing involved next-generation sequencing of *BRCA1/BRCA2/RAD51C/RAD51D/BRIP1* genes and 30 GWAS-validated OC SNPs. Pathogenic variants detected were reconfirmed in an NHS laboratory.

4.5. Risk Model

Epidemiological/hormonal/reproductive data affecting OC risk collected at baseline (age/OC-FH/body mass index (BMI)/tubal ligation/hormone-replacement therapy (HRT)/oral contraceptive pill (OCP) use/endometriosis/parity) were combined with genetic information in a risk prediction algorithm (RPA) to provide a personalised predicted lifetime OC risk (till 80 years). Model validation (personal communication) [5] was undertaken in prospective datasets and cancers accrued in the UK OC screening trial cohorts [5,29,30]. Following RPA assessment, all participants were stratified into risk categories by lifetime OC risk (low risk: <5%; intermediate risk: ≥5%–<10%; high risk: ≥10%).

4.6. Test Result Management

High/intermediate-risk (and an equivalent number of randomly selected low-risk) individuals received their result at a face-to-face post test risk stratification counselling appointment. Identified pathogenic/likely pathogenic variant heterozygotes were referred to an NHS regional genetics clinic for confirmatory testing and to established NHS risk management services. Other low-risk individuals received results via post. Variants of uncertain significance (VUS) results were not returned.

4.7. Assessment of Demographics, Outcomes and Follow Up

Sociodemographic, family history, perceived risk/limitation (4-point Likert scale), telephone helpline and DA evaluation data were collected using customised questionnaires. Anxiety and depression were assessed with the Hospital Anxiety and Depression Scale (HADS) [31]. Distress was assessed using the Impact of Events Scale (IES) [32]. General cancer risk perception was measured by two items. Comparative risk: 'Compared with other people of your age/sex, do you think your chances of getting cancer in your life are: much-lower, lower, about-the-same, higher, much-higher?' An additional risk item: 'On a scale from 0 to 100, where 0 is no chance at all and 100 is absolutely certain, what are the chances you will get cancer sometime during your lifetime?'. OC worry was assessed by the Cancer Worry Scale (CWS) [33]. Generic QoL was measured with the EQ-5D-5L questionnaire [34]. Satisfaction and regret were measured by the Decision Regret Satisfaction Scale (DRS) and one additional 5-point Likert scale item, 'I am satisfied with the decision I have made' [35]. Smoking, diet and physical activity were evaluated. Data were gathered at baseline following consent and post results delivery (seven days/three months/six months).

4.8. Statistical Analysis

Descriptive statistics were used for baseline characteristics/telephone helpline/DA/follow-up questionnaire data. The Wilcoxon rank sum test and Fisher's exact test evaluated differences in means and proportions correspondingly.

As outcome data from the HADS/EQ-5D-5L/IES/CWS/CRP/DRS questionnaires were collected over multiple time points, linear random-effects mixed models were used to allow for individual baseline-level variability. Each scale was analysed, with the outcome as a continuous response variable. Models included a group effect and time effect. Models were adjusted for FH of OC/BC (positive/negative), age, income (in £10,000 increments), marital status (cohabiting/living with partner/married versus divorced/separated/single/widowed), ethnicity (Caucasian versus non-Caucasian) and religion (Muslim/Christian/Jewish/no religion/other (Hindu/Buddhist/Sikh)). Linear random-effects mixed models were used to model trends in DA scores for participants viewing the DA on multiple occasions.

Post modelling, three contrast tests were considered (each on three degrees of freedom). We assessed (a) overall time effects, i.e., whether the overall mean values at seven days, three months and six months from baseline were jointly different from the baseline level, (b) between-group differences over time (whether the mean group differences between those 'with' and 'without' a FH of OC at seven days, three months and six months from baseline were jointly different from the baseline level) and (c) within-group differences over time (whether mean values at seven days, three months and six months from baseline were jointly different from the baseline level within the groups 'with' and 'without' FH of OC). Statistical analysis used Stata-13.0 (Stata-Corp-LP, TX, https://www.stata.com/) and R version 3.5.1 (https://www.r-project.org/).

5. Conclusions

Our current health care systems remain primarily centred on improving disease diagnosis and treatment rather than prevention. Prevention of chronic disease, cancer being the second most common cause, is a major challenge for our health systems. PGT and personalised OC risk stratification can spur CSG detection and maximise precision prevention to reduce OC burden. We have shown that population-based personalised OC risk stratification is feasible and acceptable, has high satisfaction, reduces cancer worry/risk perception, and does not negatively impact on psychological health/quality of life. Further research and implementation studies evaluating the impact, clinical efficacy, long-term psychological, and socioethical consequences and cost effectiveness of this strategy are needed. This includes evaluation through large implementation studies of real-world health outcomes. Future implementation of such a strategy will require varying levels of workforce expansion/upskilling and reorganisation of health service infrastructure covering aspects of genetic testing and downstream care including screening and prevention pathways. PGT is an exciting and evolving field and personalised OC risk stratification offers a new paradigm for precision prevention in OC.

Table S1: Perceived benefits, risks, limitations or panel genetic testing/ovarian cancer risk assessment measured at baseline; Table S2: Decision aid question responses for women who consented and who did not consent to this study; Table S3: Mean scores at repeat viewings for participants who viewed the decision aid on multiple occasions; Table S4: Linear random-effects mixed models for trends in decision aid scores in participants viewing the decision aid on multiple occasions; Figure S1: Distributions of the remaining lifetime ovarian cancer risks given by different model versions.

Author Contributions: All authors have read and agree to the published version of the manuscript. Conception of study: I.J. and R.M. Design and development: R.M. and I.J. Trial management: R.M., F.G., I.J., U.M., L.S., M.A., M.K., J.K., and A.G.-M. Genetic testing: A.W., Y.W., C.L., J.D., A.D., and A.L. (Andrew Lee). Decision aid development: S.S., A.L. (Anne Lanceley), J.W., L.S., and R.M. Risk modelling: A.C.A., X.Y., U.M., R.M., and F.G. Data acquisition: F.G., R.M., X.L., S.G., N.L., D.C., and M.K. Data analysis: F.G., O.B., and R.M. Preparation of tables: F.G., O.B., and R.M. Initial draft of manuscript: F.G., R.M., O.B., and R.L.

Acknowledgments: This study is supported by researchers at the Cancer Research UK Barts Centre, Queen Mary University of London (C16420/A18066). We are particularly grateful to the women who participated in this study. We are grateful to the entire medical, nursing, and administrative staff who work on the PROMISE Feasibility Study.

References

1. Kuchenbaecker, K.B.; Hopper, J.L.; Barnes, D.R.; Phillips, K.A.; Mooij, T.M.; Roos-Blom, M.J.; Jervis, S.; van Leeuwen, F.E.; Milne, R.L.; Andrieu, N.; et al. Risks of Breast, Ovarian, and Contralateral Breast Cancer for BRCA1 and BRCA2 Mutation Carriers. *JAMA* **2017**, *317*, 2402–2416. [CrossRef] [PubMed]
2. Yang, X.; Song, H.; Leslie, G.; Engel, C.; Hahnen, E.; Auber, B.; Horváth, J.; Kast, K.; Niederacher, D.; Turnbull, C.; et al. Ovarian and breast cancer risks associated with pathogenic variants in RAD51C and RAD51D. *JNCI: J. Natl. Cancer Inst.* **2020**. [CrossRef] [PubMed]
3. Ramus, S.J.; Song, H.; Dicks, E.; Tyrer, J.P.; Rosenthal, A.N.; Intermaggio, M.P.; Fraser, L.; Gentry-Maharaj, A.; Hayward, J.; Philpott, S.; et al. Germline Mutations in the BRIP1, BARD1, PALB2, and NBN Genes in Women With Ovarian Cancer. *J. Natl. Cancer Inst.* **2015**, *107*. [CrossRef] [PubMed]
4. Jervis, S.; Song, H.; Lee, A.; Dicks, E.; Harrington, P.; Baynes, C.; Manchanda, R.; Easton, D.F.; Jacobs, I.; Pharoah, P.P.; et al. A risk prediction algorithm for ovarian cancer incorporating BRCA1, BRCA2, common alleles and other familial effects. *J. Med. Genet.* **2015**. [CrossRef]

5. Yang, X.; Leslie, G.; Gentry-Maharaj, A.; Ryan, A.; Intermaggio, M.; Lee, A.; Kalsi, J.K.; Tyrer, J.; Gaba, F.; Manchanda, R.; et al. Evaluation of polygenic risk scores for ovarian cancer risk prediction in a prospective cohort study. *J. Med. Genet.* **2018**. [CrossRef]
6. Pearce, C.L.; Stram, D.O.; Ness, R.B.; Stram, D.A.; Roman, L.D.; Templeman, C.; Lee, A.W.; Menon, U.; Fasching, P.A.; McAlpine, J.N.; et al. Population distribution of lifetime risk of ovarian cancer in the United States. *Cancer Epidemiol. Biomark. Prev.* **2015**, *24*, 671–676. [CrossRef]
7. Childers, C.P.; Childers, K.K.; Maggard-Gibbons, M.; Macinko, J. National Estimates of Genetic Testing in Women With a History of Breast or Ovarian Cancer. *J. Clin. Oncol.* **2017**, *35*, 3800–3806. [CrossRef]
8. Manchanda, R.; Blyuss, O.; Gaba, F.; Gordeev, V.S.; Jacobs, C.; Burnell, M.; Gan, C.; Taylor, R.; Turnbull, C.; Legood, R.; et al. Current detection rates and time-to-detection of all identifiable BRCA carriers in the Greater London population. *J. Med Genet.* **2018**. [CrossRef]
9. Manchanda, R.; Loggenberg, K.; Sanderson, S.; Burnell, M.; Wardle, J.; Gessler, S.; Side, L.; Balogun, N.; Desai, R.; Kumar, A.; et al. Population testing for cancer predisposing BRCA1/BRCA2 mutations in the Ashkenazi-Jewish community: A randomized controlled trial. *J. Natl. Cancer Inst.* **2015**, *107*, 379. [CrossRef]
10. Gabai-Kapara, E.; Lahad, A.; Kaufman, B.; Friedman, E.; Segev, S.; Renbaum, P.; Beeri, R.; Gal, M.; Grinshpun-Cohen, J.; Djemal, K.; et al. Population-based screening for breast and ovarian cancer risk due to BRCA1 and BRCA2. *Proc. Natl. Acad. Sci. USA* **2014**, *111*, 14205–14210. [CrossRef]
11. Manchanda, R.; Patel, S.; Gordeev, V.S.; Antoniou, A.C.; Smith, S.; Lee, A.; Hopper, J.L.; MacInnis, R.J.; Turnbull, C.; Ramus, S.J.; et al. Cost-effectiveness of Population-Based BRCA1, BRCA2, RAD51C, RAD51D, BRIP1, PALB2 Mutation Testing in Unselected General Population Women. *J. Natl. Cancer Inst.* **2018**, *110*, 714–725. [CrossRef] [PubMed]
12. Manchanda, R.; Gaba, F. Population Based Testing for Primary Prevention: A Systematic Review. *Cancers* **2018**, *10*, 424. [CrossRef] [PubMed]
13. Manchanda, R.; Burnell, M.; Gaba, F.; Desai, R.; Wardle, J.; Gessler, S.; Side, L.; Sanderson, S.; Loggenberg, K.; Brady, A.F.; et al. Randomised trial of population-based BRCA testing in Ashkenazi Jews: Long-term outcomes. *BJOG* **2019**. [CrossRef] [PubMed]
14. Manchanda, R.; Legood, R.; Burnell, M.; McGuire, A.; Raikou, M.; Loggenberg, K.; Wardle, J.; Sanderson, S.; Gessler, S.; Side, L.; et al. Cost-effectiveness of population screening for BRCA mutations in Ashkenazi jewish women compared with family history-based testing. *J. Natl. Cancer Inst.* **2015**, *107*, 380. [CrossRef] [PubMed]
15. Meisel, S.F.; Fraser, L.S.M.; Side, L.; Gessler, S.; Hann, K.E.J.; Wardle, J.; Lanceley, A.; PROMISE Study Team. Anticipated health behaviour changes and perceived control in response to disclosure of genetic risk of breast and ovarian cancer: A quantitative survey study among women in the UK. *BMJ Open* **2017**, *7*, e017675. [CrossRef] [PubMed]
16. Meisel, S.F.; Freeman, M.; Waller, J.; Fraser, L.; Gessler, S.; Jacobs, I.; Kalsi, J.; Manchanda, R.; Rahman, B.; Side, L.; et al. Impact of a decision aid about stratified ovarian cancer risk-management on women's knowledge and intentions: A randomised online experimental survey study. *BMC Public Health* **2017**, *17*, 882. [CrossRef] [PubMed]
17. Manchanda, R.; Burnell, M.; Gaba, F.; Sanderson, S.; Loggenberg, K.; Gessler, S.; Wardle, J.; Side, L.; Desai, R.; Brady, A.F.; et al. Attitude towards and factors affecting uptake of population-based BRCA testing in the Ashkenazi Jewish population: A cohort study. *BJOG* **2019**, *126*, 784–794. [CrossRef]
18. Manchanda, R.; Burnell, M.; Loggenberg, K.; Desai, R.; Wardle, J.; Sanderson, S.C.; Gessler, S.; Side, L.; Balogun, N.; Kumar, A.; et al. Cluster-randomised non-inferiority trial comparing DVD-assisted and traditional genetic counselling in systematic population testing for BRCA1/2 mutations. *J. Med. Genet.* **2016**, *53*, 472–480. [CrossRef]
19. Manchanda, R.; Patel, S.; Antoniou, A.C.; Levy-Lahad, E.; Turnbull, C.; Evans, D.G.; Hopper, J.L.; Macinnis, R.J.; Menon, U.; Jacobs, I.; et al. Cost-effectiveness of population based BRCA testing with varying Ashkenazi Jewish ancestry. *Am. J. Obstet. Gynecol.* **2017**, *217*. [CrossRef]
20. Nelson, H.D.; Fu, R.; Goddard, K.; Mitchell, J.P.; Okinaka-Hu, L.; Pappas, M.; Zakher, B. *Risk Assessment, Genetic Counseling, and Genetic Testing for BRCA-Related Cancer: Systematic Review to Update the U.S. Preventive Services Task Force Recommendation*; Agency for Healthcare Research and Quality: Rockville, MD, USA, 2013.
21. Metcalfe, K.A.; Poll, A.; Llacuachaqui, M.; Nanda, S.; Tulman, A.; Mian, N.; Sun, P.; Narod, S.A. Patient satisfaction and cancer-related distress among unselected Jewish women undergoing genetic testing for BRCA1 and BRCA2. *Clin. Genet.* **2010**, *78*, 411–417. [CrossRef]

22. Sivell, S.; Iredale, R.; Gray, J.; Coles, B. Cancer genetic risk assessment for individuals at risk of familial breast cancer. *Cochrane Database Syst. Rev.* **2007**, Cd003721. [CrossRef]
23. Kerber, R.A.; Slattery, M.L. Comparison of self-reported and database-linked family history of cancer data in a case-control study. *Am. J. Epidemiol.* **1997**, *146*, 244–248. [CrossRef] [PubMed]
24. Rebbeck, T.R.; Kauff, N.D.; Domchek, S.M. Meta-analysis of risk reduction estimates associated with risk-reducing salpingo-oophorectomy in BRCA1 or BRCA2 mutation carriers. *J. Natl. Cancer Inst.* **2009**, *101*, 80–87. [CrossRef] [PubMed]
25. Manchanda, R.; Legood, R.; Antoniou, A.C.; Gordeev, V.S.; Menon, U. Specifying the ovarian cancer risk threshold of 'premenopausal risk-reducing salpingo-oophorectomy' for ovarian cancer prevention: A cost-effectiveness analysis. *J. Med. Genet.* **2016**, *53*, 591–599. [CrossRef]
26. Manchanda, R.; Legood, R.; Antoniou, A.C.; Pearce, L.; Menon, U. Commentary on changing the risk threshold for surgical prevention of ovarian cancer. *BJOG* **2018**. [CrossRef]
27. Manchanda, R.; Legood, R.; Pearce, L.; Menon, U. Defining the risk threshold for risk reducing salpingo-oophorectomy for ovarian cancer prevention in low risk postmenopausal women. *Gynecol. Oncol.* **2015**, *139*, 487–494. [CrossRef]
28. Meisel, S.F.; Side, L.; Fraser, L.; Gessler, S.; Wardle, J.; Lanceley, A. Population-based, risk-stratified genetic testing for ovarian cancer risk: A focus group study. *Public Health Genom.* **2013**, *16*, 184–191. [CrossRef]
29. Jacobs, I.J.; Menon, U.; Ryan, A.; Gentry-Maharaj, A.; Burnell, M.; Kalsi, J.K.; Amso, N.N.; Apostolidou, S.; Benjamin, E.; Cruickshank, D.; et al. Ovarian cancer screening and mortality in the UK Collaborative Trial of Ovarian Cancer Screening (UKCTOCS): A randomised controlled trial. *Lancet* **2016**. [CrossRef]
30. Rosenthal, A.N.; Fraser, L.S.M.; Philpott, S.; Manchanda, R.; Burnell, M.; Badman, P.; Hadwin, R.; Rizzuto, I.; Benjamin, E.; Singh, N.; et al. Evidence of Stage Shift in Women Diagnosed With Ovarian Cancer During Phase II of the United Kingdom Familial Ovarian Cancer Screening Study. *J. Clin. Oncol.* **2017**, *35*, 1411–1420. [CrossRef]
31. Zigmond, A.S.; Snaith, R.P. The hospital anxiety and depression scale. *Acta Psychiatr. Scand.* **1983**, *67*, 361–370. [CrossRef]
32. Horowitz, M.; Wilner, N.; Alvarez, W. Impact of Event Scale: A measure of subjective stress. *Psychosom. Med.* **1979**, *41*, 209–218. [CrossRef] [PubMed]
33. Lerman, C.; Daly, M.; Masny, A.; Balshem, A. Attitudes about genetic testing for breast-ovarian cancer susceptibility. *J. Clin. Oncol.* **1994**, *12*, 843–850. [CrossRef] [PubMed]
34. Herdman, M.; Gudex, C.; Lloyd, A.; Janssen, M.; Kind, P.; Parkin, D.; Bonsel, G.; Badia, X. Development and preliminary testing of the new five-level version of EQ-5D (EQ-5D-5L). *Qual. Life Res.* **2011**, *20*, 1727–1736. [CrossRef] [PubMed]
35. Madalinska, J.B.; Hollenstein, J.; Bleiker, E.; van Beurden, M.; Valdimarsdottir, H.B.; Massuger, L.F.; Gaarenstroom, K.N.; Mourits, M.J.; Verheijen, R.H.; van Dorst, E.B.; et al. Quality-of-life effects of prophylactic salpingo-oophorectomy versus gynecologic screening among women at increased risk of hereditary ovarian cancer. *J. Clin. Oncol.* **2005**, *23*, 6890–6898. [CrossRef] [PubMed]

8

Identifying Ovarian Cancer in Symptomatic Women

Garth Funston [1,*], Victoria Hardy [1], Gary Abel [2], Emma J. Crosbie [3,4], Jon Emery [1,5], Willie Hamilton [2] and Fiona M. Walter [1,5]

1 The Primary Care Unit, Department of Public Health and Primary Care, University of Cambridge, Cambridge CB1 8RN, UK; veh29@medschl.cam.ac.uk (V.H.); jon.emery@unimelb.edu.au (J.E.); fmw22@medschl.cam.ac.uk (F.M.W.)
2 University of Exeter Medical School, University of Exeter, Exeter EX1 1TX, UK; G.A.Abel@exeter.ac.uk (G.A.); W.Hamilton@exeter.ac.uk (W.H.)
3 Gynaecological Oncology Research Group, Division of Cancer Sciences, University of Manchester, Manchester M13 9WL, UK; emma.crosbie@manchester.ac.uk
4 Department of Obstetrics and Gynaecology, Manchester University NHS Foundation Trust, Manchester Academic Health Sciences Centre, Manchester M13 9WL, UK
5 Centre for Cancer Research and Department of General Practice, University of Melbourne, Melbourne, VIC 3000, Australia
* Correspondence: gf272@medschl.cam.ac.uk

Simple Summary: Most women with ovarian cancer are diagnosed after they develop symptoms—identifying symptomatic women earlier has the potential to improve outcomes. Tools, ranging from simple symptom checklists to diagnostic prediction models that incorporate tests and risk factors, have been developed to help identify women at increased risk of undiagnosed ovarian cancer. In this review, we systematically identified studies evaluating these tools and then compared the reported diagnostic performance of tools. All included studies had some quality concerns and most tools had only been evaluated in a single study. However, four tools were evaluated in multiple studies and showed moderate diagnostic performance, with relatively little difference in performance between tools. While encouraging, further large and well-conducted studies are needed to ensure these tools are acceptable to patients and clinicians, are cost-effective and facilitate the early diagnosis of ovarian cancer.

Abstract: In the absence of effective ovarian cancer screening programs, most women are diagnosed following the onset of symptoms. Symptom-based tools, including symptom checklists and risk prediction models, have been developed to aid detection. The aim of this systematic review was to identify and compare the diagnostic performance of these tools. We searched MEDLINE, EMBASE and Cochrane CENTRAL, without language restriction, for relevant studies published between 1 January 2000 and 3 March 2020. We identified 1625 unique records and included 16 studies, evaluating 21 distinct tools in a range of settings. Fourteen tools included only symptoms; seven also included risk factors or blood tests. Four tools were externally validated—the Goff Symptom Index (sensitivity: 56.9–83.3%; specificity: 48.3–98.9%), a modified Goff Symptom Index (sensitivity: 71.6%; specificity: 88.5%), the Society of Gynaecologic Oncologists consensus criteria (sensitivity: 65.3–71.5%; specificity: 82.9–93.9%) and the QCancer Ovarian model (10% risk threshold—sensitivity: 64.1%; specificity: 90.1%). Study heterogeneity precluded meta-analysis. Given the moderate accuracy of several tools on external validation, they could be of use in helping to select women for ovarian cancer investigations. However, further research is needed to assess the impact of these tools on the timely detection of ovarian cancer and on patient survival.

Keywords: ovarian cancer; symptoms; early detection; risk assessment; diagnostic prediction model; triage tool; ovarian cancer symptoms

1. Introduction

Ovarian cancer is the eighth most common cancer to affect women worldwide, accounting for over 384,000 deaths in 2018 [1]. Outcomes are strongly linked to stage at diagnosis, with five-year survivals of 90% and 4% for UK women diagnosed at stages I and IV, respectively [2]. Given this, large ovarian cancer screening trials have been conducted, but these have so far failed to demonstrate a significant reduction in long-term mortality [3,4]. In the absence of effective screening programs, the majority of ovarian cancers are diagnosed following symptomatic presentation [5,6], and a focus has been placed on the early detection of symptomatic disease [7].

While once regarded as a 'silent killer', many studies have demonstrated that a range of symptoms are more common in women with ovarian cancer than in control subjects and that symptoms occur at all stages of the disease [8]. Clinical guidelines in countries around the world recommend that patients presenting with symptoms of possible ovarian cancer undergo investigation, although debate remains over which symptoms are indicative of disease and should be included in guidelines [7]. To facilitate the early detection of symptomatic cancer, researchers have developed a number of symptom-based checklists for use either when patients first present in the clinical setting or in 'symptom-triggered screening' programs, in which symptoms are proactively solicited [9–11]. More sophisticated tools, which can take the form of diagnostic prediction models [12], have also been developed to incorporate test results and ovarian cancer risk factors alongside symptoms, in a bid to improve tool performance. Several of these tools have been incorporated into clinical computer systems, which, then, automatically alert the clinician to consider ovarian cancer investigations when relevant symptoms are present or when the risk of undiagnosed cancer reaches a certain level. However, the relative limitations and merits of the various available tools remain unclear. In this systematic review, we aimed to identify and compare the diagnostic performances of symptom-predicated tools for the detection of ovarian cancer.

2. Methods

2.1. Eligibility Criteria and Searches

This review was conducted and is reported in accordance with the Preferred Reporting Items for Systematic Reviews and Meta-Analysis (PRISMA) guidelines (Table S1); a study protocol was registered with PROSPERO [CRD42020149879]. We searched MEDLINE, EMBASE and Cochrane CENTRAL for keywords relating to ovarian cancer, symptoms and prediction/diagnostic tools to identify papers published between 1 January 2000 and 3 March 2020 (Text S1). The start date was chosen to predate the publication of key ovarian cancer symptom papers [13,14]. No language restrictions or restrictions on methodological design were applied. No restrictions were placed on study setting, so studies conducted in the general population or in primary, secondary, or tertiary care were all eligible for inclusion. Reference lists of included papers were screened to identify any additional relevant papers.

Studies were included if they (a) described the development and or evaluation of a multivariable tool designed to identify patients with undiagnosed ovarian cancer and (b) provided the sensitivity and specificity of the tool or gave sufficient data to allow these metrics to be calculated. For the purposes of this review, we defined a multivariable tool as a combination of three or more variables used to detect or predict the risk of undiagnosed ovarian cancer. This broad definition encompasses traditional multivariable diagnostic prediction models and clinical prediction rules [12,15]. We considered variable 'checklists', in which any one variable in the list needed to be present for a positive result, to be a form of multivariable tool. As the focus of this review was on symptom-based tools, the tool under investigation had to include at least one symptom for a study to be eligible. No other restrictions were placed on the type of variable that could be included in a tool. Studies on tools intended to estimate future risk of developing ovarian cancer rather than the current risk of having an undiagnosed ovarian cancer were excluded, as were studies on tools that solely provide an indication of the risk of relapse or recurrence. We excluded studies in which all participants had a pelvic mass—as this represents a highly selected high-risk population—and studies undertaken solely in paediatric (<18 years) populations. Non-primary research studies were also excluded.

2.2. Study Selection

The online Rayyan software was used to facilitate abstract screening and study selection [16]. Following removal of duplicates, two reviewers (G.F. and V.H.) independently screened titles and abstracts against eligibility criteria. Potentially eligible papers identified at the screening stage were obtained and the full texts were independently examined against eligibility criteria by two reviewers (G.F. and V.H.). Any disagreements were resolved by consensus.

2.3. Data Extraction and Synthesis

Data extraction was performed by one reviewer (G.F.) and checked against full-text papers by a second reviewer (V.H.) to ensure accuracy. Using a predeveloped template, information was extracted on study characteristics (year of publication and location), study design (methodology, population, data source and outcome definition), tools (variables and tool development methods), and tool performance metrics (sensitivity, specificity and other diagnostic metrics). Where a study evaluated multiple tools, data relating to each tool were extracted separately.

Sensitivity and specificity were used to compare tool accuracy. For diagnostic prediction models, area under the receiver operator characteristic curve (AUC) was used to compare discrimination (the ability of a tool to identify those with a condition from those without a condition) and calibration (agreement between estimated and observed outcomes). Due to the marked heterogeneity of included studies in terms of the study designs, populations, variable definitions, outcome definitions and use of different tool thresholds, and the failure of multiple studies to report numbers of patients with true positive/true negative/false positive/false negative results, we were unable to perform any meta-analyses. Instead, performance characteristics were summarised in tabular form and using a narrative synthesis approach. When synthesising data, we paid particular attention to several study and tool characteristics. First, the source of participant recruitment. For example, whether controls were recruited from the general population or after entry into healthcare, as symptoms may be more common in clinical controls than population controls, which could influence measures of tool sensitivity and specificity [17]. Second, whether the measures of tool accuracy were obtained directly from the patient sample in which the tool was developed (apparent performance), by applying internal validation methods, such as splitting the sample into development and validation sets or using cross-validation techniques (internal validation), or from a separate analysis in a distinct population (external validation) [12]. Tools usually exhibit poorer diagnostic performance in external validation studies than when evaluated in the original development sample, and external validation of tools is recommended before they are used in clinical practice [12]. Third, we considered whether tools consisted solely of symptoms or symptoms in addition to other variables, as this is likely to impact the clinical utility of the tool.

2.4. Risk of Bias Assessment

The Quality Assessment of Diagnostic Accuracy Studies 2 (QUADAS-2) tool was used to assess the risk of bias and applicability of the included studies [18]. QUADAS-2 includes signalling questions (intended to identify areas of potential bias or concern over study applicability) covering four domains: (1) patient selection, (2) index test(s), (3) reference standard and (4) flow and timing. Each domain was rated as having "high", "low" or "unclear" (where insufficient information is provided) risk of bias. Domains 1–3 were also rated for applicability as "high", "low" or "unclear" concern. Two reviewers (G.F. and V.H.) independently assessed each study using QUADAS-2. Ratings were compared and disagreements were resolved by consensus.

3. Results

3.1. Study Selection

In total, 2331 records were identified from database searches, of which 708 were duplicates. Two additional records were identified from examination of reference lists. A total of 1625 titles and abstracts were screened, and 35 full-text papers were examined. Sixteen studies met the eligibility criteria and were included (Figure 1).

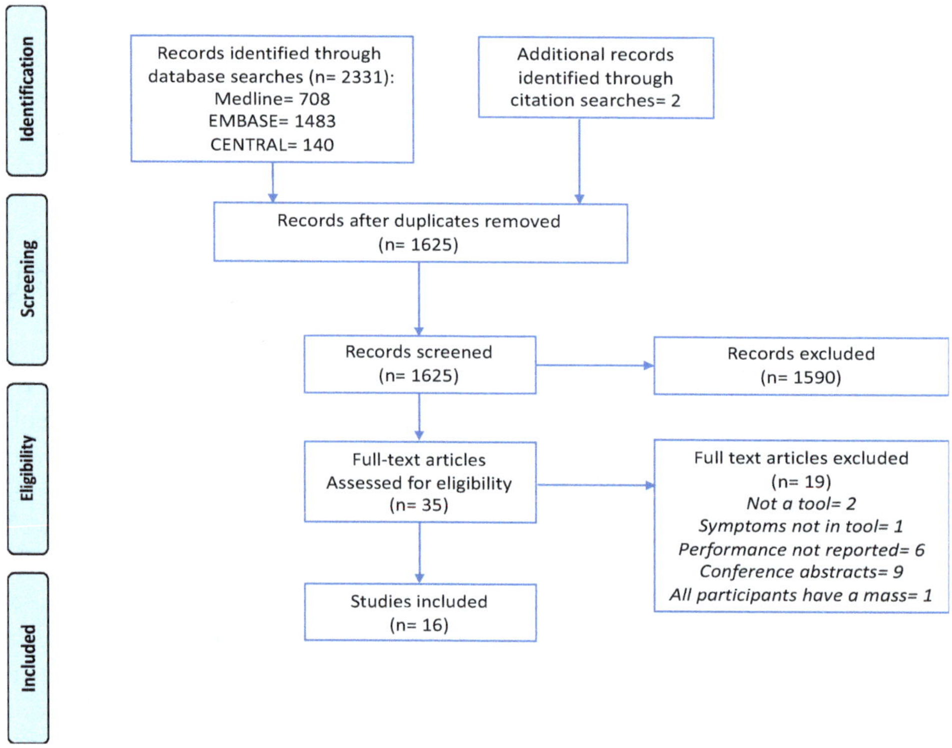

Figure 1. Preferred Reporting Items for Systematic Reviews and Meta-Analysis (PRISMA) flow diagram illustrating the study selection process.

3.2. Study Characteristics

The characteristics of the included studies are summarised in Table 1 and additional exclusion criteria are detailed in Supplementary Material Table S2. Three studies were population-based [19–21], five studies were based in a primary care setting [14,22–25], four studies were entirely hospital-based [26–29] and four studies were hospital-based but also recruited controls from screening studies [30–33]. All population- and hospital-based studies were of case-control design. Two of the studies that recruited from the hospital setting included a proportion of controls with benign ovarian pathology [26,28]. Three of the five primary care studies were of cohort design [22–24], and the remaining two were of case-control design [14,25]. The studies used a variety of data sources for variables, including pre-existing routinely collected primary care data ($n = 6$), information from surveys or patient interviews ($n = 11$) and blood samples ($n = 4$). Study sizes varied markedly, with 75–1,908,467 participants and 24–1885 women with ovarian cancer per study. While all studies used ovarian cancer as an outcome, how this was defined differed, with some only including invasive epithelial cancer or specifically stating that they excluded borderline tumours [19–21,26–29], and others apparently including both invasive and borderline epithelial tumours or all ovarian cancers [14,22–25,30–33]. One study included ovarian cancer alongside other common cancers in a composite outcome, but tool performance characteristics for each cancer were given separately [23]. Seven studies developed entirely new tools [14,19,22,23,25,30,33], six modified existing tools [26–29,31,32] and eight externally validated existing tools [20,21,24,26–29,33].

Table 1. Study characteristics.

Author, Date, Country	Design		Objective			Primary Outcome	Candidate Variable Data Sources	Participants	Study Sample
	Case Control	Cohort	Develop New Tool	Modify Existing Tool	Externally Validate Existing Tool				
Population based									
Lurie, 2009, USA	•		•			Primary invasive ovarian carcinoma	In-person patient interviews using a structured survey	Cases: Women aged 19–88 years histologically-confirmed primary invasive ovarian carcinoma (1993–2007) Controls: Aged ≥ 18 years, Hawaii resident ≥ 1 year, randomly selected from statutory state survey Frequency-matched to cases (1:1) by age, ethnicity, interview time	Cases: 432 Controls: 491
Rossing, 2010, USA	•				•	Primary invasive epithelial OC [a]	In-person interviews	Cases: Residents in western Washington State, aged 35–74 years, diagnosed with a primary invasive epithelial ovarian tumour (January 2002–December 2005) Controls: Selected by random digit dialling with stratified sampling in 5-year age categories, 1-year calendar intervals and two (urban vs. suburban or rural) county strata	Cases: 594 Controls: 1313
Jordan, 2010, Australia	•				•	Invasive epithelial OC	Patient survey	Cases: Aged 20–79 years with suspected OC, subsequently diagnosed with invasive epithelial OC (January 2002–June 2005) Controls: Frequency-matched based on age (5-year groups) and state of residence identified from electoral roll [34]	Cases: 1215 Controls: 1456
Primary care population									
Hamilton, 2009, England	•		•			Primary OC, including borderline	Researcher-coded GP records	Cases: Aged ≥ 40 years with primary OC diagnosed between 2000 and 2007 Controls: Matched on age, sex and GP practice	Cases: 212 Controls: 1060
Hippisley-Cox, 2012, England and Wales		•	•			OC (NOS)	QResearch database [35]	Aged 30–84 years, registered with GP practices between 1 January 2000 and 30 September 2010	Development (2/3)—1,158,723 women with 976 OCs Validation (1/3)—608,862 women with 538 OCs

Table 1. *Cont.*

Author, Date, Country	Design		Objective			Primary Outcome	Candidate Variable Data Sources	Participants	Study Sample
	Case Control	Cohort	Develop New Tool	Modify Existing Tool	Externally Validate Existing Tool				
Hippisley-Cox, 2013, England and Wales		•	•			OC (NOS) and 10 other cancers	QResearch database [35]	Aged 25–89 years, registered with GP practices between 1 January 2000 and 1 April 2012	Development (2/3)—1,240,864 women with 1279 OCs Validation (1/3)—667,603 women with 606 OCs
Grewal, 2013, England	•		•			Primary OC, including borderline	Researcher-coded GP records	Cases: Aged ≥ 40 years with primary OC diagnosed between 2000 and 2007 Controls: Matched on age, sex and GP practice	Cases: 212 Controls: 1060
Collins, 2013, UK		•			•	OC (NOS)	THIN database [36]	Women aged 30–84 years registered with GP practices between 1 January 2000 and 30 June 2008	1,054,818 women with 735 cancers
Hospital + screening populations									
Goff, 2007, USA	•		•			OC, including borderline	Patient survey	Cases: Women with a pelvic mass recruited in secondary care prior to OC diagnosis Controls: (a) Healthy 'high-risk' [b] women enrolled in a screening study [37], (b) women who presented for pelvic/abdominal US	Development Cases: 74 Controls: 243 Validation Cases: 75 Controls: 245
Andersen, 2008, USA	•			•		OC (NOS)	Patient survey, blood sample	Cases: Women with a pelvic mass, recruited prior to OC diagnosis Controls: Healthy 'high risk' [b] women enrolled in a screening study [37]	Cases: 75 Controls: 254
Andersen, 2010, USA	•			•		OC (NOS)	Patient survey, blood sample	Cases: Women with a pelvic mass recruited in secondary care prior to OC diagnosis Controls: Healthy 'high risk' [b] women enrolled in a screening study [37], frequency matched to cases on age (</>50 years)	Cases: 74 Controls: 137
Lim, 2012, UK	•		•		•	OC, including borderline	(a) Survey, (b) telephone interview, (c) GP notes	Cases: Women aged 50–79 years with primary OC recruited prior to diagnosis (February 2006–February 2008) Controls: Screening trial participants [38], frequency matched on year of birth and agreement to a telephone interview	Cases: 194 [c] Controls: 268 [c]

Table 1. *Cont.*

Author, Date, Country	Design		Objective			Primary Outcome	Candidate Variable Data Sources	Participants	Study Sample
	Case Control	Cohort	Develop New Tool	Modify Existing Tool	Externally Validate Existing Tool				
Hospital based population									
Kim, 2009, Korea	•			•	•	Epithelial OC (NOS)	Patient survey, blood sample	Cases: OC diagnosis Controls: Women with benign ovarian cysts recruited prior to surgery and those undergoing routine pap smear	Cases: 116 Controls: 209 (Benign: 74, Pap smear: 135)
Macuks, 2011, Latvia	•			•	•	Epithelial OC (NOS)	Patient survey, blood sample	Cases: Women with epithelial OC recruited prior to surgery/diagnosis Controls: Age-matched 'healthy women' attending a gynaecology outpatient clinic [d]	Cases: 24 Controls: 31 [d]
Shetty, 2015, India	•			•	•	OC, excluding borderline	Patient survey	Cases: Women admitted to hospital for investigation and subsequently diagnosed with OC Controls: (a) Women with benign ovarian pathology; (b) those undergoing a 'gynaecological check-up'	Cases: 74 Controls: 218 (benign: 144, gynaecological check-up: 74)
Jain, 2018, India	•			•	•	OC, excluding borderline	Patient survey, blood sample	Cases: Women undergoing surgery for a pelvic mass, subsequently diagnosed with ovarian cancer Controls: First-degree healthy relatives of cases	Cases: 45 Controls: 90

[a] Data collected on borderline tumours but not included in their tool performance evaluation. [b] Women with high-risk family histories consistent with a possible BRCA1/2 mutation in their families, participating in the Ovarian Cancer Early Detection Study (OCEDS) [37]. [c] Numbers varied by study component: questionnaire (191 cases, 268 controls), telephone interview (111 cases, 125 controls) and GP notes (171 cases, 227 controls). [d] Controls with benign gynaecological disease were also included in study but are excluded from the review, as performance was examined separately to healthy controls and no overall specificity measure was given. Study design and Objectives denoted by "•". Abbreviations: OC = Ovarian cancer; NOS = Not otherwise specified; GP = General practice; US = Ultrasound.

3.3. *Risk of Bias*

The main potential sources of bias were identified in the "patient selection" and the "index test" domains (Figure 2). As the case-control design can lead to overestimation of test performance [18], 13 studies were flagged as being at high risk of bias for patient selection. Key potential sources of bias identified for studies in the "index test" domain included failing to pre-define the tool threshold and retrospectively administering the tool after the outcome had been determined, e.g., questioning participants after the ovarian cancer diagnosis had been made. The risk of bias was generally judged as low for the "reference standard" and "flow and timing" domains. However, all primary care studies were flagged as being at high risk of bias in the "reference standard" domain as they relied on general practitioner (GP) records to identify ovarian cancer diagnoses, supplemented in two studies by death registration data [22,23] rather than hospital or cancer registry histological diagnoses. Concern over the applicability of studies was judged as low, save for the "reference standard" domain of one study which used a composite cancer outcome [23].

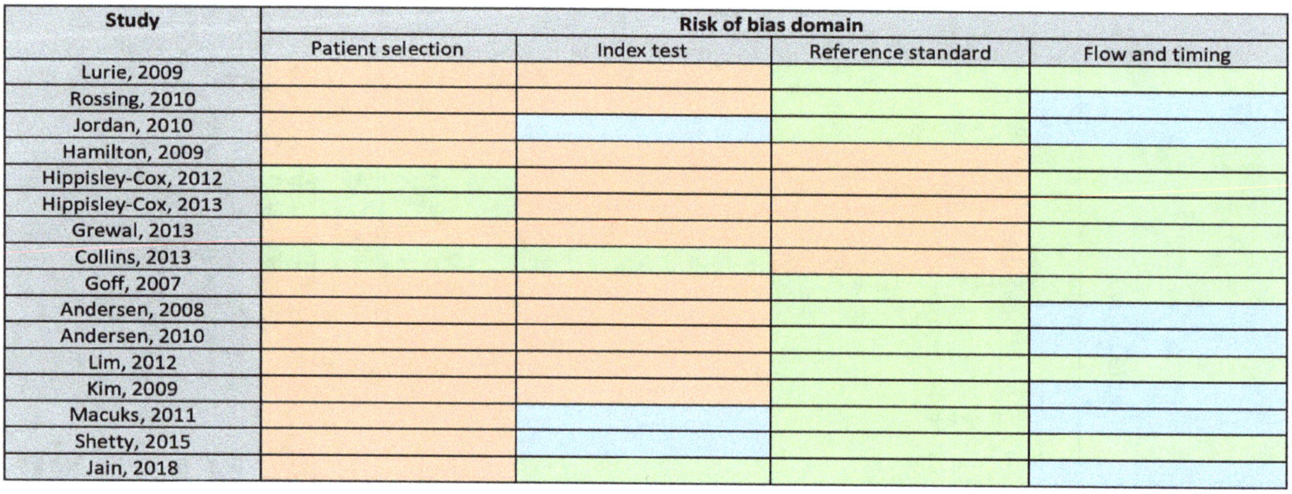

Figure 2. QUADAS-2 Risk of Bias Assessment. Green = "low", orange = "high", blue = "unclear" risk of bias.

4. Tool Variables

The studies evaluated a total of 21 distinct tools, of which five were diagnostic prediction models developed using appropriate statistical methods from which variable weights were derived [12]. We grouped variables included in the tools into four categories: (1) patient demographics, (2) personal and family medical history, (3) symptoms and (4) test results (Table 2). By definition, all tools included symptoms, with 14 including only symptoms. Four tools incorporated demographics, two incorporated personal and family medical history and six incorporated test results. Five symptoms (abdominal pain, pelvic pain, distension, bloating and appetite loss) were included in more than half (≥11) of the tools and a further six symptoms (feeling full quickly, difficulty eating, postmenopausal bleeding, urinary frequency, palpable abdominal mass/lump and rectal bleeding) were included in at least a quarter (≥6) of the tools. Six tools were based on an existing tool—the Goff Symptom Index (SI)—which was modified to include additional symptom or test result variables. Specifications of each tool, including how variables were defined, are included in the Supplementary Material Table S3.

Table 2. Variables included in the final tools.

Tool (Study, Year)	Demographics		Personal/Family History		Symptoms														Test Results		
	Age	Other	PMH	FH	Abdo. Pain	Pelvic Pain	Increase Abdo. Size/Distens.	Bloat.	Appetite Loss	Feeling Full	Difficulty Eating	Weight Loss	Postmen. Bleeding	Rectal Bleeding	Palpable Abdo. Mass/lump	Urinary Freq.	Other		Hb	CA125	HE4
Symptom checklists																					
Goff SI (Goff, 2007)					•	•	•	•		•	•										
Modified Goff SI 1 (Kim, 2009)					•	•	•	•		•	•					•	Urinary urgency				
Lurie 7-SI (Lurie, 2009					•	•	•	•	•						•	•	Bowel symptoms, difficulty emptying bladder, dysuria, fatigue, abnormal vaginal bleed.				
Lurie 5-SI (Lurie, 2009)					•	•	•								•	•	Difficulty emptying bladder, dysuria, abnormal vaginal bleed.				
Lurie 4-SI (Lurie, 2009)					•	•	•								•		Abnormal vaginal bleed.				
Lurie 3-SI (Lurie, 2009)							•								•		Abnormal vaginal bleed.				
Hamilton SI (Hamilton, 2009)					•		•	•	•				•	•		•					
SGO consensus criteria * (Rossing, 2010)					•	•		•		•						•	Urinary urgency				
Lim SI 1 (Lim, 2012)					•	•	•	•	•	•		•			•						
Lim SI 2 (Lim, 2012)					•	•	•		•						•		Vaginal discharge				
Hippisley-Cox SI (Hippisley-Cox, 2012)					•		•		•			•	•	•							

Table 2. *Cont.*

Tool (Study, Year)	Demographics		Personal/Family History		Symptoms													Test Results		
Modified Goff SI 2 (Shetty, 2015)					•	•	•	•	•	•	•	•				•	Urinary urgency			
	Age	Other	PMH	FH	Abdo. Pain	Pelvic Pain	Increase Abdo. Size/Distens.	Bloat.	Appetite Loss	Feeling Full	Difficulty Eating	Weight Loss	Postmen. Bleeding	Rectal Bleeding	Palpable Abdo. Mass/lump	Urinary Freq.	Other	Hb	CA125	HE4
Augmented symptom checklists																				
Goff SI + CA125 (Andersen, 2008)					•	•	•	•		•	•								•	
Goff SI + HE4 (Andersen, 2010)					•	•	•	•		•	•									•
Goff SI + HE4 + CA125 (Andersen, 2010)					•	•	•	•		•	•								•	•
Goff SI + CA125 + menopause (Macuks, 2011)		Menopause			•	•	•	•		•	•								•	
Prediction models																				
QCancer Ovarian (Hippisley-Cox, 2012)	•			OC	•		•		•			•	•	•				•		
QCancer Female (Hippisley-Cox, 2013)	•	Townsend score, smoking, alcohol, BMI	T2DM, COPD, endomet. hyperplasia or polyp, chronic pancreatitis	OC, GI cancer, breast cancer	•		•		•			•	•	•			Difficulty swallowing, heartburn/indigestion, blood in urine, blood in vomit, blood when cough, irregular menstrual bleeding, vaginal bleeding after sex, breast lump, breast skin tethering or nipple discharge, breast pain, lump in neck, night sweats, venous thromboembolism, CIBH, constipation, cough, unexplained bruising	•		

Table 2. *Cont.*

Tool (Study, Year)	Demographics		Personal/Family History		Symptoms													Test Results		
	Age	Other	PMH	FH	Abdo. Pain	Pelvic Pain	Increase Abdo. Size/Distens.	Bloat.	Appetite Loss	Feeling Full	Difficulty Eating	Weight Loss	Postmen. Bleeding	Rectal Bleeding	Palpable Abdo. Mass/lump	Urinary Freq.	Other	HE4	CA125	Hb
OC Score A (Grewal, 2013)					•		•	•	•				•	•		•				
OC Score B (Grewal, 2013)					•		•	•	•				•	•		•				
OC Score C (Grewal, 2013)	•				•		•	•	•				•	•		•				

* Consensus statement released by the Society of Gynaecologic Oncologists (SGO), the Gynaecologic Cancer Foundation and the American Cancer Society. The presence of a variable within a model is denoted by "•". The terms used to describe a given symptom varied subtly between studies—full details of each tool, including symptom terminology and duration and frequency criteria, are included in Supplementary Material Table S3. Abbreviations: PMH = past medical history; FH = family history; Abdo. = abdominal; Distens. = distension; Bloat. = bloating; Postmen. = postmenopausal; bleed. = bleeding; Freq. = frequency; Hb = haemoglobin; CA125 = cancer antigen 125; HE4 = human epididymis protein 4; SI = symptom index; OC = ovarian cancer; BMI = body mass index; endomet. = endometrial; T2DM = type 2 diabetes mellites; COPD = chronic obstructive pulmonary disease; GI = gastrointestinal; CIBH = change in bowel habit.

4.1. *Evaluation of Tool Performance*

The diagnostic performance of the included tools is summarised in Table 3. Measures of diagnostic performance for the majority of the tools were obtained directly from the patient sample with which the tool was developed (apparent performance) or by applying internal validation methods, such as splitting the sample into development and validation sets (internal validation), with only four tools—the Society of Gynaecologic Oncology (SGO) consensus criteria, Goff SI, QCancer Ovarian, Modified Goff SI 1—undergoing independent validation with an external dataset. Although the Goff SI in combination with CA125 was evaluated in several studies, the CA125 thresholds used varied markedly, so no studies were considered to have externally validated the same combination. There was overlap in evaluation of tools between healthcare settings, but no tool evaluated in primary care was evaluated in another setting or vice versa.

The most widely studied tool was the Goff SI, which was evaluated in nine studies [20,21,26,27,29–33], but two of these used data from subsets of women in the original tool development study [31,32]. Apparent deviations from the original Goff SI in how variables were defined were noted in several studies (Table S4). The Goff SI was the only tool to be externally validated in groups of women recruited from more than one setting.

4.2. *Tool Diagnostic Accuracy*

4.2.1. Hospital Setting

All but two tools evaluated in hospital populations incorporated the Goff SI. Two of these underwent external evaluation—the original Goff SI and a modified version incorporating additional symptoms (Modified Goff SI 1). The Goff SI, which was externally validated in six studies, demonstrated sensitivities which ranged from 56.9% to 83.3% (an outlier result) and specificities from 48.3% (an outlier result) to 98.9%. A modified version of the Goff SI (Modified Goff SI 1) demonstrated a sensitivity of 71.6% and a specificity of 88.5% in a single external validation study.

Augmenting symptom checklists with baseline risk factors and test results generally led to a reduction in sensitivity and an increase in specificity, or vice versa, depending on the threshold used. For example, the addition of the serum ovarian cancer biomarker CA125 to the Goff SI by Anderson et al. (2008) led to a reduction in tool sensitivity—if both variables were required to be abnormal for a positive tool result—or in tool specificity—if only one was required to be abnormal for a positive tool result [31].

4.2.2. Population Setting

In women recruited from the population setting, two symptom checklists were externally validated side by side—the Goff SI and the SGO consensus criteria. While the sensitivities and specificities of the tools differed between the studies, within each study, they were similar, with an in-study maximum difference in sensitivity of 3.4% and specificity of 2.4% between the tools.

4.2.3. Primary Care

A single tool (QCancer Ovarian), which took the form of a prediction model and combined symptom variables with demographics, family history and routine blood test results, underwent external validation in a primary care setting. When the threshold for abnormality was set to include the 5% of women at the highest predicted risk, QCancer Ovarian had a sensitivity of 43.8% and a specificity of 95%, while when the threshold was set to include women at the 10% highest risk, the sensitivity increased to 64.1% but the specificity fell to 90.1%. Several scores, developed by Grewal et al., demonstrated higher sensitivities and specificities than QCancer Ovarian at the 5% risk threshold (OC Score B $\geq$ 4) and 10% risk threshold (OC Score C $\geq$ 4), but diagnostic accuracy measures were derived from the same dataset used in score development.

Table 3. Tool diagnostic accuracy.

Tool	Study	Recruitment				Source of Accuracy Estimate			Sensitivity (95% CI)	Specificity (95% CI)	PPV	AUC (95% CI)
		Population Level	1° Care	Hospital + Screening	Hospital	Apparent Performance	Internal Validation	External Validation				
Symptom checklists												
Goff SI	Goff, 2007			•			•		≥50 yrs: 66.7 <50 yrs: 86.7	≥50 yrs: 90 <50 yrs: 86.7	-	-
	Andersen, 2008 [a]			•			•		64 (52.1–74.8)	88.2 (83.6–91.9)	-	-
	Kim, 2009				•			•	56.9	87.6	-	-
	Rossing, 2010	•						•	67.5 (65.4–69.6)	94.9 (93.9–95.8)	0.77–1.12 [b]	-
	Jordan, 2010	•						•	68.1 (65.5–70.7)	85.3	0.09 [c] (≥55 yrs: 0.21–0.31 <55 yrs: 0.04) [d]	-
	Andersen, 2010 [a]			•			•		63.5 (51.5–74.4)	88.3 (81.7–93.2)	-	-
	Macuks, 2011				•			•	83.3	48.3	-	-
	Jain, 2018				•			•	77.8	87.8	-	-
	Lim, 2012			•				•	61.4–75.7 [e]	89.6–98.9 [e]	-	-
Modified Goff SI 1	Kim, 2009				•	•			65.5	84.7	-	-
	Shetty, 2015				•			•	71.6	88.5	-	-
7-symptom Index	Lurie, 2009	•				•			85	40	-	-
5-symptom Index	Lurie, 2009	•				•			80	63	-	-
4-symptom Index	Lurie, 2009	•				•			74	77	-	-
3-symptom Index	Lurie, 2009	•				•			54	93	-	-
Hamilton SI	Hamilton, 2009		•			•			85	85	-	-
SGO consensus criteria	Rossing, 2010	•						•	65.3 (63.1–67.4)	93.9 (92.8–95)	0.63–0.92 [b]	-
	Jordan, 2010	•						•	71.5 (69–74.1)	82.9 (81–84.8)	0.08 [c] (≥55 yrs: 0.18–0.27 <55 yrs: 0.05) [d]	-
Lim SI 1	Lim, 2012			•			•		69.6–91 [e]	76–91 [e]	-	-

Table 3. *Cont.*

Tool	Study	Recruitment				Source of Accuracy Estimate			Sensitivity (95% CI)	Specificity (95% CI)	PPV	AUC (95% CI)
		Population Level	1° Care	Hospital + Screening	Hospital	Apparent Performance	Internal Validation	External Validation				
Lim SI 2	Lim, 2012			•			•		67.3–91 [e]	82.4–94 [e]	-	-
Hippisley-Cox SI	Hippisley-Cox, 2012		•				•		71.9	82.9	0.5	-
Modified Goff SI 2	Shetty, 2015				•	•			77	88.5	-	-
Augmented symptom checklists												
Goff SI or CA125 [f]	Andersen, 2008			•		•			89.3 (80.1–95.3)	83.5 (78.3–87.8)	-	-
Goff SI or CA125 (>35 U/mL)	Jain, 2018				•	•			97.8	68.9	-	-
Goff SI & CA125 (>21 U/mL)	Macuks, 2011				•	•			79.1	100	-	-
Goff SI & CA125 (>35 U/mL)	Macuks, 2011				•	•			70.8	100	-	-
Goff SI & CA125 (>65 U/mL)	Macuks, 2011				•	•			70.8	100	-	-
Goff SI or CA125 [f]	Andersen, 2010			•		•			91.9 (83.2–97)	83.2 (75.9–89)	-	-
Goff SI or HE4 [f]	Andersen, 2010			•		•			91.9 (83.2–97)	84.7 (77.5–90.3)	-	-
Any 1 of 3 (Goff SI or CA125 or HE4) [f]	Andersen, 2010			•		•			94.6 (86.7–98.5)	79.6 (71.8–86)	-	-
Any 2 of 3 (Goff SI or CA125 or HE4) [f]	Andersen, 2010			•		•			83.8 (73.4–91.3)	98.5 (94.8–99.8)	-	-
Goff SI & 1 or more of CA125 or HE4 [f]	Andersen, 2010			•		•			58.1 (46.1–69.5)	98.5 (94.8–99.8)	-	-
Goff SI & CA125 (>25 U/mL) & menopause	Macuks, 2011				•	•			50	100	-	-
Goff SI & CA125 (>35 U/mL) & menopause	Macuks, 2011				•	•			45.8	100	-	-
Goff SI & CA125 (>65 U/mL) & menopause	Macuks, 2011				•	•			45.8	100	-	-
Prediction models												

Table 3. *Cont.*

Tool	Study	Recruitment				Source of Accuracy Estimate			Sensitivity (95% CI)	Specificity (95% CI)	PPV	AUC (95% CI)
		Population Level	1° Care	Hospital + Screening	Hospital	Apparent Performance	Internal Validation	External Validation				
QCancer Ovarian (Top 10% risk)	Hippisley-Cox, 2012		•				•		63.2	90.8	0.8	084 (0.83–0.86)
	Collins, 2013		•					•	64.1	90.1	0.5	0.86 (0.84–0.87)
QCancer Ovarian (Top 5% risk)	Hippisley-Cox, 2012		•				•		42.2	95.6	1.1	-
	Collins, 2013		•					•	43.8	95	0.6	-
QCancer Ovarian (Top 1% risk)	Hippisley-Cox, 2012		•				•		13.9	99.3	2.1	-
QCancer Ovarian (Top 0.5% risk)	Hippisley-Cox, 2012		•				•		11	99.6	3.2	-
QCancer Ovarian (Top 0.1% risk)	Hippisley-Cox, 2012		•				•		3.9	99.9	5.5	-
QCancer Female (Top 10% risk)	Hippisley-Cox, 2013		•				•		61.6	90	0.6	0.84 (0.82–0.86)
OC Score A (Score ≥ 3)	Grewal, 2013		•			•			58.5	97.3	-	0.89
OC Score A (Score ≥ 4)	Grewal, 2013		•			•			57.6	97.3	-	
OC Score B (Score ≥ 3)	Grewal, 2013		•			•			75	90.1	-	0.89
OC Score B (Score ≥ 4)	Grewal, 2013		•			•			58.9	97.3	-	
OC Score C (Score ≥ 3)	Grewal, 2013		•			•			85.4	85.1	-	0.88
OC Score C (Score ≥ 4)	Grewal, 2013		•			•			72.6	91.3	-	

[a] Study used a subset of patients from Goff, 2007. [b] Calculated using external data from screening studies. [39,40]. [c] Calculated using external Australian population-level data. [d] Calculated using external data from US and UK screening studies and Australian population-level data. [41,42]. [e] Sensitivity and specificity varied by data collection method (questionnaire, telephone interview, GP notes). [f] Biomarker level (CA125, HE4) dichotomised at 95th percentile in control group—levels above that deemed abnormal. The Recruitment setting and the source of accuracy estimate are denoted by "•". Abbreviations: OC = ovarian cancer; CI = confidence interval; AUC = area under the receiver operator characteristic curve; PPV = positive predictive values; yrs = years.

Discrimination was reported for five tools (Table 3), all of which had similar AUCs within the 'good' range (0.84–0.89), with QCancer Ovarian exhibiting an AUC of 0.86 on external validation. Tool calibration was assessed for QCancer tools by graphically comparing the predicted cancer risk at two years with the observed risk by predicted risk deciles [22–24]. Authors reported good calibration on internal validation. On external validation, QCancer Ovarian had reasonable calibration but overpredicted risk, particularly in older women [24].

4.2.4. Positive Predictive Values

The three cohort studies conducted in primary care reported positive predictive values (PPV) for QCancer tools at a range of thresholds (Table 3). The PPVs at any given risk threshold were similar—for example, values ranged from 0.5 to 0.8% when the threshold was set to identify the 10% of women at highest risk. Two case control studies (Rossing et al. and Jordan et al.) used external disease prevalence figures from screening studies and available population-level statistics to estimate the PPVs of the Goff SI and SGO consensus criteria—if they were to be used in general populations. The tools had similar estimated PPVs within each study, but PPVs were higher in Rossing et al. (0.63–1.12%) than in Jordan et al. (<55 years: 0.04–0.05%, ≥55 years: 0.18–0.31%).

5. Discussion

To our knowledge, this is the first systematic review to compare the diagnostic performance of existing symptom-based tools for ovarian cancer detection. We identified 21 symptom-based tools designed to help identify women with undiagnosed ovarian cancer. These tools comprised simple symptom checklists, checklists which included both symptoms and tests and more complex diagnostic prediction models which incorporated symptoms, test results and baseline risk factors. While the diagnostic performances of most tools were evaluated solely within the study development datasets, four tools were independently externally validated, with one being validated in multiple population settings. Externally validated tools demonstrated similar moderate diagnostic performances. Our findings should inform future studies evaluating the clinical impact of validated symptom-based tools when implemented in clinical practice.

5.1. Study Strengths and Limitations

The main strengths of this study were its systematic approach, broad search strategy and liberal eligibility criteria, which enabled us to identify and compare the performances of a wide variety of tools. However, the identified studies were extremely heterogeneous in their designs, populations, variable definitions, outcome definitions and thresholds, which ultimately precluded any meaningful meta-analyses. For example, although the Goff SI was evaluated in nine studies, there was overlap between the participants in three studies, control groups ranged from apparently healthy general population participants to hospital gynaecology patients (with or without benign pathology), ovarian cancer definitions differed and deviations in the parameters of the SI itself, in terms of symptom duration and frequency criteria, were noted in several studies. While meta-analysis was not deemed appropriate, our results demonstrate how the Goff SI performs under different conditions. An additional limitation was that all included studies were at high risk of bias in at least one QUADAS-2 domain, which limits the conclusions that can be drawn.

5.2. Comparison of Tools

Although all tools were symptom-based and designed to help identify women with ovarian cancer, they varied markedly in the symptoms they included. This mirrors discrepancies in the literature and within national guidelines as to which symptoms are associated with the disease and probably reflects differences in study methodologies and study populations [7]. Despite this, the symptoms with the highest positive likelihood ratios for ovarian cancer in a recent systematic review (distension, bloating, abdominal or pelvic pain) were incorporated into the majority of tools [8]. The more cancer-associated symptoms that are included in a checklist, the higher the sensitivity of the tool is likely to be, but at the cost of reducing specificity, as demonstrated by several of the included studies [19,26,33]. This was cited by Goff et al. as a rationale for not including urinary symptoms in the Goff SI [30]. Ultimately, variation in which additional symptoms a tool includes may have limited impact on tool performance; on external validation, two studies reported similar diagnostic accuracy metrics for the Goff SI and the SGO criteria (which differed on several symptoms), and on internal validation, Lim et al. concluded that changing several of the symptoms made relatively little difference to tool diagnostic accuracy [33].

In multiple studies, symptom checklists were augmented by ovarian cancer biomarkers with the aim of improving tool diagnostic accuracy. This approach naturally led to a reduction in tool specificity (where either symptoms or an abnormal test resulted in a positive tool) or sensitivity (where symptoms and an abnormal test were needed for a positive tool). If ovarian cancer biomarkers are to be included alongside symptoms within tools, this loss of performance could be avoided by incorporating them within prediction models, as per the inclusion of anaemia in QCancer Ovarian. As the prediction model threshold can be set at a desired risk level, biomarkers, such as CA125 and HE4, could be incorporated without harming tool performance. However, this would require women to have specialist ovarian cancer markers performed in order for the tool to be used, which significantly limits clinical utility. A more practical approach would be to incorporate tools within a two-step pathway in which symptom-based tools (which do not include specialist test variables) are used to help select higher-risk women for specialist ovarian cancer tests.

Variation in the reported sensitivity and specificity of the most widely evaluated tool, the Goff SI, was noted between studies. This variation is likely to be due, in part, to the marked differences in study design, populations and outcome definitions which precluded meta-analysis across these studies. Despite these differences, in 5 of the 6 external validation studies (including two large population-based studies), the Goff SI had a sensitivity in excess of 60%, and in all but the smallest study, which included only 24 ovarian cancers and 31 controls, its specificity exceeded 85%. The sensitivities and specificities of the two other externally validated symptom checklists—the SGO consensus criteria and the modified Goff SI 1—were similar, as were those of the only externally validated diagnostic prediction model—QCancer Ovarian (applying a 10% risk threshold). Given the similarity in performance of the various existing validated tools, future research efforts may be better directed at evaluating the impact of using available tools in practice rather than developing further tools consisting of different symptom combinations.

5.3. *Clinical Relevance*

Two distinct uses for tools were identified by the authors of the included studies: (1) assessment of women presenting symptomatically in the standard clinical setting to identify those at higher risk of undiagnosed cancer and to inform decision making and further investigation, and (2) proactive 'symptom-triggered screening' programs in which women are actively screened using the tool, with further testing for ovarian cancer occurring if the tool is positive. Several of the tools identified in this review are already available for use within the standard clinical setting in the form of electronic clinical decision support tools (eCDSTs). QCancer tools are integrated within some UK general practice IT systems and alert the clinician if the risk of ovarian cancer in an individual reaches a certain level, prompting them to consider ovarian cancer as a possible diagnosis. eCDSTs have been shown to improve practitioner performance and patient care, but there are multiple barriers to their implementation and they do not always lead to improved outcomes [43,44]. Therefore, even if eCDSTs are deemed to have acceptable diagnostic accuracy, their cost-effectiveness, acceptability to patients and clinicians and their impact on timely ovarian cancer detection and survival need to be evaluated. Currently, a large, clustered, randomised control trial is seeking to help to address this by investigating the clinical impact of implementing a suite of electronic cancer risk assessment tools (including an electronic version of the Hamilton ovarian SI) in UK general practice [45]. Studies have also sought to evaluate the impact of using tools as part of 'symptom-triggered screening' programs, but none have taken the form of randomised control trials—the gold standard approach—and so findings should be interpreted with caution. In one study, 5000 women were approached in primary care clinics and screened for symptoms using the Goff SI, with further investigations performed if the Goff SI was positive [11]. However, conclusions were limited as only two ovarian cancers were identified in the study window. The Diagnosing Ovarian and Endometrial Cancer Early (DOvEE) trial also employs a proactive symptom-triggered testing approach, supported by media campaigns, in which women can self-refer and are screened for range of symptoms prior to study inclusion. Although the final DOvEE results are yet to be published, a pilot study reported that participants had lower tumour burden and more resectable disease than women diagnosed via the standard clinical pathway [9].

When considering the clinical utility of a tool, it is important to assess the proportion of women who are 'tool-positive' who ultimately have ovarian cancer, i.e., the PPV. Primary care cohort studies indicated that between 1 in 200 and 1 in 100 women who were QCancer tool-positive (5% or 10% risk) had the disease. Although these figures may appear low, evidence indicates that patients would opt for cancer testing at PPVs of 1% [46]. Further, having a positive tool result in the clinical setting does not necessarily mean that further investigation will automatically occur, as there may be a clear alternative cause for the symptoms—the tool is simply intended as a diagnostic aid to highlight the risk of ovarian cancer to the clinician. In addition, the most common follow-up tests—CA125 and transvaginal ultrasound—are relatively non-invasive, and CA125 is known to perform well when used in a symptomatic primary care population [47], although invasive investigations/surgery may ultimately be needed to determine whether ovarian cancer is present. In proactive symptom-triggered screening programs, the tool is more than just a diagnostic aid—it is the initial screening step which will dictate whether further ovarian cancer tests take place. The two population studies reporting PPVs relied on external ovarian cancer prevalence figures, but their PPV estimates were similar to that reported in the pilot DOvEE study (0.76% in women $\geq$ 50 years) [9]. Further research is needed to help determine whether, given this PPV, follow-up testing in proactive symptom-triggered testing programs is acceptable to women and improves outcomes. The definitive diagnosis of ovarian cancer often involves invasive procedures/surgery, which has contributed to patient morbidity in key ovarian cancer screening trials [3,39]. Although initial findings indicate that proactive symptom triggered testing approaches lead to minimal unnecessary surgery [9,11], large trials are needed to confirm that the implementation of symptom-based tools in clinical practice does not lead to significant excess morbidity.

6. Conclusions

Over 20 symptom-based tools have been developed in different populations to help assess women for ovarian cancer, but the majority have not been validated. Four symptom-based tools—the Goff SI, a modified version of the Goff symptom Index, SGO consensus criteria and QCancer Ovarian—have undergone independent external validation and exhibit similar sensitivities and specificities. These tools could have an important role to play in the detection of ovarian cancer, but further large well-conducted studies are needed to assess their cost-effectiveness, their acceptability, their effect on the timeliness of ovarian cancer diagnosis and their impact on clinical outcomes, including patient survival.

Author Contributions: Conceptualization, G.F.; methodology, G.F., F.M.W. and W.H.; formal analysis, G.F. and V.H.; data curation, G.F. and V.H.; writing—original draft preparation, G.F.; writing—review and editing, G.F., V.H., G.A., E.J.C., W.H., F.M.W. and J.E.; supervision, F.M.W., G.A., E.J.C. and W.H.; funding acquisition, F.M.W. and W.H. All authors have read and agreed to the published version of the manuscript.

References

1. Bray, F.; Ferlay, J.; Soerjomataram, I.; Siegel, R.L.; Torre, L.A.; Jemal, A. Global cancer statistics 2018: GLOBOCAN estimates of incidence and mortality worldwide for 36 cancers in 185 countries. *CA Cancer J. Clin.* **2018**, *68*, 394–424. [CrossRef] [PubMed]
2. Cancer Research UK. Ovarian Cancer Survival Statistics. Available online: http://www.cancerresearchuk.org/health-professional/cancer-statistics/statistics-by-cancer-type/ovarian-cancer/survival#heading-Three (accessed on 20 May 2020).
3. Jacobs, I.J.; Menon, U.; Ryan, A.; Gentry-Maharaj, A.; Burnell, M.; Kalsi, J.K.; Amso, N.N.; Apostolidou, S.; Benjamin, E.; Cruickshank, D.; et al. Ovarian cancer screening and mortality in the UK Collaborative Trial of Ovarian Cancer Screening (UKCTOCS): A randomised controlled trial. *Lancet* **2016**, *387*, 945–956. [CrossRef]
4. Pinsky, P.F.; Yu, K.; Kramer, B.S.; Black, A.; Buys, S.S.; Partridge, E.; Gohagan, J.; Berg, C.D.; Prorok, P.C. Extended mortality results for ovarian cancer screening in the PLCO trial with median 15 years follow-up. *Gynecol. Oncol.* **2016**, *143*, 270–275. [CrossRef] [PubMed]
5. Barrett, J.; Sharp, D.J.; Stapley, S.; Stabb, C.; Hamilton, W. Pathways to the diagnosis of ovarian cancer in the UK: A cohort study in primary care. *BJOG* **2010**, *117*, 610–614. [CrossRef]
6. National Cancer Intellegence Network. Routes to Diagnosis 2006–2016 by year, V2.1a. Available online: http://www.ncin.org.uk/publications/routes_to_diagnosis (accessed on 21 May 2020).
7. Funston, G.; Melle, V.M.; Ladegaard Baun, M.-L.; Jensen, H.; Helpser, C.; Emery, J.; Crosbie, E.; Thompson, M.; Hamilton, W.; Walter, F.M. Variation in the initial assessment and investigation for ovarian cancer in symptomatic women: A systematic review of international guidelines. *BMC Cancer* **2019**, *19*, 1028. [CrossRef]
8. Ebell, M.H.; Culp, M.B.; Radke, T.J. A Systematic Review of Symptoms for the Diagnosis of Ovarian Cancer. *Am. J. Prev. Med.* **2016**, *50*, 384–394. [CrossRef]
9. Gilbert, L.; Basso, O.; Sampalis, J.; Karp, I.; Martins, C.; Feng, J.; Piedimonte, S.; Quintal, L.; Ramanakumar, A.V.; Takefman, J.; et al. Assessment of symptomatic women for early diagnosis of ovarian cancer: Results from the prospective DOvE pilot project. *Lancet Oncol.* **2012**, *13*, 285–291. [CrossRef]
10. Goff, B.A.; Lowe, K.A.; Kane, J.C.; Robertson, M.D.; Gaul, M.A.; Andersen, M.R. Symptom triggered screening for ovarian cancer: A pilot study of feasibility and acceptability. *Gynecol. Oncol.* **2012**, *124*, 230–235. [CrossRef]
11. Andersen, M.R.; Lowe, K.A.; Goff, B.A. Value of Symptom-Triggered Diagnostic Evaluation for Ovarian Cancer. *Obstet. Gynecol.* **2014**, *123*, 73–79. [CrossRef]
12. Moons, K.G.M.; Altman, D.G.; Reitsma, J.B.; Ioannidis, J.P.A.; Macaskill, P.; Steyerberg, E.W.; Vickers, A.J.; Ransohoff, D.F.; Collins, G.S. Transparent reporting of a multivariable prediction model for individual prognosis or diagnosis (TRIPOD): Explanation and elaboration. *Ann. Intern. Med.* **2015**, *162*, W1–W73. [CrossRef]
13. Goff, B.A.; Mandel, L.S.; Melancon, C.H.; Muntz, H.G. Frequency of symptoms of ovarian cancer in women presenting to primary care clinics. *JAMA* **2004**, *291*, 2705–2712. [CrossRef] [PubMed]
14. Hamilton, W.; Peters, T.J.; Bankhead, C.; Sharp, D. Risk of ovarian cancer in women with symptoms in primary care: Population based case-control study. *BMJ* **2009**, *339*, b2998. [CrossRef] [PubMed]
15. Laupacis, A.; Sekar, N.; Stiell, I.G. Clinical prediction rules: A review and suggested modifications of methodological standards. *J. Am. Med. Assoc.* **1997**, *277*, 488–494. [CrossRef]
16. Ouzzani, M.; Hammady, H.; Fedorowicz, Z.; Elmagarmid, A. Rayyan-a web and mobile app for systematic reviews. *Syst. Rev.* **2016**, *5*, 210. [CrossRef]
17. Usher-Smith, J.A.; Sharp, S.J.; Griffin, S.J. The spectrum effect in tests for risk prediction, screening, and diagnosis. *BMJ* **2016**, *353*, i3139. [CrossRef]
18. Whiting, P.F.; Rutjes, A.W.S.; Westwood, M.E.; Mallett, S.; Deeks, J.J.; Reitsma, J.B.; Leeflang, M.M.G.; Sterne, J.A.C.; Bossuyt, P.M.M. Quadas-2: A revised tool for the quality assessment of diagnostic accuracy studies. *Ann. Intern. Med.* **2011**, *155*, 529–536. [CrossRef]
19. Lurie, G.; Thompson, P.J.; McDuffie, K.E.; Carney, M.E.; Goodman, M.T. Prediagnostic symptoms of ovarian carcinoma: A case-control study. *Gynecol. Oncol.* **2009**, *114*, 231–236. [CrossRef]
20. Rossing, M.A.; Wicklund, K.G.; Cushing-Haugen, K.L.; Weiss, N.S. Predictive value of symptoms for early detection of ovarian cancer. *J. Natl. Cancer Inst.* **2010**, *102*, 222–229. [CrossRef]
21. Jordan, S.J.; Coory, M.D.; Webb, P.M. Re: Predictive Value of Symptoms for Early Detection of Ovarian Cancer. *JNCI J. Natl. Cancer Inst.* **2010**, *102*, 1599–1601. [CrossRef]

22. Hippisley-Cox, J.; Coupland, C. Identifying women with suspected ovarian cancer in primary care: Derivation and validation of algorithm. *BMJ* **2012**, *344*, d8009. [CrossRef]
23. Hippisley-Cox, J.; Coupland, C. Symptoms and risk factors to identify women with suspected cancer in primary care: Derivation and validation of an algorithm. *Br. J. Gen. Pract.* **2013**, *63*, e11–e21. [CrossRef]
24. Collins, G.S.; Altman, D.G. Identifying women with undetected ovarian cancer: Independent and external validation of QCancer® (Ovarian) prediction model. *Eur. J. Cancer Care (Engl.)* **2013**, *22*, 423–429. [CrossRef]
25. Grewal, K.; Hamilton, W.; Sharp, D. Ovarian cancer prediction: Development of a scoring system for primary care. *BJOG An Int. J. Obstet. Gynaecol.* **2013**, *120*, 1016–1019. [CrossRef]
26. Kim, M.-K.; Kim, K.; Kim, S.M.; Kim, J.W.; Park, N.-H.; Song, Y.-S.; Kang, S.-B. A hospital-based case-control study of identifying ovarian cancer using symptom index. *J. Gynecol. Oncol.* **2009**, *20*, 238–242. [CrossRef]
27. Macuks, R.; Baidekalna, I.; Donina, S. Diagnostic test for ovarian cancer composed of ovarian cancer symptom index, menopausal status and ovarian cancer antigen CA125. *Eur. J. Gynaecol. Oncol.* **2011**, *32*, 286–288.
28. Shetty, J.; Priyadarshini, P.; Pandey, D.; Manjunath, A.P. Modified Goff Symptom Index: Simple triage tool for ovarian malignancy. *Sultan Qaboos Univ. Med. J.* **2015**, *15*, e370–e375. [CrossRef]
29. Jain, S.; Danodia, K.; Suneja, A.; Mehndiratta, M.; Chawla, S. Symptom index for detection of ovarian malignancy in indian women: A hospital-based study. *J. Indian Acad. Clin. Med.* **2018**, *19*, 27–32.
30. Goff, B.A.; Mandel, L.S.; Drescher, C.W.; Urban, N.; Gough, S.; Schurman, K.M.; Patras, J.; Mahony, B.S.; Robyn Andersen, M. Development of an ovarian cancer symptom index: Possibilities for earlier detection. *Cancer* **2007**, *109*, 221–227. [CrossRef]
31. Andersen, M.R.; Goff, B.A.; Lowe, K.A.; Scholler, N.; Bergan, L.; Dresher, C.W.; Paley, P.; Urban, N. Combining a symptoms index with CA 125 to improve detection of ovarian cancer. *Cancer* **2008**, *113*, 484–489. [CrossRef]
32. Andersen, M.R.; Goff, B.A.; Lowe, K.A.; Scholler, N.; Bergan, L.; Drescher, C.W.; Paley, P.; Urban, N. Use of a Symptom Index, CA125, and HE4 to predict ovarian cancer. *Gynecol. Oncol.* **2010**, *116*, 378–383. [CrossRef] [PubMed]
33. Lim, A.W.W.; Mesher, D.; Gentry-Maharaj, A.; Balogun, N.; Jacobs, I.; Menon, U.; Sasieni, P. Predictive value of symptoms for ovarian cancer: Comparison of symptoms reported by questionnaire, interview, and general practitioner notes. *J. Natl. Cancer Inst.* **2012**, *104*, 114–124. [CrossRef] [PubMed]
34. Merritt, M.A.; Green, A.C.; Nagle, C.M.; Webb, P.M.; Bowtell, D.; Chenevix-Trench, G.; Green, A.; Webb, P.; DeFazio, A.; Gertig, D.; et al. Talcum powder, chronic pelvic inflammation and NSAIDs in relation to risk of epithelial ovarian cancer. *Int. J. Cancer* **2008**, *122*, 170–176. [CrossRef] [PubMed]
35. QResearch The QResearch Database. Available online: https://www.qresearch.org (accessed on 8 January 2019).
36. THIN® The Health Improvement Network. Available online: https://www.the-health-improvement-network.com/en/ (accessed on 9 November 2020).
37. Lowe, K.A.; Shah, C.; Wallace, E.; Anderson, G.; Paley, P.; McIntosh, M.; Andersen, M.R.; Scholler, N.; Bergan, L.; Thorpe, J.; et al. Effects of personal characteristics on serum CA125, mesothelin, and HE4 levels in healthy postmenopausal women at high-risk for ovarian cancer. *Cancer Epidemiol. Biomark. Prev.* **2008**, *17*, 2480–2487. [CrossRef]
38. Menon, U.; Gentry-Maharaj, A.; Hallett, R.; Ryan, A.; Burnell, M.; Sharma, A.; Lewis, S.; Davies, S.; Philpott, S.; Lopes, A.; et al. Sensitivity and specificity of multimodal and ultrasound screening for ovarian cancer, and stage distribution of detected cancers: Results of the prevalence screen of the UK Collaborative Trial of Ovarian Cancer Screening (UKCTOCS). *Lancet Oncol.* **2009**, *10*, 327–340. [CrossRef]
39. Buys, S.S.; Partridge, E.; Greene, M.H.; Prorok, P.C.; Reding, D.; Riley, T.L.; Hartge, P.; Fagerstrom, R.M.; Ragard, L.R.; Chia, D.; et al. Ovarian cancer screening in the Prostate, Lung, Colorectal and Ovarian (PLCO) cancer screening trial: Findings from the initial screen of a randomized trial. *Am. J. Obstet. Gynecol.* **2005**, *193*, 1630–1639. [CrossRef]
40. Jacobs, I.; Prys Davies, A.; Bridges, J.; Stabile, I.; Fay, T.; Lower, A.; Grudzinskas, J.G.; Oram, D. Prevalence screening for ovarian cancer in postmenopausal women by CA 125 measurement and ultrasonography. *Br. Med. J.* **1993**, *306*, 1030–1034. [CrossRef]
41. *Cancer Incidence Projections Australia 2002 to 2011*; Australian Institute of Health and Welfare; Australasian Association of Cancer Registries; National Cancer Strategies Group: Canberra, Australia, 2005.
42. *Australian Demographic Statistics*; Australian Bureau of Statistics D: Canberra, Australia, 2007.
43. Chima, S.; Milley, K.; Reece, J.C.; Milton, S.; McIntosh, J.G.; Emery, J.D. Decision support tools to improve cancer diagnostic decision making in primary care: A systematic review. *Br. J. Gen. Pract.* **2019**, *69*, e809–e818. [CrossRef]

44. Chiang, P.C.; Glance, D.; Walker, J.; Walter, F.M.; Emery, J.D. Implementing a qcancer risk tool into general practice consultations: An exploratory study using simulated consultations with Australian general practitioners. *Br. J. Cancer* **2015**, *112*, S77–S83. [CrossRef]
45. Hamilton, W. Electronic Risk Assessment for Cancer for Patients in General Practice (ISRCTN22560297). Available online: http://www.isrctn.com/ISRCTN22560297 (accessed on 30 October 2020).
46. Banks, J.; Hollinghurst, S.; Bigwood, L.; Peters, T.J.; Walter, F.M.; Hamilton, W. Preferences for cancer investigation: A vignette-based study of primary-care attendees. *Lancet Oncol.* **2014**, *15*, 232–240. [CrossRef]
47. Funston, G.; Hamilton, W.; Abel, G.; Crosbie, E.J.; Rous, B.; Walter, F.M. The diagnostic performance of CA125 for the detection of ovarian and non-ovarian cancer in primary care: A population-based cohort study. *PLoS Med.* **2020**, *17*, e1003295. [CrossRef]

Rare Germline Genetic Variants and the Risks of Epithelial Ovarian Cancer

Marina Pavanello [1,2,†], Isaac HY Chan [1,†], Amir Ariff [1,2], Paul DP Pharoah [3], Simon A. Gayther [4,5] and Susan J. Ramus [1,2,*]

1 School of Women's and Children's Health, Faculty of Medicine, University of New South Wales, Sydney 2052, Australia; m.pavanello@student.unsw.edu.au (M.P.); isaac.chan@unsw.edu.au (I.H.C.); amir.ariff@unsw.edu.au (A.A.)
2 Adult Cancer Program, Lowy Cancer Research Centre, University of New South Wales, Sydney 2052, Australia
3 Strangeways Research Laboratory, University of Cambridge, Cambridge CB1 8RN, UK; pp10001@medschl.cam.ac.uk
4 Center for Cancer Prevention and Translational Genomics, Cedars Sinai Medical Center, Los Angeles, CA 90048, USA; simon.gayther@cshs.org
5 Applied Genomics, Computation and Translational Core, Cedars Sinai Medical Center, Los Angeles, CA 90048, USA
* Correspondence: s.ramus@unsw.edu.au
† These authors have contributed equally to this work.

Simple Summary: Several genes have been confirmed as risk genes for epithelial ovarian cancer (EOC). There are five main types of EOC, with different molecular changes and clinical characteristics, suggesting they should be considered different diseases. This review summarises the contribution of rare inherited mutations to EOC susceptibility, focussing on the frequency in each EOC type. Susceptibility genes can have a major clinical impact, reducing ovarian cancer incidence by screening of family members to detect women at higher risk than the general population. They can also lead to the development of new targeted treatments.

Abstract: A family history of ovarian or breast cancer is the strongest risk factor for epithelial ovarian cancer (EOC). Germline deleterious variants in the *BRCA1* and *BRCA2* genes confer EOC risks by age 80, of 44% and 17% respectively. The mismatch repair genes, particularly *MSH2* and *MSH6*, are also EOC susceptibility genes. Several other DNA repair genes, *BRIP1*, *RAD51C*, *RAD51D*, and *PALB2*, have been identified as moderate risk EOC genes. EOC has five main histotypes; high-grade serous (HGS), low-grade serous (LGS), clear cell (CCC), endometrioid (END), and mucinous (MUC). This review examines the current understanding of the contribution of rare genetic variants to EOC, focussing on providing frequency data for each histotype. We provide an overview of frequency and risk for pathogenic variants in the known susceptibility genes as well as other proposed genes. We also describe the progress to-date to understand the role of missense variants and the different breast and ovarian cancer risks for each gene. Identification of susceptibility genes have clinical impact by reducing disease-associated mortality through improving risk prediction, with the possibility of prevention strategies, and developing new targeted treatments and these clinical implications are also discussed.

Keywords: ovarian cancer risk; rare germline variants; susceptibility genes

1. Introduction

Epithelial ovarian cancer (EOC) is the seventh most common cancer in women worldwide, with over 295,000 incident cases each year, and is the leading cause of mortality relating to gynaecological malignancies, with 184,000 deaths each year [1]. Typically, EOCs are stratified into five main histological subtypes: High grade serous, which account for up to 70% of all EOC cases, endometrioid (~10%), clear cell (~10%), mucinous (~3%), and low-grade serous carcinomas (<5%) [2]. The five different histotypes have different risk factors and molecular characteristics. The inherited genetics of each histotype is also likely to be different.

The prognosis of ovarian cancer is poor, with a five-year survival rate of just 47% [3]. Ovarian cancer is difficult to diagnose early in its disease course, and 80% of cases are diagnosed after extensive metastasis at stage III or IV, which carry a five-year survival rate of 41% and 20% respectively [3]. However, outcomes are good if ovarian cancer is detected early, with an 89% five-year survival in stage I cancers [3]. Screening for ovarian cancer is of limited utility and no studies investigating ovarian cancer screening have shown a significant impact of screening on mortality [4,5]. As a result, population-based screening for ovarian cancer is not recommended in the guidelines of any major society. As the prognosis of EOC is related to its stage at diagnosis, the ability to use genetic information to predict EOC risk and intervene before disease development would reduce overall mortality and morbidity in ovarian cancer [6].

A family history of EOC confers an increase in relative risk (RR) of ovarian cancer of 2.96. The known EOC risk genes explain less than half of the excess familial risk for EOC, suggesting that there are still undiscovered ovarian cancer predisposing genes to be found [7,8]. The known ovarian cancer predisposing genes are from two different DNA repair pathways. The homologous recombination (HR) DNA repair pathway and the mismatch repair (MMR) DNA pathway. The majority of the genes are part of the HR DNA repair pathway. *BRCA1* and *BRCA2* have been confirmed as highly penetrant predisposition genes for EOC [9]. Several other genes—*BRIP1*, *RAD51C*, *RAD51D*, and *PALB2*, recently described as moderate risk genes, are also part of this pathway [10–12]. The mismatch repair genes *MLH1*, *MSH2*, *MSH6*, and *PSM2* are also confirmed moderate risk EOC susceptibility genes [13]. The frequency of disease-associated variants in these genes is different for the different EOC histotypes. Thirty-seven common variants have been identified for ovarian cancer, using genome-wide association studies (GWAS) [14,15]. The ability to derive accurate risk estimates for ovarian cancer from genetic information in asymptomatic women has significant implications for ovarian cancer management.

This review aims to summarise the progress to date in efforts to understand the contribution of rare genetic variants to ovarian cancer and histotype specific differences, as well as the clinical implications of these discoveries. In the first part of this review, we describe germline protein truncating variants (insertion/deletions or nonsense) in confirmed EOC susceptibility genes, followed by an overview of the role of missense variants in these genes. Lastly, we described germline protein truncating variants in other proposed genes that have not been validated as EOC susceptibility genes.

2. Protein Truncating Variants in Confirmed Susceptibility Genes

2.1. BRCA1 and BRCA2

These two major breast/ovarian cancer susceptibility genes encode proteins that work in DNA replication pathways to avoid double-strand DNA damage. Deleterious protein truncating variants include small insertions and deletions and single base changes, as well as large genomic alterations, which account for approximately 10% of *BRCA1* variants [16]. Several deleterious missense variants have also been described.

The prevalence and penetrance of deleterious variants in *BRCA1* and *BRCA2* has been extensively studied in ovarian cancer patients. The case ascertainment, either from families with a history of breast or ovarian cancer or from the general ovarian cancer population, has a major impact on the results. The presence of founder mutations in the population also affects the prevalence and has important implications for clinical testing. The presence of founder mutations can allow for cheap and rapid testing and the potential for population screening. In the Ashkenazi Jewish population, there are three *BRCA* founder mutations (185delAG and 5382insC in *BRCA1* and 6174delT in *BRCA2*) that accounts for almost all mutations present in this population [17]. In the Icelandic population, there is a single founder mutation, 999del5, in the *BRCA2* gene. Most of the breast and ovarian cancer cases in Icelandic families have this *BRCA2* founder mutation, while mutations in *BRCA1* are very rare [18]. Founder mutations in the *BRCA* genes have also been reported in many other populations, including Russians [19,20], Polish [21], Norwegian [22], Finnish [23], Japanese [24], and Chinese [25]. While some mutations are restricted to isolated regions or certain populations, others are common across different countries, such as *BRCA1* 5382insC mutation that is common in many European populations [17].

Early studies of cases selected for a family history of breast or ovarian cancer found that 24–76% had deleterious variants in *BRCA1* and 1–17% had deleterious variants in *BRCA2* [17]. Recent studies using clinical testing laboratory data have reported the prevalence of *BRCA1/2* pathogenic variants in 5020 and 7489 cases from the USA [26,27], 4409 cases from France [28], and 3230 cases from a meta-analysis of 48 multi-gene panel testing-based studies [29]. In these studies, the frequency of germline pathogenic variants in *BRCA1* in ovarian cancer cases were 5.1%, 3.6%, 3.7%, and 8.6%, respectively, and 3.9%, 3.3%, 4.0%, and 4.5% in *BRCA2* [26–29].

Testing of unselected ovarian cancer cases in non-Ashkenazi Jewish populations shows that the frequency of deleterious *BRCA1* and *BRCA2* variants ranged from 3–10% and 0.6–6%, respectively [17]. Recent population-based studies from Table 1 found that 3.8–11.1% of cases have *BRCA1* deleterious variants and 4.3–6.4% had *BRCA2* deleterious variants.

In a large prospective study of *BRCA* carriers ascertained through family clinics, the cumulative risk, by age 80, of ovarian cancer in women with pathogenic variants in *BRCA1* and *BRCA2* was estimated to be 44% (95% confidence interval (CI), 36–53%) and 17% (95% CI, 11–25%), respectively [9]. The histotypes of ovarian cancer diagnosed in the study were not described [9]. Breast cancer was also assessed and the cumulative risk at the age of 80 years was estimated to be 72% (95% CI, 65–79%) for *BRCA1* carriers and 69% (95% CI, 61–77%) for *BRCA2* [9]. Variants in these *BRCA* genes are also associated with increased risk of pancreatic cancer [30] and high-grade prostate cancer [31].

Four studies, with cases unselected for age or family history, provided information on histotype (Table 1). Due to the small numbers of the much rarer histotypes (END, CCC, LGS, and MUC), the frequencies of germline pathogenic variants varied significantly. In an effort to estimate the frequency in these rarer histotypes, we have combined the results across studies. This showed that the frequency of deleterious variants in *BRCA1* were approximately 7.8% in HGS, 3% in END, 3.6% in CCC, 3.7% in LGS, and <1% in MUC [32–35]. In *BRCA2*, deleterious variants were seen in approximately 5.9% of HGS cases, 2.9% of END, 0.9% of CCC, 2.0% of LGS, and <1% of MUC [33–35] (Table 1). According to these data, both genes have a higher frequency of variants in the HGS histotype compared to the non-HGS histotypes, and a much lower frequency in mucinous cases. Available cumulative risks from these retrospective studies are comparable to the prospective study previously mentioned [9] (Table 1).

Ovarian cancer patients with deleterious variants in *BRCA1* and *BRCA2* are characterized by genomic instability within their tumours. They have a better response to platinum-based chemotherapies, resulting in improved five-year overall survival. Five-year overall survival for non-carriers was reported to be 36% (95% CI 34–38) compared to 44% (95% CI 40–48) for *BRCA1*-carriers and 52% (95% CI 46–58) for *BRCA2*-carriers [36]. However, this survival advantage was not present when follow-up was extended to 10 years [37,38].

Identifying pathogenic variants associated with increased risk of ovarian cancer has major clinical implications. Due to the magnitude of ovarian cancer risk associated with variants in *BRCA1* and *BRCA2*, risk-reducing salpingo-oophorectomy (RRSO) is currently recommended as a prevention strategy for *BRCA1* carriers by age 35 to 40 years, once the woman's childbearing is complete, and for *BRCA2* carriers by age 40 to 45 [39].

Table 1. Frequency of germline pathogenic variants in *BRCA1/2* in epithelial ovarian cancer (EOC) histotypes, in cases from population studies.

Gene	Study	Cases Carriers/Total (Frequency)							Controls Carriers/Total (Frequency)		OR (95% CI)	Cumulative Risk (95% CI) [a]
		HGS	END	CCC	LGS	MUC	Mixed/ Unk [b]	All EOC	Matched	Publicly Available		
BRCA1	Walsh et al., 2011 [34]	31/242 ** (12.8%)	2/23 (8.7%)	1/17 (5.9%)	**	-	6/78 (7.7%)	40/360 (11.1%)	-	-	NC	NC
	Alsop et al., 2012 † [32]	74/709 ** (10.4%)	7/119 (5.9%)	4/63 (6.3%)	**	-	3/110 (2.7%)	88/1001 (8.79%)	-	-	NC	NC
	Song et al., 2014 ^ [33]	58/1105 * (5.2%)	3/322 (0.9%)	3/192 (1.6%)	6/172 (3.5%)	1/157 (0.6%)	13/274 (4.7%)	84/2222 (3.78%)	1/1528 (0.07%)	-	60 # (10–2100)	61% (15–99%)
	Norquist et al., 2016 [35]	155/1498 (10.3%)	4/77 (5.2%)	4/58 (6.9%)	3/70 (4.3%)	0/16 (0%)	16/196 (8.2%)	142/1915 (7.41%)	-	114/36276 (0.31%)	48.9 (24–100)	NC
	Total	**278/3554 (7.82%)**	**16/541 (2.95%)**	**12/330 (3.63%)**	**9/242 (3.72%)**	**1/173 (0.58%)**	**38/658 (5.77%)**	**354/5498 (6.43%)**	**1/1528 (0.07%)**	-	-	-
BRCA2	Walsh et al., 2011 [34]	18/242 ** (7.4%)	0/23 (0%)	0/17 (0%)	**	-	5/78 (6.4%)	23/360 (6.38%)	-	-	NC	NC
	Alsop et al., 2012 † [32]	44/709 ** (6.2%)	3/119 (2.5%)	0/63 (0%)	**	-	6/110 (5.4%)	53/1001 (5.29%)	-	-	NC	NC
	Song et al., 2014 ^ [33]	64/1105 * (5.8%)	10/322 (3.1%)	3/192 (1.6%)	4/172 (2.3%)	1/157 (0.6%)	12/274 (4.4%)	94/2222 (4.23%)	4/1528 (0.26%)	-	17 # (6.3–63)	24% (10–62%)
	Norquist et al., 2016 [35]	85/1498 (5.7%)	3/77 (3.9%)	0/58 (0%)	1/70 (1.4%)	0/16 (0%)	9/196 (4.6%)	98/1915 (5.11%)	-	149/36276 (0.41%)	14 (8.2–23.8)	NC
	Total	**211/3554 (5.93%)**	**16/541 (2.95%)**	**3/330 (0.91%)**	**5/242 (2.0%)**	**1/173 (0.57%)**	**32/658 (4.86%)**	**268/5498 (4.87%)**	**4/1528 (0.26%)**	-	-	-

-: Not available, NC: Not calculated due to no controls or not described, ** Frequency of serous combined, * Frequency of HGS and serous undifferentiated, # Odds ratio (OR) for the matched controls analysis, [a] Risks based on all cases combined, [b] Mixed/Unknown includes some other histotypes, † Mucinous ovarian cancer cases were excluded, ^ Not screened for large genomic alterations. Bold: highlight info.

Furthermore, understanding the role of *BRCA1/2* variants in ovarian cancer has allowed for the development of targeted therapies, namely PARP (poly[adenosine diphosphate–ribose] polymerase) inhibitors, which improve progression-free survival in selected women with ovarian cancer. Approximately 50% of HGS cases present defects in DNA repair mechanisms due to pathogenic variants in the homologous recombination deficiency (HRD) genes, such as *BRCA1/2*, or due to functional inactivation through methylation [40]. PARPi have shown highly efficacious activity particularly in women with platinum-sensitive disease carrying *BRCA1/2* variants, or women with other homologous recombination deficiencies [41–43]. Improved activity has also been seen in women with recurrent disease regardless of their *BRCA* status [44]. As *BRCA1/2* status affects clinical management of affected women, current guidelines recommend *BRCA1/2* testing in all non-mucinous ovarian cancer cases [39].

2.2. *BRIP1*

The protein encoded by *BRIP1* is part of the Fanconi anaemia group (FANCJ) and is involved in the repair of DNA double-strand breaks by homologous recombination. *BRIP1* was described as a candidate risk gene by Walsh et al. that identified germline loss-of-function variants in 1% of ovarian cancer cases not selected for age or family history [34]. Pathogenic germline variants in *BRIP1* are the most common mutation found in ovarian cancer after *BRCA1/2* with a frequency of approximately 1% of the EOC cases [11].

The contribution of germline protein truncating variants in *BRIP1* have not yet been assessed in prospective studies. Ramus et al. described a relative risk associated with protein truncating variants in *BRIP1* of 11.2 (95% CI 3.2–34.1), with an estimated cumulative risk of 5.8% (95% CI 3.6–9.1%) by the age of 80 years [11] (Table 3). The association between protein truncating variants in *BRIP1* and risk of ovarian cancer has been confirmed in other analyses (associated risks ranged from 2.6 to 6.4 [27–29,35,45]) (Tables 2 and 3). The frequency of protein truncating variants in population-based studies, separated by ovarian cancer histotypes are given in Table 3, and the frequency in the other retrospective studies, mostly family studies or with women referred to clinical testing, are given in Table 2. Some of the studies in Table 2 have included predicted deleterious missense changes that cannot be separated from the totals, and these are indicated.

Three studies have reported the frequency of protein truncating variants in *BRIP1* by ovarian cancer histotype. Combining these data show that approximately 1.2% of HGS and END cases and 0.8% of LGS cases had protein truncating variants in *BRIP1* [11,34,35] (Table 3). No variants were observed in CCC and MUC, but the total number of cases examined were low. Additional studies are needed to further assess the contribution of germline protein truncating variants in *BRIP1* in the ovarian cancer histotypes.

Available data for *BRIP1* consistently have shown an increased risk of ovarian cancer, with cumulative risk estimated to be approximately 6% by age of 80, and the National Comprehensive Cancer Network, USA, now recommends RRSO for women, starting from ages 45 to 50 [39].

2.3. *RAD51C and RAD51D*

RAD51C and *RAD51D* are homologous recombination genes, which encode proteins that interact with *BRCA1/2* and participate in the DNA repair process. Ovarian cancer risk attributed to protein truncating variants in *RAD51C* and *RAD51D* was first described by Meindl et al. in 2010 and Loveday et al. in 2011 [46,47].

Song et al. and Norquist et al. provided the frequency of protein truncating variants in the *RAD51C/D* genes in population-based studies by ovarian cancer histotypes [35,48] (Table 3). Combining their data, approximately 0.4–0.5% of HGS, END and CCC cases and 0.2% of LGS had protein truncating variants in *RAD51C*. For *RAD51D*, 0.5% of HGS cases and 0.9% of END cases had protein truncating variants. These variants were not detected in CCC, LGS, and MUC cases, although so far, the number of cases of these histotypes in the datasets are low. The frequency of deleterious variants in family-based studies that combined all EOC cases are given in Table 2. The estimated risk associated with *RAD51C/D* described in the two population-studies were OR 5.2 (95% CI 1.1–24) and 3.4 (95% CI 1.5–7.6) for *RAD51C* and 12.0 (95% CI 1.5–90) and 10.9 (95% CI 4.6–26) for *RAD51D* (Table 3) [35,48]. Three additional case-control studies which included only individuals referred to clinical testing estimated a risk of OR 4.9 (95%CI 3.0–8.0), OR 14.6 (95% CI 5.3 –29.5), and SRR 5.12 (95% CI 3.7–6.9) for *RAD51C*. For *RAD51D*, associated risks were OR 4.78 (95% CI 2.1–10.7), OR 11.8 (95% CI 1.1–40), and SRR 6.34 (95% CI 3.1–11.3) (Table 2) [26–28].

More recently, Yang et al. performed a study of 125 families with pathogenic variants in *RAD51C* and 60 families with pathogenic variants in *RAD51D* and confirmed an increased risk of ovarian cancer associated with pathogenic variants in both genes (*RAD51C*, RR 7.55, 95% CI 5.6–10.2 and *RAD51D*, RR 7.6, 95% CI 5.6–10.3) [10]. The cumulative risk of having ovarian cancer by age 80 was estimated to be 11% (95% CI 6–21%) for *RAD51C* and 13% (95% CI 7–23%) for *RAD51D* based on their segregation analysis [10] (Table 2). *RAD51C/D* were also shown to be associated with breast cancer with cumulative risk of 21% (95% CI 15–29%) and 20% (95% CI 14–28%) for these genes by the age of 80 years, respectively [10].

There is no consensus about the EOC risk threshold for surgical prevention, although the acceptability of RRSO for women with a lifetime risk greater than 10% is well-established. It has been recently suggested that this threshold should be lower and was demonstrated that prophylactic surgery is cost-effective for women at lifetime risk of 5% [49–51]. Considering the current cumulative risk estimates for *RAD51C* and *RAD51D*, women carrying pathogenic variants in these genes could be offered preventive surgery starting from ages 45 to 50, once childbearing is complete.

2.4. PALB2

PALB2 is a confirmed breast cancer susceptibility gene with a cumulative risk estimated to be 44% by 80 years [52], and therefore clinical testing for germline pathogenic variants in this gene is part of breast cancer standard of care. *PALB2* is needed to recruit *BRCA2* in the HR DNA repair pathway [53].

Initial analysis of 3227 EOC cases and 3444 matched-controls suggested that larger numbers of samples were required to determine if *PALB2* was an ovarian cancer susceptibility gene (p 0.08) [11]. Evidence of risk association was observed in case-control analysis of 1915 EOC cases compared to publicly available controls with the OR estimated to be 4.4 (95% CI 2.1–9.1) [35]. Recently, *PALB2* has been confirmed as a risk gene by targeted sequencing in 5123 HGS cases and 5202 controls, WES data from 829 cases and 913 controls, and genotyping data from an independent set of ~14,000 EOC cases and 29,000 controls [54]. The odds ratio was estimated to be 3.01 (95% CI 1.59–5.68) [54] (Table 3).

Histotype data are only available from the first two studies, and combined show that approximately 0.4% of HGS cases had protein truncating variants in *PALB2* (Table 3). A lower frequency was found for LGS (0.2%) and no variants were found in END and MUC. In contrast CCC cases had a frequency of 2.4%. The total number of non-HGS cases examined to date, particularly for CCC, is very low, thus larger numbers are needed to establish the true frequency of *PALB2* pathogenic variants in the rarer histotypes.

An increased risk of ovarian cancer has recently been confirmed in a study of 976 individuals with protein truncating variants in *PALB2* from 524 families, where complex segregation analysis adjusted for ascertainment was performed. The relative risk was estimated to be 2.91 (95% CI 1.4–6.0) [12] (Table 2). Cumulative risks were estimated to be approximately 5% (95% CI 2–10%) by the age of 80 years in the family-based study [12] and 3.2% (95% CI 1.8–5.7%) by the same age in the case-control study previously described [54]. Discussions in the clinical community on whether or not these women should be eligible for prophylactic surgery are still ongoing.

Yang et al. also showed that protein truncating variants in *PALB2* were associated with increased risk of female and male breast cancer (RR 7.18 95% CI 5.8–8.8 and 7.34 95% CI 1.2–42.8, respectively) and pancreatic cancer (RR 2.37 95% CI 1.2–4.5) [12].

Table 2. Frequency of germline pathogenic variants in *BRIP1*, *RAD51C*, *RAD51D*, and *PALB2*, in EOC cases from family history studies.

Gene	Study	Type of Study	Cases Carriers/Total (Frequency)	Controls (Carriers/Total Frequency)		Risk (95% CI)	Cumulative Risk (95% CI)
			All EOC	Matched	Publicly Available		
BRIP1	Lilyquist et al., 2017 ¶ [27]	Clinical testing lab	58/6294 (0.92%)	-	ExAC	SRR: 4.99 (3.8–6.4)	NC
	Kurian et al., 2017 ¶ [26]	Clinical testing lab	36/5020 (0.71%)	161/64,649 (0.24%)	-	OR: 2.62 (1.7–3.9)	NC
	Castera et al., 2018 ¶ [28]	Genetic counselling	21/4408 (0.48%)	-	72/36,276 [a] (0.20%)	OR: 3.77 (0.7–9.4)	NC
	Suszynska et al., 2020 [45]	Meta-analysis ^	200/22,494 (0.89%)	-	209/115,375 [b] (0.18%)	OR: 4.94 (4.0–6.0)	NC
RAD51C	Meindl et al., 2010 [46]	Family study	6/480 families	-	-	NC	NC
	Lilyquist et al., 2017 ¶ [27]	Clinical testing lab	44/6294 (0.7%)	-	ExAC	SRR: 5.12 (3.7–6.9)	NC
	Kurian et al., 2017 ¶ [26]	Clinical testing lab	32/5020 (0.6%)	72/64,649	-	OR: 4.98 (3.0–8.0)	NC
	Castera et al., 2018 ¶ [28]	Genetic counselling	23/4309 (0.5%)	-	43/36,276 [a] (0.12%)	OR: 14.6 (5.3–29.5)	NC
	Suszynska et al., 2019 [29]	Meta-analysis ^^	21/3791 (0.6%)	-	-	OR: 4.3 (2.5–7.5)	NC
	Yang et al., 2020 [10]	*RAD51C* families #	125 families	-	-	RR: 7.55 (5.6–10.2)	11% (15–29%)
	Suszynska et al., 2020 [45]	Meta-analysis ^	149/23,802 (0.62%)	-	130/115,475 [b] (0.11%)	OR: 5.59 (4.4–7.0)	NC
RAD51D	Loveday et al., 2011 [47]	Family study	8/911 families	1/1060 (0.09%)	-	RR: 6.30 (2.8–13.8)	NC
	Lilyquist et al., 2017 ¶ [27]	Clinical testing lab	11/5743 (0.2%)	-	ExAC	SRR: 6.34 (3.1–11.3)	NC
	Kurian et al., 2017 ¶ [26]	Clinical testing lab	9/5020 (0.2%)	40/64,649 (0.06%)	-	OR: 4.78 (2.1–10.7)	NC
	Castera et al., 2018 ¶ [28]	Genetic counselling	9/4011 (0.2%)	-	18/36,276 [a] (0.05%)	OR: 11.8 (1.1–40)	NC
	Suszynska et al., 2019 [29]	Meta-analysis ^^	19/3258 (0.6%)	-	-	OR: 11.6 (5.9–23)	NC
	Yang et al., 2020 [10]	*RAD51D* families #	60 families	-	-	RR: 7.6 (5.6–10.3)	13% (7–23%)
	Suszynska et al., 2020 [45]	Meta-analysis ^	94/22,787 (0.45%)	-	72/120,688 [b] (0.06%)	OR: 6.9 (5.1–9.4)	NC
PALB2	Yang et al., 2020 [12]	*PALB2* families #	524 families	-	-	RR: 2.91 (1.4–6.0)	5% (2–10%)

Abbreviations: RR —Relative risk; OR—odds ratio; SRR—Standardized risk ratio; PVs—Pathogenic variants; -: Not available, NC: Not calculated, [a] ExAC NFE non-TCGA, [b] gnomAD NFE non-TCGA, ¶ deleterious missense changes included, ^ [45] Overlapped with 6 studies included in this review; ^^ [29] Overlapped with 1 study included in this review; # Segregation analysis. Bold: highlight info.

Table 3. Frequency of germline protein truncating variants in *BRIP1*, *RAD51C*, *RAD51D*, and *PALB2* in EOC histotypes, in cases from population studies.

Gene	Study	Cases Carriers/Total (Frequency)							Controls Carriers/Total (Frequency)		Risk (95% CI)	Cumulative Risk (95% CI) [a]
		HGS	END	CCC	LGS	MUC	Mixed/ Unk [b]	All EOC	Matched	Publicly Available		
BRIP1	Walsh et al., 2011 [34]	2/242 ** (0.8%)	1/23 (4.3%)	0/17 (0%)	**	-	1/78 (1.3%)	4/360 (1.1%)	-	-	NC	NC
	Ramus et al., 2015 [11]	26/2535 * (1.0%)	0/65 (0%)	0/25 (0%)	4/416 (0.9%)	0/26 (0%)	0/160 (0%)	30/ 3227 (0.92%)	3/3444 (0.09)	-	RR: 11.2 [#] (3.2–34.1)	5.8% (3.6–9.1%)
	Norquist et al., 2016 [35]	22/1498 (1.5%)	1/77 (1.3%)	0/58 (0%)	0/70 (0%)	0/16 (0%)	3/196 (1.5%)	26/1915 (1.36%)	-	60/36276 [c] (0.17%)	OR: 6.4 (3.8–10.6)	NC
	Total	**50/4275 (1.17%)**	**2/165 (1.21%)**	**0/100 (0%)**	**4/486 (0.82%)**	**0/42 (0%)**	**4/434 (0.9%)**	**60/5502 (1.1%)**	**3/3444 (0.09%)**	-	-	-
RAD51C	Song et al., 2015 [†] [48]	10/1806 * (0.6%)	1/383 (0.3%)	1/225 (0.4%)	1/405 (0.2%)	0/166 (0%)	1/444 (0.2%)	14/3429 (0.40%)	2/2772 (0.07%)	-	OR: 5.2 [#] (1.1–24)	5.2% ¶ (1.1–22%)
	Norquist et al., 2016 [†] [35]	7/1498 (0.5%)	1/77 (1.3%)	0/58 (0%)	0/70 (0%)	0/16 (0%)	3/196 (1.5%)	11/1915 (0.57%)	-	39/36276 [c] (0.11%)	OR: 3.4 (1.5–7.6)	NC
	Total	**17/3304 (0.51%)**	**2/460 (0.43%)**	**1/283 (0.35%)**	**1/475 (0.21%)**	**0/182 (0%)**	**4/640 (0.62%)**	**25/5344 (0.47%)**	**2/2772 (0.07%)**	-	-	-
RAD51D	Song et al., 2015 [48]	9/1806 * (0.5%)	3/383 (0.8%)	0/225 (0%)	0/405 (0%)	0/166 (0%)	0/444 (0%)	12/3429 (0.35%)	1/2772 (0.04%)	-	OR: 12 [#] (1.5–90)	12%¶ (1.5–60%)
	Norquist et al., 2016 [35]	7/1498 (0.5%)	1/77 (1.3%)	0/58 (0%)	0/70 (0%)	0/16 (0%)	3/196 (1.5%)	11/1915 (0.57%)	-	14/36276 [c] (0.04%)	OR: 10.9 (4.6–26.0)	NC
	Total	**16/3304 (0.48%)**	**4/460 (0.87%)**	**0/283 (0%)**	**0/475 (0%)**	**0/182 (0%)**	**3/640 (0.47%)**	**23/5344 (0.43%)**	**1/2772 (0.04%)**	-	-	-
PALB2	Ramus et al., 2015 [11]	6/2535 * (0.24%)	0/65 (0%)	1/25 (4%)	1/416 (0.24%)	0/26 (0%)	1/160 (0.62%)	9/3227 (0.28%)	3/3444 (0.09%)	-	NC	NC
	Norquist et al., 2016 [35]	9/1498 (0.60%)	0/77 (0%)	1/58 (1.7%)	0/70 (0%)	0/16 (0%)	2/196 (1.0%)	12/1915 (0.62%)	-	39/36276 [c] (0.10%)	OR: 4.4 (2.1–9.1)	NC
	Song et al., 2019 [54]	18/5123 (0.35%)	-	-	-	-	-	18/5123 (0.35%)	6/5202 (0.12%)	-	OR: 3.01 [#] (1.6–5.7)	3.2% (1.8–5.7%)
	Total ^	**15/4033 (0.37%)**	**0/142 (0%)**	**2/83 (2.4%)**	**1/486 (0.2%)**	**0/42 (0%)**	**3/356 (0.84%)**	**21/5142 (0.41%)**	**3/3444 (0.09%)**	-	-	-

Abbreviations: RR—Relative risk; OR—odds ratio; SRR—Standardized risk ratio; -: Not available, NC: Not calculated due to no controls or not described, ** Frequency of serous combined, * Frequency of HGS and serous undifferentiated, [#] OR for the matched controls analysis, [†] Studies included one known deleterious missense variant [55], [a] Risks based on all cases combined, [b] Mixed/Unknown includes some other histotypes, [c] ExAC NFE-nonTCGA, ¶ Cumulative risks by age 70, ^ Total does not include Song et al., 2019 [54], study as extensive overlap with Ramus et al., 2015 [11]. Bold: highlight info.

2.5. Mismatch Repair (MMR) Genes

Germline protein truncating and known deleterious missense variants in four MMR genes are associated with Lynch syndrome, which is an inherited disorder that increases the risk of many types of cancers including colon, endometrial, ovarian, pancreatic, small-bowel, and ureteric. In ovarian cancer cases from Lynch syndrome families, deleterious variants in the MMR genes were mostly seen in END and CCC cases and were more prevalent in the *MSH2* and *MSH6* genes [56]. This histotype-specific characteristic has been confirmed by population-based cohorts of EOC [33,34].

Germline deleterious MMR gene variants in ovarian cancer cases appear to be very rare, which may partly be because they are associated with the rare histotypes of disease [33]. Three studies have described MMR gene mutation frequencies by ovarian cancer histotypes [33–35] (Table 4).

We have combined the data across studies to provide an estimate of the frequency in these rarer histotypes (Table 4). Deleterious variants in these genes were more frequent in END and CCC cases than HGS. No variants were reported in MUC or LGS cases, although some studies combined HGS and LGS cases. Variants were more frequently found in *MSH6* than the other genes, with CCC and END cases both having greater than 1% frequency.

Five other case-control studies have investigated MMR frequencies between 2000 and 7500 EOC cases, four of which included data from commercial laboratories where clinical grade testing was performed in women with hereditary cancer risk [26–28,57], while another was a meta-analysis [29]. These studies have estimated the OR for mutation carriers of these genes. For *MLH1* carriers the OR was 3 (95% CI, 1.47–6.59) [26], for *MSH2* carriers, OR data from different studies ranged from 2 to 14 [26–29], and for *MSH6* carriers, ranged from 2 to 9 [26–29,57]. For the MMR genes combined, the OR was estimated to be 2.3 (95% CI, 0.83–8.2) with a cumulative risk of ovarian cancer by age 80 years of 3.7% (95% CI, 1.4–13%) in cases from a population-based study [33].

A Lynch syndrome prospective study had estimated the cumulative risk of ovarian cancer as a unique disease to be 10% (95% CI 4.8–15.4%) for *MLH1* carriers by the age of 75 years, 17% (95% CI 5.7–28.0%) for *MSH2* carriers, and 13% (95% CI 0.1–31.2%) for *MSH6* carriers [13]. The risk in the different EOC histotypes was not reported [13], although it is known that they are mostly seen in END and CCC cases.

The cumulative risk of endometrial cancer by the age of 75 years was estimated to be 43% (95% CI 33.1–52.3%), 57% (95% CI 41.8–71.6%), and 46% (95% CI 27.3–65.0%) for *MLH1*, *MSH2*, and *MSH6* carriers, respectively [13]. Due to the increased risk of both ovarian and endometrial cancer in women with Lynch syndrome, discussion about RRSO with hysterectomy is recommended. MMR carriers from these Lynch syndrome families were also reported to have an increased risk of colorectal, upper gastrointestinal, urinary tract, prostate, and brain cancers [13].

3. Missense Variants in Confirmed Susceptibility Genes

Protein truncating variants have been classified as deleterious, however a relatively large number of missense variants, including some rare predicted pathogenic missense variants have also been identified in these genes. Determining if any of these missense variants are also pathogenic is important for patient management and risk prediction in families.

3.1. BRCA1/2 and MMR Genes

Over many years, due to efforts of commercial labs, independent research groups, and large consortia, many missense variants of unknown significance (VUS) or unclassified variants (UV) have been reclassified as either pathogenic or benign. However, there are still many variants that remain unclassified. Large-scale consortia efforts, such as the Evidence-based Network for the Interpretation of Germline Mutant Alleles (ENIGMA) are in the process of investigating and classifying these variants in the *BRCA1/2* genes and the interpretation of the results of genetic testing for reporting and counselling [58].

Table 4. Frequency of germline pathogenic variants in the mismatch repair (MMR) genes in EOC histotypes, in cases from population studies.

Gene	Study	Cases Carriers/Total (Frequency)							Controls Carriers/Total (Frequency)
		HGS	END	CCC	LGS	MUC	Mixed/Unk [a]	All EOC	Matched
MLH1	Song et al., 2014 [33]	0/1105 * (0%)	0/322 (0%)	1/192 (0.52%)	0/172 (0%)	0/157 (0%)	0/274 (0%)	1/2222 (0.04%)	2/1528 (0.13%)
	Norquist et al., 2016 [35]	0/1498 (0%)	0/77 (0%)	0/58 (0%)	0/70 (0%)	0/16 (0%)	1/196 [b] (0.51%)	1/1915 (0.05%)	-
	Total	**0/2603 (0%)**	**0/399 (0%)**	**1/250 (0.40%)**	**0/242 (0%)**	**0/173 (0%)**	**1/470 (0.21%)**	**2/4137 (0.04%)**	**2/1528 (0.13%)**
MSH2	Song et al., 2014 [33]	1/1105 * (0.09%)	0/322 (0%)	1/192 (0.52%)	0/172 (0%)	0/157 (0%)	0/274 (0%)	2/2222 (0.09%)	0/1528 (0%)
	Total	**1/1105 (0.09%)**	**0/322 (0%)**	**1/192 (0.52%)**	**0/172 (0%)**	**0/157 (0%)**	**0/274 (0%)**	**2/2222 (0.09%)**	**0/1528 (0%)**
MSH6	Walsh et al., 2011 [34]	0/242 ** (0%)	2/23 (8.7%)	0/17 (0%)	**	-	0/78 (0%)	2/360 (0.55%)	-
	Song et al., 2014 [33]	4/1105 * (0.36%)	2/322 (0.62%)	3/192 (1.56%)	0/172 (0%)	0/157 (0%)	0/274 (0%)	9/2222 (0.40%)	1/1528 (0.06%)
	Norquist et al., 2016 [35]	1/1498 (0.06%)	2/77 (2.59%)	0/58 (0%)	0/70 (0%)	0/16 (0%)	0/196 (0%)	3/1915 (0.15%)	-
	Total	**5/2845 (0.17%)**	**6/422 (1.42%)**	**3/267 (1.12%)**	**0/242 (0%)**	**0/173 (0%)**	**0/548 (0%)**	**14/4497 (0.31%)**	**1/1528 (0.06%)**
PMS2	Song et al., 2014 [33]	0/1105 * (0%)	1/322 (0.31%)	0/192 (0%)	0/172 (0%)	0/157 (0.6%)	0/274 (0%)	1/2222 (0.04%)	0/1528 (0%)
	Norquist et al., 2016 [35]	4/1498 (0.3%)	0/77 (0%)	0/58 (0%)	0/70 (0%)	0/16 (0%)	0/196 (0%)	4/1915 (0.20%)	-
	Total	**4/2603 (0.15%)**	**1/399 (0.25%)**	**0/250 (0%)**	**0/242 (0%)**	**0/173 (0%)**	**0/470 (0%)**	**5/4137 (0.12%)**	**0/1528 (0%)**
All 4 genes	**Total [$]**	**10/2845 (0.35%)**	**7/422 (1.65%)**	**5/267 (1.87%)**	**0/242 (0%)**	**0/173 (0%)**	**1/548 (0.18%)**	**23/4497 (0.51%)**	**3/1528 (0.19%)**

-: Not available, ** serous combined, * HGS and serous undifferentiated, [a] Mixed/Unknown includes some other histotypes, [b] *MLH1* variant found in carcinosarcoma, [$] Totals did not include overlapped studies. Bold: highlight info.

To date, the National Institutes of Health (NIH) repository, ClinVar, has reported approximately 7000 pathogenic or likely pathogenic variants and 7400 VUS in *BRCA1/2* genes (mostly missense changes, but also in-frame deletions and insertions, and intronic and exonic variants that may affect splicing efficiency) [59]. The same clinical challenge occurs in patients with variants in the MMR genes, approximately 30% of all variants are classified as VUS [60].

Individual studies may include analysis of missense variants using bioinformatic tools such as SIFT [61], PolyPhen-2 [62], and Provean [63] to predict the functional effect of variants. Association between predicted deleterious rare missense variants and ovarian cancer risk can be assessed using burden tests, such as the rare admixture maximum likelihood test (RAML), that accounts for differences in risk of each associated variant [64]. Song et al. have performed this type of analysis in 131 predicted deleterious missense variants in *BRCA1/2* and the MMR genes (*MLH1*, *MSH2*, *MSH6*, and *PMS2*) and found little evidence for ovarian cancer risk association between these variants in any of the six genes [33].

3.2. *BRIP1*, *RAD51C/D* and *PALB2*

Missense variants in the moderate-risk genes recently confirmed as susceptibility genes in ovarian cancer need further investigation to determine if any are likely to be pathogenic. Some studies have included predicted deleterious missense variants in estimating mutation frequencies.

Ramus et al. used SIFT, PolyPhen-2, and Provean scores to predict if uncommon (minor allele frequency (MAF) < 1%) and rare (MAF < 0.1%) missense variants were potentially deleterious and identified 35 for *BRIP1* and 26 in *PALB2*. They performed the RAML burden test and found an increased risk association for uncommon and rare missense variants in *BRIP1*, but not for *PALB2* [11,54].

In *RAD51C/D*, Song et al. performed the RAML test for 28 rare predicted deleterious missense variants (12 in *RAD51C* and 16 in *RAD51D*) [48]. Evidence for an association of rare predicted deleterious missense variants with an increased risk of ovarian cancer was observed in both genes [48] (Table 5).

The data from the RAML burden test suggest that some of the predicted deleterious missense variants in *BRIP1*, *RAD51C*, and *RAD51D* likely increase disease risk, but it does not indicate how many or which ones. There is no evidence for specific missense variants.

Table 5. Predicted deleterious missense variants in known moderate risk genes for EOC.

Genes	Study	Cases Del Missense/Total (Frequency)	Predicted Deleterious	Evidence of Risk from RAML
BRIP1	Ramus et al., 2015 [11]	35/3227 [a] (1.1%)	SIFT, PolyPhen-2 and Provean	Yes (All EOC, but stronger in HGS)
	Suszynska et al., 2020 [45]	2 */22494	Described in ClinVar	-
RAD51C	Song et al., 2015 [11]	12/3429 [b] (0.32%)	SIFT, PolyPhen-2 and Provean	Yes (All EOC, but stronger in HGS)
	Lilyquist et al., 2017 [27]	2 $/6294	Described in ClinVar	-
	Norquist et al., 2016 [35]	1 #/1915 [c]	Functional assay [65]	-
	Suszynska et al., 2020 [45]	3 ^/22,494	Described in ClinVar	-
RAD51D	Song et al., 2015 [11]	16/3429 (0.46%)	SIFT, PolyPhen-2 and Provean	Yes (Only in HGS)
	Suszynska et al., 2020 [45]	1 ¶/22,494	Described in ClinVar	-
PALB2	Ramus et al., 2015 [11]	26/3227 (0.80%)	SIFT, PolyPhen-2 and Provean	No
	Song et al., 2019 [54]	40/5123 [a] (0.78%)	SIFT, PolyPhen-2 and Provean	No

-: Not available, [a] All variants reported in HGS, [b] One variant found in LGS – (histotype not available for the other variants), [c] Variant found in a serous carcinoma. *ClinVar reported variants:* * p.Gln169 = and p.Ala349Pro; $ p.C135Y and p.L138F; # p.Q143R; ^ p.Cys135Tyr, p.Cys135Ser and p.Leu138Phe; ¶ p.Ser207Leu.

4. Deleterious Variants in Other Proposed Susceptibility Genes

4.1. FANCM

FANCM is part of the Fanconi anemia group together with *BRCA2*, *BRIP1* and *PALB2* (also known as *FANCD1*, *FANCJ*, and *FANCN*). A case-control study was performed by Dicks et al. where *FANCM* targeted sequencing was performed in 3107 HGS cases, 1491 cases of other histotypes, and 3368 unaffected matched controls [66]. A significantly higher frequency of protein truncating variants was found in the HGS cases compared to the controls (p 0.008) and no evidence of association was observed with other histotypes (p 0.82) [66]. The relative risk for HGS was estimated to be 2.5 (95% CI 1.3–5) with lifetime average risk of 3.8% (80% CI 2.2–4.5%) [66]. Lifetime risk was increased when known ovarian cancer risk factors such as common risk alleles and lifestyle factors were taken into account (4.6% (80% CI 3.1–7.0%) and 5.2% (80% CI 3.4–7.8%), respectively) [66]. Additionally, the RAML test was performed for 243 uncommon predicted deleterious missense variants (effect given by at least two of the three function prediction programs Polyphen-2, Provean, and SIFT), but there was no difference in the frequency of these variants in cases compared to controls [66].

Although this study had shown evidence of association between germline protein truncating variants in *FANCM* and moderate increase in risk of HGS ovarian cancer, larger and prospective studies are still needed to confirm this.

4.2. ATM

ATM is a candidate ovarian cancer susceptibility gene due to its role in breast [67] and pancreatic cancer [68]. Germline heterozygous pathogenic *ATM* variants are associated with fivefold higher risk of breast cancer by the age of 50 years [67] and some rare variants have been shown to have penetrance as high as the *BRCA2* gene [69].

In ovarian cancer, case-control studies mainly enriched for a family history of breast or ovarian cancer, have suggested that pathogenic or likely pathogenic variants in *ATM* might be associated with moderate increased risk (OR 1.69, 95% CI 1.2–2.4 [26]; Standardized risk ratio (SRR) 2.25, 95% CI 1.7–3 [27]; OR 1.97, 95% CI 1.3–3 [29]; OR 2.4, 95% CI 1.2–4.7 [35]; OR 2.85, 95% CI 1.3–6.3 [57]), however the cumulative lifetime risk has been estimated to be lower than 3%.

4.3. BARD1 and NBN

The *BARD1* and *NBN* genes were included in breast/ovarian cancer genetic panel tests, due to their breast cancer risk, despite the ovarian cancer risk for deleterious variants in these genes being unknown. The *BARD1* encoded protein interacts closely with the *BRCA1* protein due to sharing the N-terminal RING finger and the BRCA1 C-terminal domains. Interaction between these genes affects double-strand break repair and apoptosis suggesting that this protein may play an important role in *BRCA1* tumour suppression [70]. Consequently, *BARD1* was considered a potential candidate susceptibility gene for ovarian cancer. However, Ramus et al. found no significant differences in *BARD1* deleterious variants frequency in a cohort of ~3200 ovarian cancer cases compared with ~3400 matched-controls (p 0.39) [11]. Several additional case-control studies confirmed that no evidence of association was observed between ovarian cancer risk and pathogenic variants in *BARD1* (OR 0.59, 95% CI 0.21–1.68 [26]; SSR 1.28, 95% CI 0.55–2.51 [27]; OR 1.4, 95% CI 0.7–2.9 [29]). A moderate increase in breast cancer risk has been suggested but more evidence is needed to validate these findings [70,71].

The *NBN* encoded protein interacts with *MRE11A* and *RAD50* encoded proteins as a large complex, which interacts with the protein produced by the *ATM* gene. These combined proteins have an important role in identifying broken strands of DNA and repairing it. Due to its essential function in the DNA repair pathway and because this gene is commercially available in gene testing panels for ovarian cancer, case-controls studies have examined if they are susceptibility genes. However, most studies have not found a higher frequency of pathogenic variants in *NBN*, *MRE11A*, or *RAD50* in cases compared to controls (*NBN*: *p* 0.61 [11] and 0.09 [35]; *MRE11A*: *p* 1.0 [35]; *RAD50*: *p* 0.63 [35]) and therefore no evidence of association with risk was observed in any of these 3 genes.

4.4. *CHECK2*

Germline pathogenic variants in *CHECK2* (a cell cycle checkpoint regulator) are associated with an increased risk of breast cancer [72] and *CHECK2* was proposed to be a candidate gene for ovarian cancer risk on that basis. A prospective study had shown that in estrogen receptor–positive breast cancer, CHEK2*1100delC heterozygosity was associated with increased risk of early death, breast cancer–specific death, and risk of a second breast cancer [72]. However, numerous retrospective case-control studies did not find an association between pathogenic variants in *CHECK2* and an increased risk of ovarian cancer [26,27,35].

4.5. *Other Genes*

TP53 was suggested as a potential candidate susceptibility gene for ovarian cancer from a case only study [34] and from a whole-exome sequencing analysis where protein truncating variants were identified at a greater frequency in ovarian cancer cases compared to publicly available controls (OR 18.5; 95% CI, 2.6–808.1) [34,57]. This gene has not been validated in other targeted sequencing and WES studies [26,35].

Other candidate genes selected for targeted sequencing validation in cases and controls have shown weak evidence of association with ovarian cancer risk for protein truncating variants in *POLK*, *SLX4* (also known as *FANCP*), and *FBXO10*, but further studies are required to confirm this [54]. Several Fanconi Anaemia genes (*FANCA*, *FANCB*, *FANCC*, *FANCD2*, *FANCE*, *FANCG*, *FANCI*, and *FANCL*) have been tested in these case-control studies but a risk association has not been detected [54]. A large number of other genes have been examined and not been shown to be ovarian cancer risk genes [48,57,66].

5. Discussion

We have presented a comprehensive review of the contribution of rare genetic variants to ovarian cancer, with a focus on the relationship between genetic variation and ovarian cancer histotypes, using data mostly only presented as supplementary in the original papers.

For *BRCA1/2*, deleterious germline variants are more common in HGS (8% for *BRCA1* and 6% for *BRCA2*), but there is a significant frequency of variants in END (3% for both genes), CCC (3% for *BRCA1* and 1% for *BRCA2*), and LGS (3% for *BRCA1* and 2% for *BRCA2*) patients. Consequently, the current guidelines recommend *BRCA1/2* testing in all non-mucinous ovarian cancer cases. For the MMR genes, the frequency of deleterious germline variants is higher in END and CCC patients, with variants in *MSH6* being more common than variants in *MLH1*, *MSH2*, and *PMS2* (greater than 1% in *MSH6* and approximately or less than 0.5% in *MLH1/MSH2/PMS2*). For *BRIP1*, the frequency of protein truncating variants seems to be similar for HGS and END (approximately 1.2%), but slightly lower for LGS cases (0.8%). For *RAD51C*, a slightly higher frequency of variants in the HGS cases is observed (0.5%), and frequencies range from 0.2 to 0.4% in END, CCC, and LGS. No variants in MUC were found. In contrast, a higher frequency of protein truncating variants in END cases is seen for *RAD51D* (0.9%), compared to the HGS cases (0.5%). No variants were detected in CCC, LGS, or MUC. A higher frequency of protein truncating variants in CCC is seen in *PALB2*, compared to 0.4% in HGS and 0.2% in LGS. However, larger numbers of the non-HGS cases are needed to confirm these frequencies especially in the moderate risk genes that have been recently confirmed as susceptibility genes for ovarian cancer.

The role of individual missense variants in the known ovarian cancer genes is not yet known. Work by the ENIGMA consortium is underway to identify deleterious missense variants in *BRCA1* and *BRCA2*, and ongoing efforts will be required for other genes [58].

The frequency of large genomic alternations (insertions, deletions, and rearrangements) have been examined in *BRCA1/2* and the MMR genes [17,73]. These types of changes make up 8–40% of *BRCA1* mutations, depending on the population [17]. We do not yet know how frequent they are in the *BRIP1*,

RAD51C, *RAD51D*, and *PALB2* genes, and this could affect prevalence estimates. These types of changes cannot be detected with the methods currently used for targeted sequencing in clinical panel testing.

As outcomes in ovarian cancer are linked to its stage at diagnosis, the ability to identify women at risk earlier or before diagnosis has important clinical implications. The use of multigene panel testing has allowed women to be tested for multiple genetic variants associated with increased cancer risk, enabling personalised risk estimates to be developed [74,75]. While screening for ovarian cancer has not been shown to reduce mortality, RRSO can be offered to women at a sufficiently high risk of developing ovarian cancer [4,5].

There has been some debate as to what level of lifetime cancer risk justifies prophylactic surgical intervention. Traditionally, a threshold of greater than 10% lifetime ovarian cancer risk was used, allowing for RRSO in women carrying *BRCA1*, *BRCA2*, or mismatch repair gene mutations, which confer lifetime ovarian cancer risk well in excess of 10% [76]. The more recent discovery of moderate penetrance genes has prompted formal studies into risk thresholds for invention, and recent analyses have suggested that offering RRSO to women with a lifetime risk as low as 4–5% can be cost-effective [50]. On that basis, women carrying variants in *BRIP1*, *RAD51C*, and *RAD51D* may also be offered RRSO [77,78].

The best approach to managing patients with genetic variants that do not sufficiently increase ovarian cancer risk to justify RRSO but increase risk to higher than that of the general population is not yet known. While it is plausible that targeting these women for screening may allow for detection of cancers at an earlier stage, this has not been studied. Studies investigating the impact of ovarian cancer screening using ultrasonographic and biochemical methods in both the general population, and high-risk groups (greater than 10% risk on the basis of family history or presence of genetic variants) have been associated with stage-shift, but have not been shown to significantly reduce mortality [5,79].

Genetic testing is fraught with ethical, legal, and psychosocial implications for patients, and the rate of advancement in our understanding of cancer genetics often outstrips our ability to use information in the clinic [80,81]. It is important to note that genetic susceptibility to EOC cancer does not exist in isolation, and variants conferring increased ovarian cancer risk also often increase the risk of developing other cancers—most notably breast cancer in *BRCA1* and *BRCA2*, and colon cancer in Lynch syndrome. Furthermore, breast and ovarian cancer genes are often combined into a single panel test, potentially uncovering variants in genes for which pathogenicity is disputed. As an example, *PALB2* is associated with a lifetime breast cancer risk of 53%, but also lifetime risks of 5% and 2–3% for ovarian and pancreatic malignancies, respectively [12]. While a 53% lifetime breast cancer risk is clearly clinically actionable, the risk of ovarian and pancreatic cancers associated with *PALB2* exists in an area of clinical uncertainty. The opposite is seen for deleterious variants in *BRIP1*, with an increased risk of ovarian cancer but no increase in breast cancer risk. For these reasons, all women undergoing genetic testing for familial susceptibility to ovarian cancer should receive appropriate pre- and post-test counselling, and follow-up with relevant clinical services. Genetic information should be applied cautiously in the clinic, after careful evaluation of the available literature, as some genes included on so called "ovarian cancer" panel tests have now been shown not to increase ovarian cancer risk [82,83] (Table 6). The risks of ovarian and breast cancer for genes in the double-strand DNA break repair pathway are shown in Figure 1.

Current testing guidelines do not recommend population-based genetic testing for ovarian cancer, however population-based testing approaches may be effective in groups with a small number of common founder mutations such as the three *BRCA1/2* variants in Ashkenazi Jews [86,87]. With the decreasing costs of sequencing methods, these approaches may also become cost effective in other populations. Population-based genetic testing has many issues, including cultural and psychosocial, that need to be investigated [87]. The majority of the genetic studies in ovarian cancer have been performed in white populations, and work on other ethnic groups is ongoing [88].

Table 6. Summary of the frequency of deleterious variants by EOC histotype for each homologous recombination (HR) gene and the MMR genes, and a comparison of risk and clinical management for ovarian and breast cancer patients.

Genes	Frequency (%)					Risk Est. ^		Risk Level		Clinical Management $	
	HGS	END	CCC	LGS	MUC	EOC	BC	EOC	BC	EOC	BC
BRCA1	7.8	2.9	3.6	3.7	<1	60	72% *	Very high	Very high	RRSO age 35 to 45 PARPi	RRM age 25 to 40
BRCA2	5.9	2.9	<1	2	<1	17	69% *	High	Very high		
MMR	<1	1.6	1.9	0	0	2.3	-	Mod	None	RRSO with hysterectomy for LS	No increased risk
BRIP1	1.2	1.2	0	<1	0	11.2	-	Mod	None	RRSO age 45 to 50 no consensus	Insufficient evidence
RAD51C	<1	<1	<1	<1	0	5.2	1.9	Mod	None		
RAD51D	<1	<1	0	0	0	12	1.8	Mod	None		
PALB2	<1	0	2.4	<1	0	3.0	7.2	Low	Mod	Insufficient evidence	Annual mammography/breast MRI age 30 no consensus
TP53	Insufficient data					Insuf	Insuf	Low	Mod	Insufficient evidence	Insufficient evidence
CHEK2	No increased risk					-	3.0	None	Low	No increased risk	Annual mammography/breast MRI age 40 no consensus
ATM	No increased risk					-	2.8	None	Low		
NBN	No increased risk					-	2.7	None	Low		
RAD50	No increased risk					-	Insuf	None	Low	No increased risk	Insufficient evidence
MRE11A	No increased risk					-	Insuf	None	Low		

Abbreviations: BC—breast cancer; RRM—Risk-reducing mastectomy; LS—Lynch Syndrome; MRI—Magnetic Resonance Imaging; Insuf—Insufficient. ^ From Tables 1, 3 and 4. EOC *BRCA1/2* from ref [33], MMR from ref [33], *BRIP1* from ref [11], *RAD51C/D* from ref [48], *PALB2* from ref [54]. BC *BRCA1/2* from ref [9], *RAD51C/D* from ref [10], *PALB2* from ref [12], *CHEK2/ATM/NBN* from ref [84]. $ *BRCA1/2* from refs [39,85], MMR from ref [13], *BRIP1/RAD51C/D* from ref [49], *PALB2/CHEK2/ATM/NBN* from refs [77,84]. * Cumulative risk data by the age of 80.

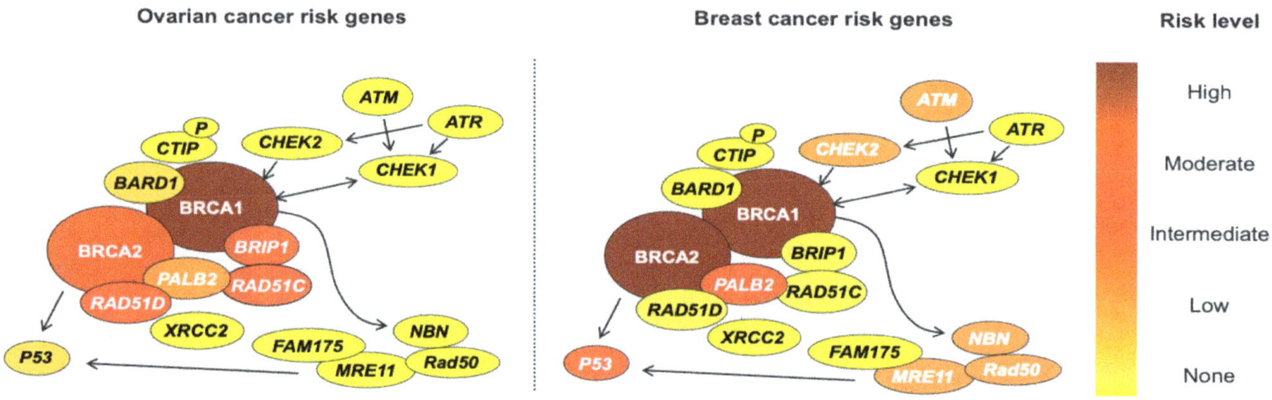

Figure 1. Susceptibility genes present in the double-strand DNA break repair pathway for ovarian and breast cancer and its different correspondent risks levels in each disease.

Identifying ovarian cancer genes has translated to novel therapeutic options for patients. PARP inhibitors, which target double-stranded DNA repair in cells with deficient homologous recombination, including cells with dysfunctional BRCA DNA repair pathways, have been shown to improve progression free survival (PFS) in serous and endometrioid ovarian cancers [89–92]. The impact of PARP inhibitors on PFS is most dramatic in patients with mutations in *BRCA1* and *BRCA2*, but can also benefit women without BRCA mutations if they are found to have deficiencies in homologous recombination, such as variants in the DNA repair genes discussed above [92]. However, improvements in PFS do not necessarily translate to improved overall survival, and the impact of PARP inhibitors on the overall survival endpoint has not yet been reported [92].

To date, ovarian cancer has largely been treated as a single entity. However, as outlined above, the five main histotypes of epithelial ovarian cancer appear to be characterised by distinct genetic mutations. The tumours also have different molecular profiles, and patients have different treatment responses [93]. Therefore, it has become increasingly clear that ovarian cancer represents not just a single disease but encompasses a number of distinct cancers. Most of our understanding of ovarian cancer genes relates to high-grade serous tumours, as they represent the majority of ovarian cancers. Identifying genetic variants contributing to non-serous ovarian cancers has posed an ongoing challenge for researchers, as finding rare variants for rare cancers requires studies with sample sizes that are not yet feasible.

Despite significant advancements in our understanding of the genetic epidemiology of ovarian cancer, the known ovarian cancer risk variants explain less than half of the excess familial risk for ovarian cancer [8]. Efforts to identify novel genetic variants associated with ovarian cancer are ongoing. The discovery of new genetic variants should be accompanied by efforts to accurately quantify the exact magnitude of increased risk associated with that variant. Case-control studies, the most commonly used study design in gene discovery, are only able to generate relative risks, from which absolute risks are extrapolated.

Prospective population-based studies, which have been used to provide gold-standard estimates of lifetime cancer risk in *BRCA1*, *BRCA2*, and the mismatch repair genes, would provide more accurate risk estimates for moderate penetrance ovarian cancer genes, but are costly, and require long-term investment. Segregation analysis from large international consortia has been used to calculate ovarian cancer risks in *RAD51C*, *RAD51D*, and *PALB2*, and could be applied to other moderate risk ovarian cancer genes [10,12].

Genetic association studies, by their design, are unable to establish a causal relationship between germline variant status and cancer phenotype. The discovery of novel ovarian cancer risk genes should be followed-up by further efforts to characterise the functional mechanisms by which they contribute to cancer development and identify potential therapeutic targets.

6. Conclusions

Ovarian cancer is the most lethal gynaecological malignancy, and an improved understanding of the contribution of rare genetic variants to the development of ovarian cancer allows for better clinical management of at-risk women. Based on the best available evidence, variants in *BRCA1*, *BRCA2*, *BRIP1*, *RAD51C*, *RAD51D*, and the mismatch repair genes confer ovarian cancer risks that warrant the consideration of risk-reducing surgery. The best approach for managing women with deleterious variants in ovarian cancer genes that do not warrant prophylactic surgery requires further investigation.

References

1. Bray, F.; Ferlay, J.; Soerjomataram, I.; Siegel, R.L.; Torre, L.A.; Jemal, A. Global cancer statistics 2018: GLOBOCAN estimates of incidence and mortality worldwide for 36 cancers in 185 countries. *CA Cancer J. Clin.* **2018**, *68*, 394–424. [CrossRef]
2. Prat, J. Ovarian carcinomas: Five distinct diseases with different origins, genetic alterations, and clinicopathological features. *Virchows Arch.* **2012**, *460*, 237–249. [CrossRef]
3. Torre, L.A.; Trabert, B.; DeSantis, C.E.; Miller, K.D.; Samimi, G.; Runowicz, C.D.; Gaudet, M.M.; Jemal, A.; Siegel, R.L. Ovarian cancer statistics, 2018. *CA Cancer J. Clin.* **2018**, *68*, 284–296. [CrossRef]
4. Buys, S.S.; Partridge, E.; Black, A.; Johnson, C.C.; Lamerato, L.; Isaacs, C.; Reding, D.J.; Greenlee, R.T.; Yokochi, L.A.; Kessel, B.; et al. Effect of screening on ovarian cancer mortality: The Prostate, Lung, Colorectal and Ovarian (PLCO) Cancer Screening Randomized Controlled Trial. *JAMA* **2011**, *305*, 2295–2303. [CrossRef]
5. Jacobs, I.J.; Menon, U.; Ryan, A.; Gentry-Maharaj, A.; Burnell, M.; Kalsi, J.K.; Amso, N.N.; Apostolidou, S.; Benjamin, E.; Cruickshank, D.; et al. Ovarian cancer screening and mortality in the UK Collaborative Trial of Ovarian Cancer Screening (UKCTOCS): A randomised controlled trial. *Lancet* **2016**, *387*, 945–956. [CrossRef]
6. Jayson, G.C.; Kohn, E.C.; Kitchener, H.C.; Ledermann, J.A. Ovarian cancer. *Lancet* **2014**, *384*, 1376–1388. [CrossRef]
7. Thomas, D.M.; James, P.A.; Ballinger, M.L. Clinical implications of genomics for cancer risk genetics. *Lancet Oncol.* **2015**, *16*, e303–e308. [CrossRef]
8. Jervis, S.; Song, H.; Lee, A.; Dicks, E.; Tyrer, J.; Harrington, P.; Easton, D.F.; Jacobs, I.J.; Pharoah, P.P.; Antoniou, A.C. Ovarian cancer familial relative risks by tumour subtypes and by known ovarian cancer genetic susceptibility variants. *J. Med. Genet.* **2014**, *51*, 108–113. [CrossRef]
9. Kuchenbaecker, K.B.; Hopper, J.L.; Barnes, D.R.; Phillips, K.A.; Mooij, T.M.; Roos-Blom, M.J.; Jervis, S.; van Leeuwen, F.E.; Milne, R.L.; Andrieu, N.; et al. Risks of Breast, Ovarian, and Contralateral Breast Cancer for BRCA1 and BRCA2 Mutation Carriers. *JAMA* **2017**, *317*, 2402–2416. [CrossRef]
10. Yang, X.; Song, H.; Leslie, G.; Engel, C.; Hahnen, E.; Auber, B.; Horváth, J.; Kast, K.; Niederacher, D.; Turnbull, C.; et al. Ovarian and Breast Cancer Risks Associated With Pathogenic Variants in RAD51C and RAD51D. *J. Natl. Cancer Inst.* **2020**, *112*. [CrossRef]
11. Ramus, S.J.; Song, H.; Dicks, E.; Tyrer, J.P.; Rosenthal, A.N.; Intermaggio, M.P.; Fraser, L.; Gentry-Maharaj, A.; Hayward, J.; Philpott, S.; et al. Germline Mutations in the BRIP1, BARD1, PALB2, and NBN Genes in Women With Ovarian Cancer. *J. Natl. Cancer Inst.* **2015**, *107*. [CrossRef]
12. Yang, X.; Leslie, G.; Doroszuk, A.; Schneider, S.; Allen, J.; Decker, B.; Dunning, A.M.; Redman, J.; Scarth, J.; Plaskocinska, I.; et al. Cancer Risks Associated with Germline PALB2 Pathogenic Variants: An International Study of 524 Families. *J. Clin. Oncol.* **2020**, *38*, 674–685. [CrossRef]
13. Møller, P.; Seppälä, T.T.; Bernstein, I.; Holinski-Feder, E.; Sala, P.; Gareth Evans, D.; Lindblom, A.; Macrae, F.; Blanco, I.; Sijmons, R.H.; et al. Cancer risk and survival in path_MMR carriers by gene and gender up to 75 years of age: A report from the Prospective Lynch Syndrome Database. *Gut* **2018**, *67*, 1306–1316. [CrossRef]

14. Kar, S.P.; Berchuck, A.; Gayther, S.A.; Goode, E.L.; Moysich, K.B.; Pearce, C.L.; Ramus, S.J.; Schildkraut, J.M.; Sellers, T.A.; Pharoah, P.D.P. Common Genetic Variation and Susceptibility to Ovarian Cancer: Current Insights and Future Directions. *Cancer Epidemiol. Biomark. Prev.* **2018**, *27*, 395. [CrossRef]
15. Phelan, C.M.; Kuchenbaecker, K.B.; Tyrer, J.P.; Kar, S.P.; Lawrenson, K.; Winham, S.J.; Dennis, J.; Pirie, A.; Riggan, M.J.; Chornokur, G.; et al. Identification of 12 new susceptibility loci for different histotypes of epithelial ovarian cancer. *Nat. Genet.* **2017**, *49*, 680–691. [CrossRef]
16. Ramus, S.J.; Harrington, P.A.; Pye, C.; DiCioccio, R.A.; Cox, M.J.; Garlinghouse-Jones, K.; Oakley-Girvan, I.; Jacobs, I.J.; Hardy, R.M.; Whittemore, A.S.; et al. Contribution of BRCA1 and BRCA2 mutations to inherited ovarian cancer. *Hum. Mutat.* **2007**, *28*, 1207–1215. [CrossRef]
17. Ramus, S.J.; Gayther, S.A. The Contribution of BRCA1 and BRCA2 to Ovarian Cancer. *Mol. Oncol.* **2009**, *3*, 138–150. [CrossRef]
18. Johannesdottir, G.; Gudmundsson, J.; Bergthorsson, J.T.; Arason, A.; Agnarsson, B.A.; Eiriksdottir, G.; Johannsson, O.T.; Borg, A.; Ingvarsson, S.; Easton, D.F.; et al. High Prevalence of the 999del5 Mutation in Icelandic Breast and Ovarian Cancer Patients. *Cancer Res.* **1996**, *56*, 3663–3665.
19. Gayther, S.A.; Harrington, P.; Russell, P.; Kharkevich, G.; Garkavtseva, R.F.; Ponder, B.A. Frequently occurring germ-line mutations of the BRCA1 gene in ovarian cancer families from Russia. *Am. J. Hum. Genet.* **1997**, *60*, 1239–1242.
20. Sokolenko, A.P.; Rozanov, M.E.; Mitiushkina, N.V.; Sherina, N.Y.; Iyevleva, A.G.; Chekmariova, E.V.; Buslov, K.G.; Shilov, E.S.; Togo, A.V.; Bit-Sava, E.M.; et al. Founder mutations in early-onset, familial and bilateral breast cancer patients from Russia. *Fam. Cancer* **2007**, *6*, 281–286. [CrossRef] [PubMed]
21. Menkiszak, J.; Gronwald, J.; Górski, B.; Jakubowska, A.; Huzarski, T.; Byrski, T.; Foszczyńska-Kłoda, M.; Haus, O.; Janiszewska, H.; Perkowska, M.; et al. Hereditary ovarian cancer in Poland. *Int. J. Cancer* **2003**, *106*, 942–945. [CrossRef]
22. Heimdal, K.; Maehle, L.; Apold, J.; Pedersen, J.C.; Møller, P. The Norwegian founder mutations in BRCA1: High penetrance confirmed in an incident cancer series and differences observed in the risk of ovarian cancer. *Eur. J. Cancer* **2003**, *39*, 2205–2213. [CrossRef]
23. Sarantaus, L.; Huusko, P.; Eerola, H.; Launonen, V.; Vehmanen, P.; Rapakko, K.; Gillanders, E.; Syrjäkoski, K.; Kainu, T.; Vahteristo, P.; et al. Multiple founder effects and geographical clustering of BRCA1 and BRCA2 families in Finland. *Eur. J. Hum. Genet.* **2000**, *8*, 757–763. [CrossRef]
24. Sekine, M.; Nagata, H.; Tsuji, S.; Hirai, Y.; Fujimoto, S.; Hatae, M.; Kobayashi, I.; Fujii, T.; Nagata, I.; Ushijima, K.; et al. Mutational analysis of BRCA1 and BRCA2 and clinicopathologic analysis of ovarian cancer in 82 ovarian cancer families: Two common founder mutations of BRCA1 in Japanese population. *Clin. Cancer Res.* **2001**, *7*, 3144–3150.
25. Khoo, U.S.; Chan, K.Y.; Cheung, A.N.; Xue, W.C.; Shen, D.H.; Fung, K.Y.; Ngan, H.Y.; Choy, K.W.; Pang, C.P.; Poon, C.S.; et al. Recurrent BRCA1 and BRCA2 germline mutations in ovarian cancer: A founder mutation of BRCA1 identified in the Chinese population. *Hum. Mutat.* **2002**, *19*, 307–308. [CrossRef]
26. Kurian, A.W.; Hughes, E.; Handorf, E.A.; Gutin, A.; Allen, B.; Hartman, A.-R.; Hall, M.J. Breast and Ovarian Cancer Penetrance Estimates Derived from Germline Multiple-Gene Sequencing Results in Women. *JCO Precis. Oncol.* **2017**, *1*, 1–12. [CrossRef]
27. Lilyquist, J.; LaDuca, H.; Polley, E.; Davis, B.T.; Shimelis, H.; Hu, C.; Hart, S.N.; Dolinsky, J.S.; Couch, F.J.; Goldgar, D.E. Frequency of mutations in a large series of clinically ascertained ovarian cancer cases tested on multi-gene panels compared to reference controls. *Gynecol. Oncol.* **2017**, *147*, 375–380. [CrossRef]
28. Castéra, L.; Harter, V.; Muller, E.; Krieger, S.; Goardon, N.; Ricou, A.; Rousselin, A.; Paimparay, G.; Legros, A.; Bruet, O.; et al. Landscape of pathogenic variations in a panel of 34 genes and cancer risk estimation from 5131 HBOC families. *Genet. Med.* **2018**, *20*, 1677–1686. [CrossRef]
29. Suszynska, M.; Klonowska, K.; Jasinska, A.J.; Kozlowski, P. Large-scale meta-analysis of mutations identified in panels of breast/ovarian cancer-related genes—Providing evidence of cancer predisposition genes. *Gynecol. Oncol.* **2019**, *153*, 452–462. [CrossRef]
30. Iqbal, J.; Ragone, A.; Lubinski, J.; Lynch, H.T.; Moller, P.; Ghadirian, P.; Foulkes, W.D.; Armel, S.; Eisen, A.; Neuhausen, S.L.; et al. The incidence of pancreatic cancer in BRCA1 and BRCA2 mutation carriers. *Br. J. Cancer* **2012**, *107*, 2005–2009. [CrossRef]

31. Pritchard, C.C.; Mateo, J.; Walsh, M.F.; De Sarkar, N.; Abida, W.; Beltran, H.; Garofalo, A.; Gulati, R.; Carreira, S.; Eeles, R.; et al. Inherited DNA-Repair Gene Mutations in Men with Metastatic Prostate Cancer. *N. Engl. J. Med.* **2016**, *375*, 443–453. [CrossRef]
32. Alsop, K.; Fereday, S.; Meldrum, C.; deFazio, A.; Emmanuel, C.; George, J.; Dobrovic, A.; Birrer, M.J.; Webb, P.M.; Stewart, C.; et al. BRCA mutation frequency and patterns of treatment response in BRCA mutation-positive women with ovarian cancer: A report from the Australian Ovarian Cancer Study Group. *J. Clin. Oncol.* **2012**, *30*, 2654–2663. [CrossRef]
33. Song, H.; Cicek, M.S.; Dicks, E.; Harrington, P.; Ramus, S.J.; Cunningham, J.M.; Fridley, B.L.; Tyrer, J.P.; Alsop, J.; Jimenez-Linan, M.; et al. The contribution of deleterious germline mutations in BRCA1, BRCA2 and the mismatch repair genes to ovarian cancer in the population. *Hum. Mol. Genet.* **2014**, *23*, 4703–4709. [CrossRef]
34. Walsh, T.; Casadei, S.; Lee, M.K.; Pennil, C.C.; Nord, A.S.; Thornton, A.M.; Roeb, W.; Agnew, K.J.; Stray, S.M.; Wickramanayake, A.; et al. Mutations in 12 genes for inherited ovarian, fallopian tube, and peritoneal carcinoma identified by massively parallel sequencing. *Proc. Natl. Acad. Sci. USA* **2011**, *108*, 18032–18037. [CrossRef]
35. Norquist, B.M.; Harrell, M.I.; Brady, M.F.; Walsh, T.; Lee, M.K.; Gulsuner, S.; Bernards, S.S.; Casadei, S.; Yi, Q.; Burger, R.A.; et al. Inherited Mutations in Women with Ovarian Carcinoma. *JAMA Oncol.* **2016**, *2*, 482–490. [CrossRef]
36. Bolton, K.L.; Chenevix-Trench, G.; Goh, C.; Sadetzki, S.; Ramus, S.J.; Karlan, B.Y.; Lambrechts, D.; Despierre, E.; Barrowdale, D.; McGuffog, L.; et al. Association between BRCA1 and BRCA2 Mutations and Survival in Women with Invasive Epithelial Ovarian Cancer. *JAMA* **2012**, *307*, 382–390. [CrossRef]
37. Kotsopoulos, J.; Rosen, B.; Fan, I.; Moody, J.; McLaughlin, J.R.; Risch, H.; May, T.; Sun, P.; Narod, S.A. Ten-year survival after epithelial ovarian cancer is not associated with BRCA mutation status. *Gynecol. Oncol.* **2016**, *140*, 42–47. [CrossRef]
38. McLaughlin, J.R.; Rosen, B.; Moody, J.; Pal, T.; Fan, I.; Shaw, P.A.; Risch, H.A.; Sellers, T.A.; Sun, P.; Narod, S.A. Long-Term Ovarian Cancer Survival Associated with Mutation in BRCA1 or BRCA2. *J. Natl. Cancer Inst.* **2013**, *105*, 141–148. [CrossRef]
39. National Comprehensive Cancer Network. Genetics Screening (Version 2.2019). Available online: https://www.nccn.org/professionals/physician_gls/pdf/genetics_screening.pdf (accessed on 11 June 2020).
40. Cancer Genome Atlas Research Network. Integrated genomic analyses of ovarian carcinoma. *Nature* **2011**, *474*, 609–615. [CrossRef]
41. Kaufman, B.; Shapira-Frommer, R.; Schmutzler, R.K.; Audeh, M.W.; Friedlander, M.; Balmaña, J.; Mitchell, G.; Fried, G.; Stemmer, S.M.; Hubert, A.; et al. Olaparib monotherapy in patients with advanced cancer and a germline BRCA1/2 mutation. *J. Clin. Oncol.* **2015**, *33*, 244–250. [CrossRef]
42. Swisher, E.M.; Lin, K.K.; Oza, A.M.; Scott, C.L.; Giordano, H.; Sun, J.; Konecny, G.E.; Coleman, R.L.; Tinker, A.V.; O'Malley, D.M.; et al. Rucaparib in relapsed, platinum-sensitive high-grade ovarian carcinoma (ARIEL2 Part 1): An international, multicentre, open-label, phase 2 trial. *Lancet Oncol.* **2017**, *18*, 75–87. [CrossRef]
43. Oza, A.M.; Tinker, A.V.; Oaknin, A.; Shapira-Frommer, R.; McNeish, I.A.; Swisher, E.M.; Ray-Coquard, I.; Bell-McGuinn, K.; Coleman, R.L.; O'Malley, D.M.; et al. Antitumor activity and safety of the PARP inhibitor rucaparib in patients with high-grade ovarian carcinoma and a germline or somatic BRCA1 or BRCA2 mutation: Integrated analysis of data from Study 10 and ARIEL2. *Gynecol. Oncol.* **2017**, *147*, 267–275. [CrossRef]
44. Gelmon, K.A.; Tischkowitz, M.; Mackay, H.; Swenerton, K.; Robidoux, A.; Tonkin, K.; Hirte, H.; Huntsman, D.; Clemons, M.; Gilks, B.; et al. Olaparib in patients with recurrent high-grade serous or poorly differentiated ovarian carcinoma or triple-negative breast cancer: A phase 2, multicentre, open-label, non-randomised study. *Lancet Oncol.* **2011**, *12*, 852–861. [CrossRef]
45. Suszynska, M.; Ratajska, M.; Kozlowski, P. BRIP1, RAD51C, and RAD51D mutations are associated with high susceptibility to ovarian cancer: Mutation prevalence and precise risk estimates based on a pooled analysis of ~30,000 cases. *J. Ovarian Res.* **2020**, *13*, 50. [CrossRef]
46. Meindl, A.; Hellebrand, H.; Wiek, C.; Erven, V.; Wappenschmidt, B.; Niederacher, D.; Freund, M.; Lichtner, P.; Hartmann, L.; Schaal, H.; et al. Germline mutations in breast and ovarian cancer pedigrees establish RAD51C as a human cancer susceptibility gene. *Nat. Genet.* **2010**, *42*, 410–414. [CrossRef]

47. Loveday, C.; Turnbull, C.; Ramsay, E.; Hughes, D.; Ruark, E.; Frankum, J.R.; Bowden, G.; Kalmyrzaev, B.; Warren-Perry, M.; Snape, K.; et al. Germline mutations in RAD51D confer susceptibility to ovarian cancer. *Nat. Genet.* **2011**, *43*, 879–882. [CrossRef]
48. Song, H.; Dicks, E.; Ramus, S.J.; Tyrer, J.P.; Intermaggio, M.P.; Hayward, J.; Edlund, C.K.; Conti, D.; Harrington, P.; Fraser, L.; et al. Contribution of Germline Mutations in the RAD51B, RAD51C, and RAD51D Genes to Ovarian Cancer in the Population. *J. Clin. Oncol.* **2015**, *33*, 2901–2907. [CrossRef]
49. Manchanda, R.; Legood, R.; Antoniou, A.; Pearce, L.; Menon, U. Commentary on changing the risk threshold for surgical prevention of ovarian cancer. *BJOG An. Int. J. Obstet. Gynaecol.* **2018**, *125*, 541–544. [CrossRef]
50. Manchanda, R.; Legood, R.; Antoniou, A.C.; Gordeev, V.S.; Menon, U. Specifying the ovarian cancer risk threshold of 'premenopausal risk-reducing salpingo-oophorectomy' for ovarian cancer prevention: A cost-effectiveness analysis. *J. Med. Genet.* **2016**, *53*, 591–599. [CrossRef]
51. Manchanda, R.; Legood, R.; Pearce, L.; Menon, U. Defining the risk threshold for risk reducing salpingo-oophorectomy for ovarian cancer prevention in low risk postmenopausal women. *Gynecol. Oncol.* **2015**, *139*, 487–494. [CrossRef]
52. Antoniou, A.C.; Casadei, S.; Heikkinen, T.; Barrowdale, D.; Pylkas, K.; Roberts, J.; Lee, A.; Subramanian, D.; De Leeneer, K.; Fostira, F.; et al. Breast-cancer risk in families with mutations in PALB2. *N. Engl. J. Med.* **2014**, *371*, 497–506. [CrossRef]
53. Ducy, M.; Sesma-Sanz, L.; Guitton-Sert, L.; Lashgari, A.; Gao, Y.; Brahiti, N.; Rodrigue, A.; Margaillan, G.; Caron, M.C.; Côté, J.; et al. The Tumor Suppressor PALB2: Inside out. *Trends Biochem. Sci.* **2019**, *44*, 226–240. [CrossRef]
54. Song, H.; Ramus, S.; Dicks, E.; Tyrer, J.; Intermaggio, M.; Chenevix-Trench, G.; Bowtell, D.; Traficante, N.; Brenton, J.; Goranova, T.; et al. Population based targeted sequencing of 54 candidate genes identifies PALB2 as a susceptibility gene for high grade serous ovarian cancer. *J Med Genet.* **2020**. [CrossRef]
55. Osorio, A.; Endt, D.; Fernández, F.; Eirich, K.; de la Hoya, M.; Schmutzler, R.; Caldés, T.; Meindl, A.; Schindler, D.; Benitez, J. Predominance of pathogenic missense variants in the RAD51C gene occurring in breast and ovarian cancer families. *Hum. Mol. Genet.* **2012**, *21*, 2889–2898. [CrossRef]
56. Ketabi, Z.; Bartuma, K.; Bernstein, I.; Malander, S.; Grönberg, H.; Björck, E.; Holck, S.; Nilbert, M. Ovarian cancer linked to Lynch syndrome typically presents as early-onset, non-serous epithelial tumors. *Gynecol. Oncol.* **2011**, *121*, 462–465. [CrossRef]
57. Lu, H.M.; Li, S.; Black, M.H.; Lee, S.; Hoiness, R.; Wu, S.; Mu, W.; Huether, R.; Chen, J.; Sridhar, S.; et al. Association of Breast and Ovarian Cancers with Predisposition Genes Identified by Large-Scale Sequencing. *JAMA Oncol.* **2019**, *5*, 51–57. [CrossRef]
58. Spurdle, A.B.; Healey, S.; Devereau, A.; Hogervorst, F.B.; Monteiro, A.N.; Nathanson, K.L.; Radice, P.; Stoppa-Lyonnet, D.; Tavtigian, S.; Wappenschmidt, B.; et al. ENIGMA—Evidence-based network for the interpretation of germline mutant alleles: An international initiative to evaluate risk and clinical significance associated with sequence variation in BRCA1 and BRCA2 genes. *Hum. Mutat* **2012**, *33*, 2–7. [CrossRef]
59. Li, H.; LaDuca, H.; Pesaran, T.; Chao, E.C.; Dolinsky, J.S.; Parsons, M.; Spurdle, A.B.; Polley, E.C.; Shimelis, H.; Hart, S.N.; et al. Classification of variants of uncertain significance in BRCA1 and BRCA2 using personal and family history of cancer from individuals in a large hereditary cancer multigene panel testing cohort. *Genet. Med.* **2020**, *22*, 701–708. [CrossRef]
60. Thompson, B.A.; Spurdle, A.B.; Plazzer, J.P.; Greenblatt, M.S.; Akagi, K.; Al-Mulla, F.; Bapat, B.; Bernstein, I.; Capellá, G.; den Dunnen, J.T.; et al. Application of a 5-tiered scheme for standardized classification of 2,360 unique mismatch repair gene variants in the InSiGHT locus-specific database. *Nat. Genet.* **2014**, *46*, 107–115. [CrossRef]
61. Ng, P.C.; Henikoff, S. SIFT: Predicting amino acid changes that affect protein function. *Nucleic Acids Res.* **2003**, *31*, 3812–3814. [CrossRef]
62. Adzhubei, I.; Jordan, D.M.; Sunyaev, S.R. Predicting functional effect of human missense mutations using PolyPhen-2. *Curr. Protoc. Hum. Genet.* **2013**, *76*, 7–20. [CrossRef]
63. Choi, Y.; Chan, A.P. PROVEAN web server: A tool to predict the functional effect of amino acid substitutions and indels. *Bioinformatics* **2015**, *31*, 2745–2747. [CrossRef]
64. Tyrer, J.P.; Guo, Q.; Easton, D.F.; Pharoah, P.D. The admixture maximum likelihood test to test for association between rare variants and disease phenotypes. *BMC Bioinform.* **2013**, *14*, 177. [CrossRef]

65. Bouwman, P.; van der Gulden, H.; van der Heijden, I.; Drost, R.; Klijn, C.N.; Prasetyanti, P.; Pieterse, M.; Wientjens, E.; Seibler, J.; Hogervorst, F.B.; et al. A high-throughput functional complementation assay for classification of BRCA1 missense variants. *Cancer Discov.* **2013**, *3*, 1142–1155. [CrossRef]
66. Dicks, E.; Song, H.; Ramus, S.J.; Oudenhove, E.V.; Tyrer, J.P.; Intermaggio, M.P.; Kar, S.; Harrington, P.; Bowtell, D.D.; Group, A.S.; et al. Germline whole exome sequencing and large-scale replication identifies FANCM as a likely high grade serous ovarian cancer susceptibility gene. *Oncotarget* **2017**, *8*, 50930–50940. [CrossRef]
67. Thompson, D.; Duedal, S.; Kirner, J.; McGuffog, L.; Last, J.; Reiman, A.; Byrd, P.; Taylor, M.; Easton, D.F. Cancer Risks and Mortality in Heterozygous ATM Mutation Carriers. *JNCI J. Natl. Cancer Inst.* **2005**, *97*, 813–822. [CrossRef]
68. Roberts, N.J.; Jiao, Y.; Yu, J.; Kopelovich, L.; Petersen, G.M.; Bondy, M.L.; Gallinger, S.; Schwartz, A.G.; Syngal, S.; Cote, M.L.; et al. ATM mutations in patients with hereditary pancreatic cancer. *Cancer Discov.* **2012**, *2*, 41–46. [CrossRef]
69. Goldgar, D.E.; Healey, S.; Dowty, J.G.; Da Silva, L.; Chen, X.; Spurdle, A.B.; Terry, M.B.; Daly, M.J.; Buys, S.M.; Southey, M.C.; et al. Rare variants in the ATM gene and risk of breast cancer. *Breast Cancer Res.* **2011**, *13*, R73. [CrossRef]
70. Weber-Lassalle, N.; Borde, J.; Weber-Lassalle, K.; Horváth, J.; Niederacher, D.; Arnold, N.; Kaulfuß, S.; Ernst, C.; Paul, V.G.; Honisch, E.; et al. Germline loss-of-function variants in the BARD1 gene are associated with early-onset familial breast cancer but not ovarian cancer. *Breast Cancer Res.* **2019**, *21*, 55. [CrossRef]
71. Couch, F.J.; Shimelis, H.; Hu, C.; Hart, S.N.; Polley, E.C.; Na, J.; Hallberg, E.; Moore, R.; Thomas, A.; Lilyquist, J.; et al. Associations between Cancer Predisposition Testing Panel Genes and Breast Cancer. *JAMA Oncol.* **2017**, *3*, 1190–1196. [CrossRef]
72. Weischer, M.; Nordestgaard, B.G.; Pharoah, P.; Bolla, M.K.; Nevanlinna, H.; Van't Veer, L.J.; Garcia-Closas, M.; Hopper, J.L.; Hall, P.; Andrulis, I.L.; et al. CHEK2*1100delC heterozygosity in women with breast cancer associated with early death, breast cancer-specific death, and increased risk of a second breast cancer. *J. Clin. Oncol. Off. J. Am. Soc. Clin. Oncol.* **2012**, *30*, 4308–4316. [CrossRef]
73. Gylling, A.; Ridanpää, M.; Vierimaa, O.; Aittomäki, K.; Avela, K.; Kääriäinen, H.; Laivuori, H.; Pöyhönen, M.; Sallinen, S.-L.; Wallgren-Pettersson, C.; et al. Large genomic rearrangements and germline epimutations in Lynch syndrome. *Int. J. Cancer* **2009**, *124*, 2333–2340. [CrossRef]
74. Easton, D.F.; Pharoah, P.D.; Antoniou, A.C.; Tischkowitz, M.; Tavtigian, S.V.; Nathanson, K.L.; Devilee, P.; Meindl, A.; Couch, F.J.; Southey, M.; et al. Gene-panel sequencing and the prediction of breast-cancer risk. *N. Engl. J. Med.* **2015**, *372*, 2243–2257. [CrossRef] [PubMed]
75. Prapa, M.; Solomons, J.; Tischkowitz, M. The use of panel testing in familial breast and ovarian cancer. *Clin. Med.* **2017**, *17*, 568–572. [CrossRef]
76. Menon, U.; Karpinskyj, C.; Gentry-Maharaj, A. Ovarian Cancer Prevention and Screening. *Obstet Gynecol.* **2018**, *131*, 909–927. [CrossRef]
77. Domchek, S.M.; Robson, M.E. Update on Genetic Testing in Gynecologic Cancer. *J. Clin. Oncol.* **2019**, *37*, 2501–2509. [CrossRef]
78. Manchanda, R.; Menon, U. Setting the Threshold for Surgical Prevention in Women at Increased Risk of Ovarian Cancer. *Int. J. Gynecol. Cancer* **2018**, *28*, 34–42. [CrossRef]
79. Rosenthal, A.N.; Fraser, L.S.M.; Philpott, S.; Manchanda, R.; Burnell, M.; Badman, P.; Hadwin, R.; Rizzuto, I.; Benjamin, E.; Singh, N.; et al. Evidence of Stage Shift in Women Diagnosed with Ovarian Cancer during Phase II of the United Kingdom Familial Ovarian Cancer Screening Study. *J. Clin. Oncol.* **2017**, *35*, 1411–1420. [CrossRef] [PubMed]
80. Clayton, E.W. Ethical, legal, and social implications of genomic medicine. *N. Engl. J. Med.* **2003**, *349*, 562–569. [CrossRef]
81. Mersch, J.; Brown, N.; Pirzadeh-Miller, S.; Mundt, E.; Cox, H.C.; Brown, K.; Aston, M.; Esterling, L.; Manley, S.; Ross, T. Prevalence of Variant Reclassification Following Hereditary Cancer Genetic Testing. *JAMA* **2018**, *320*, 1266–1274. [CrossRef]
82. LaDuca, H.; Stuenkel, A.J.; Dolinsky, J.S.; Keiles, S.; Tandy, S.; Pesaran, T.; Chen, E.; Gau, C.-L.; Palmaer, E.; Shoaepour, K.; et al. Utilization of multigene panels in hereditary cancer predisposition testing: Analysis of more than 2,000 patients. *Genet. Med. Off. J. Am. Coll. Med Genet.* **2014**, *16*, 830–837. [CrossRef] [PubMed]

83. Tandy-Connor, S.; Guiltinan, J.; Krempely, K.; LaDuca, H.; Reineke, P.; Gutierrez, S.; Gray, P.; Tippin Davis, B. False-positive results released by direct-to-consumer genetic tests highlight the importance of clinical confirmation testing for appropriate patient care. *Genet. Med.* **2018**, *20*, 1515–1521. [CrossRef] [PubMed]
84. Tung, N.; Domchek, S.M.; Stadler, Z.; Nathanson, K.L.; Couch, F.; Garber, J.E.; Offit, K.; Robson, M.E. Counselling framework for moderate-penetrance cancer-susceptibility mutations. *Nat. Rev. Clin. Oncol.* **2016**, *13*, 581–588. [CrossRef] [PubMed]
85. Giuliano, A.E.; Boolbol, S.; Degnim, A.; Kuerer, H.; Leitch, A.M.; Morrow, M. Society of Surgical Oncology: Position statement on prophylactic mastectomy. Approved by the Society of Surgical Oncology Executive Council, March 2007. *Ann. Surg Oncol.* **2007**, *14*, 2425–2427. [CrossRef] [PubMed]
86. Gabai-Kapara, E.; Lahad, A.; Kaufman, B.; Friedman, E.; Segev, S.; Renbaum, P.; Beeri, R.; Gal, M.; Grinshpun-Cohen, J.; Djemal, K.; et al. Population-based screening for breast and ovarian cancer risk due to *BRCA1* and *BRCA2*. *Proc. Natl. Acad. Sci. USA* **2014**, *111*, 14205–14210. [CrossRef] [PubMed]
87. Manchanda, R.; Loggenberg, K.; Sanderson, S.; Burnell, M.; Wardle, J.; Gessler, S.; Side, L.; Balogun, N.; Desai, R.; Kumar, A.; et al. Population Testing for Cancer Predisposing BRCA1/BRCA2 Mutations in the Ashkenazi-Jewish Community: A Randomized Controlled Trial. *JNCI J. Natl. Cancer Inst.* **2014**, *107*. [CrossRef] [PubMed]
88. Chen, K.; Ma, H.; Li, L.; Zang, R.; Wang, C.; Song, F.; Shi, T.; Yu, D.; Yang, M.; Xue, W.; et al. Genome-wide association study identifies new susceptibility loci for epithelial ovarian cancer in Han Chinese women. *Nat. Commun.* **2014**, *5*, 4682. [CrossRef]
89. Coleman, R.L.; Fleming, G.F.; Brady, M.F.; Swisher, E.M.; Steffensen, K.D.; Friedlander, M.; Okamoto, A.; Moore, K.N.; Efrat Ben-Baruch, N.; Werner, T.L.; et al. Veliparib with First-Line Chemotherapy and as Maintenance Therapy in Ovarian Cancer. *N. Engl. J. Med.* **2019**, *381*, 2403–2415. [CrossRef]
90. Ray-Coquard, I.; Pautier, P.; Pignata, S.; Pérol, D.; González-Martín, A.; Berger, R.; Fujiwara, K.; Vergote, I.; Colombo, N.; Mäenpää, J.; et al. Olaparib plus Bevacizumab as First-Line Maintenance in Ovarian Cancer. *N. Engl. J. Med.* **2019**, *381*, 2416–2428. [CrossRef]
91. González-Martín, A.; Pothuri, B.; Vergote, I.; DePont Christensen, R.; Graybill, W.; Mirza, M.R.; McCormick, C.; Lorusso, D.; Hoskins, P.; Freyer, G.; et al. Niraparib in Patients with Newly Diagnosed Advanced Ovarian Cancer. *N. Engl. J. Med.* **2019**, *381*, 2391–2402. [CrossRef]
92. Longo, D.L. Personalized Medicine for Primary Treatment of Serous Ovarian Cancer. *N. Engl. J. Med.* **2019**, *381*, 2471–2474. [CrossRef] [PubMed]
93. Lheureux, S.; Gourley, C.; Vergote, I.; Oza, A.M. Epithelial ovarian cancer. *Lancet* **2019**, *393*, 1240–1253. [CrossRef]

10

Economic Evaluation of Population-Based *BRCA1/BRCA2* Mutation Testing across Multiple Countries and Health Systems

Ranjit Manchanda [1,2,3,*], Li Sun [1,4], Shreeya Patel [1], Olivia Evans [1,2], Janneke Wilschut [5], Ana Carolina De Freitas Lopes [6], Faiza Gaba [1,2], Adam Brentnall [7], Stephen Duffy [7], Bin Cui [8], Patricia Coelho De Soarez [6], Zakir Husain [9,10], John Hopper [11], Zia Sadique [4], Asima Mukhopadhyay [12,13], Li Yang [8], Johannes Berkhof [5] and Rosa Legood [4]

1 Wolfson Institute for Preventive Medicine, CRUK Barts Cancer Centre, Queen Mary University of London, London EC1M 6BQ, UK; li.sun1@lshtm.ac.uk (L.S.); shreeyapatel09@hotmail.co.uk (S.P.); o.evans@qmul.ac.uk (O.E.); f.gaba@qmul.ac.uk (F.G.)
2 Department of Gynaecological Oncology, Barts Health NHS Trust, Royal London Hospital, London E1 1BB, UK
3 MRC Clinical Trials Unit at UCL, Institute of Clinical Trials & Methodology, Faculty of Population Health Sciences, University College London, London WC1V 6LJ, UK
4 Department of Health Services Research and Policy, London School of Hygiene & Tropical Medicine, London WC1H 9SH, UK; Zia.Sadique@lshtm.ac.uk (Z.S.); Rosa.Legood@lshtm.ac.uk (R.L.)
5 Department of Epidemiology and Biostatistics, Amsterdam UMC, Vrije Universiteit Amsterdam, 1081 HV Amsterdam, Netherlands; j.wilschut@amsterdamumc.nl (J.W.); h.berkhof@amsterdamumc.nl (J.B.)
6 Departamento de Medicina Preventiva, Faculdade de Medicina FMUSP, Universidade de Sao Paulo, 01246903 Sao Paulo, Brazil; acflopes@usp.br (A.C.D.F.L.); patricia.soarez@usp.br (P.C.D.S.)
7 Centre for Cancer Prevention, Wolfson Institute of Preventive Medicine, Queen Mary University of London, London EC1M 6BQ, UK; a.brentnall@qmul.ac.uk (A.B.); s.w.duffy@qmul.ac.uk (S.D.)
8 School of Public Health, Peking University, Beijing 100191, China; cuibin@bjmu.edu.cn (B.C.); lyang@bjmu.edu.cn (L.Y.)
9 Department of Humanities & Social Sciences, Indian Institute of Technology, Kharagpur, West Bengal 721302, India; dzhusain@gmail.com
10 Department of Economics, Presidency University, Kolkata 700073, India
11 Centre for Epidemiology & Biostatistics, Melbourne School of Population & Global Health, Faculty of Medicine, Dentistry & Health Sciences, University of Melbourne, Victoria 3010, Australia; j.hopper@unimelb.edu.au
12 Tata Medical Centre, Kolkata, West Bengal 700160, India; asima7@yahoo.co.in
13 Northern Institute for Cancer Research, Newcastle University, Newcastle upon Tyne NE2 4HH, UK
* Correspondence: r.manchanda@qmul.ac.uk

Abstract: Clinical criteria/Family history-based *BRCA* testing misses a large proportion of *BRCA* carriers who can benefit from screening/prevention. We estimate the cost-effectiveness of population-based *BRCA* testing in general population women across different countries/health systems. A Markov model comparing the lifetime costs and effects of *BRCA1/BRCA2* testing all general population women ≥30 years compared with clinical criteria/FH-based testing. Separate analyses are undertaken for the UK/USA/Netherlands (high-income countries/HIC), China/Brazil (upper–middle income countries/UMIC) and India (low–middle income countries/LMIC) using both health system/payer and societal perspectives. *BRCA* carriers undergo appropriate screening/prevention interventions to reduce breast cancer (BC) and ovarian cancer (OC) risk. Outcomes include OC, BC, and additional heart disease deaths and incremental cost-effectiveness ratio (ICER)/quality-adjusted life year (QALY). Probabilistic/one-way sensitivity analyses evaluate model uncertainty. For the base case, from a societal perspective, we found that population-based *BRCA* testing is cost-saving in HIC (UK-ICER = $−5639/QALY; USA-ICER = $−4018/QALY; Netherlands-ICER = $−11,433/QALY), and it appears cost-effective in UMIC (China-ICER = $18,066/QALY; Brazil-ICER = $13,579/QALY), but it is not cost-effective in LMIC (India-ICER = $23,031/QALY). From a payer perspective, population-based *BRCA* testing is highly cost-effective in HIC (UK-ICER = $21,191/QALY, USA-ICER = $16,552/QALY, Netherlands-ICER = $25,215/QALY), and it is cost-effective in UMIC (China-ICER = $23,485/QALY, Brazil−ICER = $20,995/QALY), but it is not cost-effective in LMIC (India-ICER = $32,217/QALY). *BRCA* testing costs below $172/test (ICER = $19,685/QALY), which makes it cost-effective (from a societal perspective) for LMIC/India. Population-based *BRCA* testing can prevent an additional 2319 to 2666 BC and 327 to 449 OC cases per million women than the current clinical strategy. Findings suggest that population-based *BRCA* testing for countries evaluated is extremely cost-effective across HIC/UMIC health systems, is cost-saving for HIC health systems from a societal perspective, and can prevent tens of thousands more BC/OC cases.

Keywords: BRCA; population testing; cost-effectiveness; ovarian cancer; breast cancer; cancer prevention

---

1. Introduction

Around 10–20% of ovarian cancer (OC) [1] and 6% breast cancer (BC) [2] overall are caused by inheritable *BRCA1/BRCA2* mutations. Women carrying *BRCA1/BRCA2* mutations have a 17–44% risk of OC and 69–72% risk of BC until age 80 years [3]. Most of these cancers can be prevented in unaffected *BRCA1/BRCA2* women carriers. Women can opt for risk-reducing salpingo-oophorectomy (RRSO), to reduce OC risk [4]. In *BRCA* women, RRSO reduces OC risk by 79–96% [4–6]. Additionally, they can opt for MRI/mammography screening, chemoprevention with selective estrogen-receptor modulators (SERM) or aromatase inhibitors [7]; or risk-reducing mastectomy (RRM) [8,9] to reduce their BC risk [10]. RRM reduces BC risk by 90–95% [8,9]. Mutation identification also enables women to make timely, informed reproductive/lifestyle choices and consider prenatal/pre-implantation genetic diagnosis.

Despite 25 years of *BRCA* testing and effective mechanisms for prevention, current guidelines and access to testing/treatment pathways remain complex and associated with a massive under-utilisation of genetic testing [11]. Only 20% of eligible US women have accessed/undergone genetic testing [11]. A UK analysis shows the huge majority (>97%) of *BRCA* carriers in the population remain unidentified [12]. This highlights substantial missed opportunities for early detection and primary prevention. The current approach uses established clinical-criteria/family-history (FH) based *a priori* *BRCA* probability thresholds to identify high-risk individuals eligible for *BRCA* testing. These clinical criteria/FH-based criteria are used to calculate mutation probability and have been loosened over the years. Earlier, the threshold for offering *BRCA* testing used to be 20% probability. Most countries/health systems now offer *BRCA* testing at a *BRCA* mutation probability of around 10% [13]. A number of different strategies ranging from standardised criteria to complex mathematical (Empirical/Mendelian) models have been used to calculate mutation probability and are used in clinical practice. However, this requires individuals and health practitioners to recognise and act on a significant FH. *BRCA* carriers, who are unaware of their FH, unappreciative of its risk/significance, not proactive in seeking advice, or lack a strong FH (small families/paternal inheritance/chance) get excluded. Over 50% *BRCA* carriers do not fulfil clinical criteria and are missed [14–20]. Current detection rates are inadequate to identify all *BRCA* carriers and even doubling detection rates will need 165 years to ascertain the 'clinically detectable' proportion of *BRCA* carriers [12]. Why should we wait for decades for people to develop cancer before identifying *BRCA* carriers and unaffected at-risk family members to offer prevention?

These limitations can be overcome through unrestricted/unselected population based *BRCA* testing. Falling *BRCA* testing costs, advances in computing/bioinformatics, and next-generation sequencing has made this possible. Jewish population studies show this is feasible, acceptable, has high satisfaction (91–95%), significantly reduces anxiety, doesn't harm psychological well-being or quality of life, and is extremely cost-effective [15,16,21,22]. Pilot general population studies are ongoing in the UK/Canada [23]. However, the potential applicability and scope for primary prevention transcends continents and countries. Health systems, infrastructure, costs, environment, contexts, opportunities, and capacity along with health sector priorities vary considerably across different countries, [24]. Economic evaluations of health interventions, health perspectives and cost-effectiveness thresholds differ amongst countries. Nevertheless, economic evaluation is important to weigh up costs and health effects of alternative health strategies, to help health policy decision making with respect to cost efficiency and resource allocation. For interventions to be sustainable, they need to be cost-effective and affordable. The World Bank separates countries into four income categories using Gross National Income (GNI) per capita (USA dollars): Low-income (LIC: ≤$1025), Lower–Middle Income (LMIC: $1026–$4035), Upper–Middle Income (UMIC: $4036–$12,475), and High Income (HIC: ≥$12,476). In settings of state funded universal health care coverage, the difference between government and societal perspectives is narrower than countries with a limited social security structure/net, where this gap can be significantly larger and consequences considerable. We for the first time evaluate the cost-effectiveness of population-based *BRCA*-testing (compared to clinical-criteria/family-history testing) across multiple countries/health systems: India (LMIC), Brazil (UMIC), China (UMIC), the USA (HIC), the UK (HIC), and the Netherlands (HIC). We present analyses from both health system or payer (here forth called 'payer') and societal perspectives.

2. Results

The comparison of lifetime costs and quality-adjusted life year (QALYs) of population testing and clinical-criteria/FH testing for women in different countries along with the country-specific incremental cost-effectiveness ratios (ICERs) and willingness-to-pay (WTP) thresholds are given in Table 1. Our results show that from a 'societal perspective' (using WHO guidelines), population-based *BRCA* testing is actually 'cost-saving' and contributes to better health in HIC of the UK (ICER = $–5,639/QALY; life expectancy gained = 3.0 days), USA (ICER = $–4018/QALY; life expectancy gained = 2.2 days), and The Netherlands (ICER = $–11,433/QALY; life expectancy gained = 2.8 days). It appears potentially cost-effective in UMICs of China (ICER = $18,066/QALY; life expectancy gained = 1.8 days) and cost-effective in Brazil (ICER = $13,579/QALY; life expectancy gained = 3.7 days), but it is not cost-effective in India (ICER = $23,031/QALY; life expectancy gained = 2.5 days) (LMIC) for the base case.

From a 'payer perspective' (using WHO guidelines), population-based *BRCA* testing is 'highly' cost-effective compared with clinical criteria/FH-based testing in HIC, with UK-ICER = $21,191/QALY (life expectancy gained = 3.0 days), USA-ICER = $16,552/QALY (life expectancy gained = 2.2 days), and Netherlands-ICER = $25,215/QALY (life expectancy gained = 2.8 days). In UMIC population-based *BRCA* testing is cost-effective with ICER = $23,485/QALY in China (life expectancy gained = 1.8 days) and ICER = $20,995/QALY in Brazil (life expectancy gained = 3.7 days). Population-based *BRCA* testing is not cost-effective in LMIC with ICER = $32,217/QALY in India (life expectancy gained = 2.5 days).

If we consider local, country-specific guidelines for the UK, USA, and the Netherlands, then population-based *BRCA* testing is cost-effective from the payer perspective (UK-ICER = $24,066/QALY; USA-ICER = $16,552/QALY; Netherlands-ICER = $17655/QALY), and cost-saving from the societal perspective (UK-ICER = –$3543/QALY; USA-ICER = –$4018/QALY; Netherlands ICER = –$3185/QALY). The corresponding values for life expectancy gained are 2.6 days (UK), 2.2 days (USA) and 4.2 days Netherlands. Figure 1a,b plot change in ICER/QALY with varying *BRCA* testing costs in Brazil, China and India for payer and societal perspectives. Population testing becomes potentially cost-effective (from a societal perspective) in India if the *BRCA* testing cost falls to $172/test (ICER = $19,685/QALY) (Figure 1a; Appendix D). *BRCA* testing costs need to reach $95/test (ICER = $19,670/QALY) for cost-effective population testing in India from the payer perspective (Figure 1b; Appendix D).

The lifetime population impact (reduction in BC and OC cases and deaths; and excess coronary heart disease (CHD)) of offering population *BRCA* testing for the six countries is detailed in Table 2. A population-based *BRCA* testing approach can potentially prevent an additional 2319 to 2666 BC and 327 to 449 OC cases per million women, translating to tens of thousands more BC/OC prevented across the population than the current clinical strategy.

Table 1. Baseline analysis.

Baseline Analysis Based on WHO Guidelines, Using GDP-Based Thresholds													
	Population-Based Testing				# FH-Based Testing				ICER				WTP Threshold ($/QALY)	
	Health Effects		Costs		Health Effects		Costs		Cost/LY		Cost/QALY (95% Credible Intervals)		1*GDP per Capita	3*GDP per Capita
	LY	QALY	Payer	Societal	LY	QALY	Payer	Societal	Payer	Societal	Payer	Societal		
UK	25.67	25.62	2543	18,568	25.66	25.61	2336	18,623	25,530	−6794	21,191 (14,857, 29,619)	−5639 (−11,880, 1895)	42,656	127,969
USA	25.23	25.18	7250	21,951	25.22	25.17	7122	21,982	20,997	−5097	16,552 (4435, 30,280)	−4018 (−15,947, 8764)	57,589	172,766
Netherlands	25.86	25.81	2478	24,642	25.85	25.80	2239	24,750	30,587	−13,868	25,215 (18,193, 34,069)	−11,433 (−18,054, −3689)	50,539	151,616
China	20.70	20.69	820	7687	20.70	20.68	665	7568	30,788	23,684	23,485 (13,947, 36,162)	18066 (8683, 30,653)	15,531	46,592
Brazil	24.54	24.51	834	6314	24.53	24.49	586	6153	24,496	15,844	20,995 (15,707, 27,953)	13,579 (8561, 20,180)	15,182	45,545
India	18.17	18.16	634	30,968	18.17	18.15	369	30,779	39,473	28,218	32,217 (23,982, 42,786)	23,031 (15,107, 22,112)	6574	19,722
Country-Specific Analysis Based on Local Health Economic Guidelines Where they Exist														
	Population-Based Testing				# FH-Based Testing				ICER				WTP Threshold ($/QALY)	
	Health effects		Costs		Health effects		Costs		Cost/LY		Cost/QALY (95% Credible Intervals)			
	LY	QALY	Payer	Societal	LY	QALY	Payer	Societal	Payer	Societal	Payer	Societal		
UK Π	23.55	23.51	2263	16,570	23.55	23.50	2053	16,601	29,273	−4309	24,066 (16,407, 33,590)	−3543 (−10452, 4901)	28,471	42,857
USA	25.23	25.18	7250	21,951	25.22	25.17	7122	21,982	20,997	−5097	16,552 (4435, 30,280)	−4018 (−15947, 8764)	50,000	100,000
Netherlands ∫	34.58	34.51	1968	19,109	34.57	34.49	1725	19,153	20,796	−3752	17,655 (12,948, 23,766)	−3185 (−7568, 2319)	24,390	60,976

ICER: incremental cost-effectiveness ratio, LY—life years, QALY—quality-adjusted life years, FH—family history, GDP—gross domestic product. # Reference Strategy, Costs are given in $ WTP: willingness to pay. This reflects the different cost-effective thresholds for different countries. For GDP-based thresholds: Three times GDP per capita is the threshold for being cost-effective and one time GDP per capita is the threshold for being highly cost-effective. Discount rate is 3% for costs and health effects (LYs and QALYs). For country-specific thresholds: For the UK, this is £20,000 to £30,000 [25]; For the USA, this is $50,000 to $100,000 [26]; For the Netherlands, this is: €20,000 to €50,000 [27]. Values in £s and €s have been converted to $ using PPP (purchasing power parity) [28]. Π For the UK, the discount rate is 3.5% for costs and health effects as per National Institute of Health and Care Excellence (NICE) economic evaluation guidelines [25]. ∫ For the Netherlands, the discount rate is 4% for costs and 1.5% for QALYs as per Dutch health economic analysis guidelines. Perspective: Dutch guidelines recommend a societal perspective. UK NICE guidelines recommend a payer perspective [25]. (See Appendix D for details and references). 1*GDP means 1 × GDP; 3*GDP means 3 × GDP

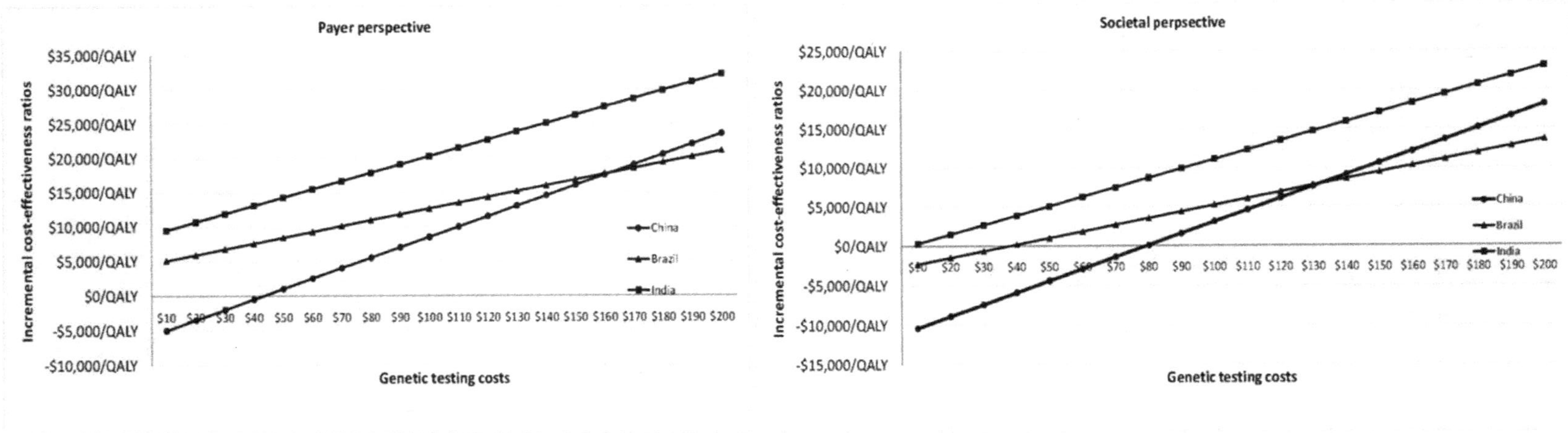

(a) (b)

Figure 1. Change in ICER/QALY with varying *BRCA* testing costs in Brazil, China, and India. (**a**) Change in ICER/QALY with varying *BRCA* testing costs in Brazil, China and India from a payer/healthcare perspective. (**b**) Change in ICER/QALY with varying *BRCA* testing costs in Brazil, China, and India from a societal perspective. The graphs depict the change in ICER/QALY at varying costs of BRCA testing for Brazil, China, and India from payer (Figure 1a) and societal (Figure 1b) perspectives. **X axis:** BRCA testing costs in US$; **Y axis:** ICER/QALY.

Table 2. Lifetime population impact of offering genetic testing for the population.

	Population-Based Testing		FH-Based Testing		Difference	
	Per Million	Actual	Per Million	Actual	Per Million	Actual
	UK (female population over 30 years = 21,760,299)					
BC cases	112,014	2,437,458	114,666	2,495,166	−2652	−57,708
OC cases	15,822	344,291	16,269	354,018	−447	−9727
BC deaths	12,985	282,557	13,258	288,498	−273	−5941
OC deaths	278	6049	550	11,968	−272	−5919
Excess CHD deaths	17	370	0	0	17	370
	USA (female population over 30 years = 101,428,241)					
BC cases	106,431	10,795,109	109,084	11,064,198	−2653	−269,089
OC cases	9985	1,012,761	10,417	1,056,578	−432	−43,817
BC deaths	8113	822,887	8285	840,333	−172	−17,446
OC deaths	235	23,836	475	48,178	−240	−24,343
Excess CHD deaths	17	1724	0	0	17	1724
	Netherlands (female population over 30 years = 5,694,479)					
BC cases	111,732	636,256	114,398	651,437	−2666	−15,181
OC cases	10,964	62,434	11,413	64,991	−449	−2557
BC deaths	11,822	67,320	12,072	68,744	−250	−1424
OC deaths	277	1577	542	3086	−265	−1509
Excess CHD deaths	17	97	0	0	17	97
	China (female population over 30 years = 422,831,894)					
BC cases	27,062	11,442,677	29,546	12,492,991	−2484	−1,050,314
OC cases	3862	1,632,977	4228	1,787,733	−366	−154,756
BC deaths	3728	1576317	4015	1,697,670	−287	−121,353
OC deaths	163	68922	369	156,025	−206	−87,103
Excess CHD deaths	12	5074	0	0	12	5074
	Brazil (female population over 30 years = 58,670,634)					
BC cases	66,227	3,885,580	68,891	4,041,879	−2664	−156,299
OC cases	5358	314,357	5787	339,527	−429	−25,170
BC deaths	12,901	756,910	13,421	787,419	−520	−30,509
OC deaths	271	15,900	539	31,623	−268	−15,724
Excess CHD deaths	17	997	0	0	17	997
	India (female population over 30 years = 298,650,697)					
BC cases	13,713	4,095,397	16,032	4,787,968	−2319	−692,571
OC cases	2826	843,987	3153	941,646	−327	−97,659
BC deaths	3796	1,133,678	4391	1,311,375	−595	−177,697
OC deaths	168	50,173	429	128,121	−261	−77,948
Excess CHD deaths	8	2389	0	0	8	2389

BC—breast cancer, CHD—coronary heart disease, FH—family history, OC—ovarian cancer. The female population data is obtained from the World Bank [29]. We used the modelling to estimate the number of BC cases, OC cases, BC deaths, OC deaths, and excess CHD deaths per million women aged 30 years in the six countries and calculated the number of cases prevented and deaths prevented. The actual numbers of cases prevented and deaths prevented were estimated based on the number of female population aged over 30 years in the six countries [29].

Scenario analyses results are given in Table 3. Different scenarios analysed include no reduction in BC risk from RRSO, nil compliance with hormone replacement therapy (HRT), reduction in RRM and RRSO rates by half, and reduced genetic testing costs of $100. Population-based *BRCA* testing remains cost-effective from payer and societal perspectives in each HIC and UMIC country at their respective WTP thresholds, even without reduction in BC risk from RRSO, no HRT uptake after RRSO, and 50% lower RRM and RRSO uptake rates (Table 3). If the *BRCA* testing costs fell to $100/test, it would be highly cost-effective from the payer perspective and cost-saving (negative ICERs) from the societal perspective for HIC; highly cost-effective from payer/societal perspectives for UMIC, and cost-effective from the societal perspective for India (LMIC). The maximum *BRCA* testing costs for population testing to remain cost-effective from the payer/societal perspectives respectively are in Appendix E. At the 3*GDP WTP threshold, these are: UK = $1254/$1520; USA = $1417/$1577; Netherlands = $1407/$1758; China = $354/$390; Brazil = $493/$582; and India = $95/$172. Using UK/USA/Netherlands guideline-based WTP thresholds, these maximum *BRCA* testing costs are UK = $365, USA = $850–$1010, and Netherlands = $800.

Results of the one-way sensitivity analysis indicate that model outcomes are not impacted much by treatment costs, utility scores, mutation prevalence, and probabilities (Appendix E). The variable with the maximum effect on ICERs is the cost of *BRCA* testing. Probabilistic sensitivity analysis (PSA) results (Figure 2) show that at the WTP thresholds in each country, a population-testing strategy is cost-effective compared to clinical-criteria/FH-testing strategy from both the payer and societal perspectives for HIC and UMIC but not LMIC countries evaluated. The PSAs were highly cost-effective for the evaluated HIC and UMIC countries. All (100%) simulations are cost-effective at the guideline-specific thresholds for the UK/USA/Netherlands from payer and societal perspectives. For the 3*GDP-based WTP threshold for China/Brazil/India, 100%/100%/22.2% for the societal perspective and 100%/100%/0% simulations for the payer perspective were cost-effective (Figure 2a,b). However, a population strategy becomes cost-effective in India (LMIC) at $172/test. At the country-specific WTP thresholds for UK/USA/Netherlands, 84.9%/100%/98.5% of simulations for the payer perspective were cost-effective, and 100% simulations for the societal perspective were cost-effective for all three countries).

Table 3. Scenario analysis.

	Population-Based Testing				FH-Based Testing				ICER				WTP	
	Health Effects		Costs		Health Effects		Costs		Cost/LY		Cost/QALY		GDP per Capita	3*GDP per Capita
	LY	QALY	Payer	Societal	LY	QALY	Payer	Societal	Payer	Societal	Payer	Societal		
Scenario: No reduction in breast cancer risk from RRSO (P9 = 1)														
UK †	25.67	25.62	2550	18,589	25.66	25.61	2336	18,626	27,692	−4729	23,188	−3960	42,656	127,969
USA ‡	25.22	25.18	7273	21,982	25.22	25.17	7125	21,986	25,474	−565	20,318	−450	57,589	172,766
Netherlands ∫	25.86	25.81	2483	24,668	25.85	25.80	2240	24,754	32,834	−11,559	27,318	−9617	50,539	151,616
China	20.70	20.69	825	7693	20.70	20.68	666	7569	32,874	25,745	25,401	19,892	15,531	46,592
Brazil	24.54	24.51	837	6321	24.53	24.49	586	6154	26,175	17,447	22,577	15,049	15,182	45,545
India	18.17	18.16	637	30,974	18.17	18.15	370	30,779	41,333	30,125	34,019	24,795	6574	19,722
Scenario: No compliance with HRT (P13 = 0)														
UK †	25.67	25.62	2542	18,569	25.66	25.61	2335	18,623	26,315	−6954	21,707	−5736	42,656	127,969
USA ‡	25.22	25.18	7250	21,951	25.22	25.17	7122	21,982	21,997	−5280	17,173	−4122	57,589	172,766
Netherlands ∫	25.86	25.81	2477	24,647	25.85	25.80	2239	24,751	31,629	−13,869	25,897	−11,356	50,539	151,616
China	20.70	20.69	812	7678	20.70	20.68	664	7566	29,975	22,722	22,750	17,246	15,531	46,592
Brazil	24.54	24.51	833	6312	24.53	24.49	586	6153	24,932	16,077	21,296	13,732	15,182	45,545
India	18.17	18.16	623	30,957	18.17	18.15	367	30,777	38,327	26,995	31,242	22,005	6574	19,722
Scenario: Half RRM uptake (p2 = 0.235) *														
UK †	25.67	25.62	2545	18,590	25.66	25.61	2336	18,627	27,301	−4834	22,648	−4010	42,656	127,969
USA ‡	25.22	25.18	7265	21,978	25.22	25.17	7125	21,987	24,248	−1503	19,122	−1185	57,589	172,766
Netherlands ∫	25.86	25.81	2480	24,671	25.85	25.80	2240	24,755	32,616	−11,449	26,879	−9435	50,539	151,616
China	20.70	20.69	826	7695	20.70	20.68	666	7569	33,440	26,362	25,453	20,066	15,531	46,592
Brazil	24.54	24.51	838	6324	24.53	24.49	587	6155	26,622	17,938	22,762	15,337	15,182	45,545
India	18.17	18.16	620	30,959	18.17	18.15	367	30,777	39,820	28,637	32,377	23,285	6574	19,722
Scenario: Half RRSO uptake (p8 = 0.275)														
UK †	25.67	25.62	2546	18,589	25.66	25.61	2336	18,628	28,209	−5272	23,325	−4359	42,656	127,969
USA ‡	25.22	25.18	7271	21,982	25.22	25.17	7127	21,989	25,917	−1205	20,308	−944	57,589	172,766
Netherlands ∫	25.86	25.81	2482	24,675	25.85	25.80	2241	24,758	33,868	−11,681	27,799	−9588	50,539	151,616
China	20.70	20.69	820	7688	20.70	20.68	665	7568	32,321	25,018	24,651	19,081	15,531	46,592
Brazil	24.54	24.51	835	6319	24.53	24.49	586	6154	26,241	17,341	22,475	14,852	15,182	45,545
India	18.17	18.16	630	30,967	18.17	18.15	369	30,779	40,490	29,175	33,037	23,805	6574	19,722

Table 3. *Cont.*

	Population-Based Testing				FH-Based Testing				ICER				WTP	
	Health Effects		Costs		Health Effects		Costs		Cost/LY		Cost/QALY		GDP per Capita	3*GDP per Capita
	LY	QALY	Payer	Societal	LY	QALY	Payer	Societal	Payer	Societal	Payer	Societal		
Scenario: Genetic testing cost of $100														
UK †	25.67	25.62	2443	18,468	25.66	25.61	2335	18,622	13,337	−18,988	11,070	−15,761	42,656	127,969
USA ‡	25.23	25.18	7150	21,851	25.22	25.17	7121	21,981	4717	−21,377	3718	−16,852	57,589	172,766
Netherlands ∫	25.86	25.81	2378	24,542	25.85	25.80	2238	24,749	17,893	−26,562	14,750	−21,897	50,539	151,616
China	20.70	20.69	721	7587	20.70	20.68	664	7567	11,165	4061	8517	3098	15,531	46,592
Brazil	24.54	24.51	735	6214	24.53	24.49	585	6152	14,741	6089	12,635	5219	15,182	45,545
India	18.17	18.16	535	30,869	18.17	18.15	368	30,778	24,832	13,577	20,267	11,081	6574	19,722

LY—life years, QALY—quality-adjusted life year, FH—family history, GDP—gross domestic product, HRT—hormone replacement therapy, ICER—incremental cost-effectiveness ratio, RRM—risk-reducing mastectomy, RRSO—risk-reducing salpingo-oophorectomy, WTP—willingness to pay. * Half the RRM uptake rate of the baseline case analysis. Baseline uptake = 47%, Half the baseline = 23.5%. # Half the RRSO uptake rate of the baseline case analysis. Baseline uptake = 55%, Half the baseline = 27.5%. † UK health-economic guideline based threshold is $28,471–$42,857/QALY. £s have been converted to $ using PPP (purchasing power parity) [28]. ‡ USA health-economic guideline based WTP threshold is $50,000–$100,000/QALY. ∫ Netherlands health-economic guideline based WTP threshold is $24,390–$60,976/QALY. €s have been converted to $ using PPP (purchasing power parity).

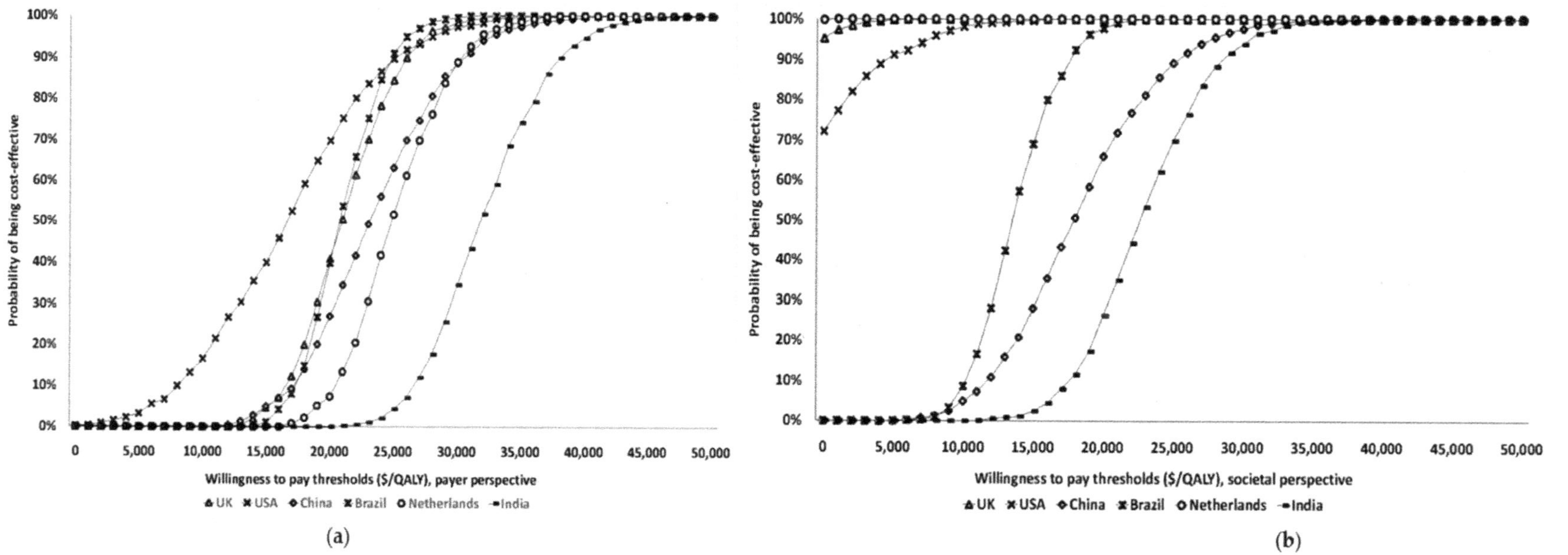

Figure 2. Cost-effectiveness acceptability curves. (**a**) Cost-effectiveness acceptability curve—payer perspective. (**b**) Cost-effectiveness acceptability curve—societal perspective. * The GDP-based (WHO) willingness-to-pay thresholds are $127,969/QALY in the UK, $172,766/QALY in the US, $151,616/QALY in the Netherlands, $46,592/QALY in China, $45,545/QALY in Brazil, and $19,722/QALY in India (Table 2). The country guideline-specific willingness-to-pay thresholds are $42,857/QALY in the UK, $100,000 in the US, and $60,976 in the Netherlands (Table 2). Probabilistic sensitivity analysis in which all model parameters/variables are varied simultaneously across their distributions to further explore model uncertainty. X-axis: Willingness-to-pay thresholds in terms of Cost ($s))/QALY; Y-axis: Proportion of simulations. The results of 1000 simulations were plotted on a cost-effectiveness acceptability curve showing the proportion of simulations (Y-axis) that indicated that the intervention was cost-effective at different willingness-to-pay thresholds (X-axis). Separate curves are plotted for the UK, USA, Netherlands, China, Brazil, and India, with different analyses provided for both payer (Figure 2a) and societal (Figure 2b) perspectives.

3. Discussion

For the first time, we explore the cost-effectiveness of population-based *BRCA* testing across countries from HIC, UMIC and LMIC health systems. We show that population-based *BRCA* testing is extremely cost-effective across HIC/UMIC health systems assessed and is potentially cost-saving for HIC health systems (UK/USA/Netherlands) if analysed from a societal perspective. Societal perspective analyses are associated with lower ICER/QALY than the payer perspective, as it incorporates additional costs linked to productivity loss. There is increasing recognition of the importance and need for economic cost-effectiveness evaluations to conform to the societal perspective and is recommended by WHO/international bodies. This is particularly important in middle/lower–income countries that lack a robust/comprehensive state-funded social security system. However, some countries such as the UK only consider a payer perspective when making health policy.

A population-based *BRCA* testing approach can potentially prevent an additional 57,708/269,089/15,181/1,050,314/156,299/692,571 BC cases and 9727/43,817/2557/154,756/25,170/97,659 OC cases in the UK/USA/Netherlands/China/Brazil/India respectively (Table 2) compared to the current clinical strategy. Given the huge under-utilisation of *BRCA* testing along with limited access and uptake associated with current treatment pathways [11,12], one could postulate that the benefit could be even higher. Our findings are important, as we show that a new population-based approach can have much broader global applicability and a far greater impact on BC/OC burden in the population than current treatment strategies. Cost-effectiveness analyses are necessary to guide policy decisions on healthcare resource allocation. Our findings support a change in paradigm toward population testing to maximise OC/BC prevention and highlights a need for further implementation research in this area.

Our results are sensitive to the cost of testing, particularly in LMIC countries. *BRCA* testing costs need to fall further for population testing to be cost-effective in LMIC countries. In India, it would become potentially cost-effective at $172/test. Although our base case analysis uses costs higher than this, we are aware of Indian providers who offer *BRCA* testing for around $140/test. Genetic testing costs have fallen considerably over the last 5 years and remain on a downward trajectory. While we have used a standard cost for *BRCA* testing that is currently available across countries, some providers may charge more than this. Our analysis of maximum cost(s) of *BRCA* testing for a population testing strategy remaining cost-effective (Appendix D) shows that these lie above what is charged by a number of providers today.

The precise definition of an appropriate cost-effectiveness threshold remains an important issue of ongoing debate. While this has been clearly defined in some (particularly HIC) health systems, a WHO-CHOICE 3*GDP threshold is considered too high by some, as it ignores opportunity costs [30]. Additionally, whilst cost-effectiveness is a key factor for allocating health budgets, it needs to be considered along with context-specific local issues, affordability, budget impact, fairness, and feasibility [31]. Some advocate against a single fixed threshold and recommend a range of thresholds for different contexts. The Norwegian health system prioritises interventions based on health benefit, resource implications, and health loss to the beneficiary if the intervention was absent (higher priority for higher health loss to the beneficiary) [32]. We provide a range of cost estimates for *BRCA* testing linked to varying potential cost-effectiveness thresholds (ICER/QALY) from payer and societal perspectives to help decision makers in UMIC and LIC. This is important, as the main model parameter impacting the overall result is the cost of *BRCA* testing (Figure 1a,b).

Our analysis has several advantages. We follow the transparency principle to facilitate the interpretation of methodology and results and use current standard of care or best practice as the comparator for measuring costs and effects. As per NICE recommendations, we use QALYs to measure health outcomes, which captures both length of life and quality of life and is generalisable across disease states. Our economic evaluation uses a lifetime horizon that is long enough to capture all costs and effects relevant to the decision problem. Additionally, costs and effects are discounted to reflect their value at the time of decision making, ensuring that the potential time preferences of the relevant population are accounted for. Our base case reflects direct health-care costs and health outcomes, and our analysis includes a societal perspective. We explore heterogeneity through scenario analyses and uncertainty and variability through extensive one-way/PSA analyses, as recommended. Our results remain robust at parameter extremes on one-way analysis (Appendix E) and with PSA (Figure 2). Our analysis uses PPP (purchasing power parity), which is a mechanism for accounting for different relative costs of goods when undertaking a comparative analysis of expenditures and incomes in different countries. Besides OC/BC outcomes, we also included excess CHD deaths from premenopausal oophorectomy [33] and incorporate costs for HRT, excess heart disease, bone health monitoring, and treatment. Our costs also include pre-test counselling for all and post-test genetic counselling for pathogenic mutations and VUS.

Similar to other modelling studies, our study has some limitations. In line with earlier analyses in high-risk and low-risk women, our base case analysis assumes a reduction in BC risk with premenopausal oophorectomy. However, recently, there has been uncertainty around the benefit of BC risk reduction from RRSO. Nonetheless, our scenario analysis shows cost-effectiveness in HIC/UMIC even without BC risk reduction (Table 3). We use established surgical prevention rates from HIC in the base-case analysis (Table 4). However, RRM/RRSO rates vary, and lower rates are reported in some populations [34]. The uptake of breast screening, chemoprevention, and risk-reducing surgery may also be influenced by socioeconomic, demographic, and cultural factors and may vary across populations [34]. Rates of screening and preventive interventions have also increased with time. Higher rates are reported in the last 10 years compared to earlier decades, as knowledge and awareness of these issues has improved. Rates could be lower in carriers ascertained from population testing, particularly in the absence of cancer burden in the family. More prospective data on the uptake of surgical prevention following population-based testing will be needed. Our scenario analyses confirm cost-effectiveness for both payer and societal perspectives, even at half of standard surgical prevention rates (Table 3). Although we incorporate a disutility for RRSO and RRM in the analysis, these procedures have potential complication rates of around 3–4% and 21%, respectively [35,36]. This needs to be part of the informed consent and decision-making process. While RRSO has been reported to have high satisfaction rates, less cancer worry, and no detriment in generic quality of life; poorer sexual function despite HRT use has been found [37]. RRM has an adverse association with body image and sexual pleasure but not with sexual activity/habit/discomfort, anxiety/depression, or generic quality of life, and overall satisfaction rates are good. Countries such as India and China lack established national breast cancer screening programmes. The uptake of mammograms is much lower in these countries. The cost-effectiveness of population testing may be higher for these countries than estimated, as the implementation of these interventions in *BRCA* carriers are likely to be more beneficial in the absence of routine mammograms in the population. In our analysis, while we included productivity loss, we did not include all indirect costs in the analysis. This may be a limitation. However, including additional indirect costs would improve cost-effectiveness, so our analysis is conservative in that respect. While our analysis covers some important/key countries across different income groups, it does not cover most countries, and therefore, these results are not generalisable globally to all countries across different (HIC/UMIC/LMIC) income groups. While the countries represented in this analysis are from four continents—North America, South America, Europe, and Asia—we do not have representation from Africa or Australia. The populations of countries in our analysis contribute approximately 45% to the global population.

Population-based *BRCA* testing implementation studies have been completed in the Jewish population [15,21,22,38], and pilot ones are being undertaken in the UK and Canadian general populations [23]. For population testing to be feasible, newer approaches for delivering pre-test information will be needed to facilitate informed decision-making. These will need to be country/region or context-specific. The best modality to deliver pre-test education within the population testing setting remains unresolved. We do not feel there will eventually be a one-size-fits-all model. Although we have costed for pre-test counselling for all in our analyses, whether formal pre-test counselling will be needed for all in the future remains uncertain. Israeli and Canadian Jewish population studies provided only 'pre-test information' and post-test genetic counselling for *BRCA* carriers, with >90% satisfaction rates [39,40]. An Australian Jewish population [41] and a UK general population study have demonstrated the feasibility of an online web-based decision aid (along with an optional telephone helpline) pre-test education and consent process [42].

A strategy for the management of variants of unknown significance (VUS) is important and will need developing. People have raised concerns at unnecessary treatment or screening/preventive intervention(s) being undertaken for VUS alone. However, VUS are currently identified through routine clinical testing, too. There is clear acceptance in clinical practice that for a VUS (class-3 variant), no clinical action should be taken based on that variant alone [43]. A key presumption inherent in a public health screening strategy is that it is not designed to identify 'all' individuals with disease, but the large/significant proportion of individuals in a clinically efficient and cost-effective manner. Therefore, some suggest an alternative option of not providing VUS results within a population-testing context [14]. We incorporate a cost for VUS counselling and management in our analysis.

Chronic disease accounts for 90% US Medicare and 70% UK health care expenditure and is a major challenge facing most health systems, with cancer being its second commonest cause. Between 2006 and 2016, the average annual age-standardised incidence rates for all cancers increased in 130 of 195 countries [44]. The leading cause for women is BC: 1.7 million cases, 535,000 deaths, 14.9 million disability adjusted life-years (DALYs) [44]. Globally breast/ovarian cancers in women are predicted to increase by 46.5%/47% and cancer deaths are predicted to increase by 58.3%/58.6% respectively over the next 20 years [45]. Population testing for *BRCA* genes can significantly increase *BRCA* carrier detection rates for maximising prevention and reducing cancer burden. It can also serve as an initial model, which subsequently informs the potential applicability of a population testing risk-stratification strategy for other cancer genes and other chronic diseases.

While developing an approach towards implementing population-based *BRCA*-testing, it is important to bear in mind the principles of population testing of disease. These were initially proposed by Wilson and Jungner [46]. Updated criteria have been suggested by the UK National Screening Committee [47], Khoury [48], the CDC (ACCE model) [49], and Burke and Zimmerman (Public Health Foundation) [50]. Analytic validity, clinical validity, clinical utility, and associated ethical, legal, and social implications remain key principles of the ACCE model, providing a framework for evaluating the applicability of a genetic test [49]. In our study, we focussed on *BRCA* testing, as testing for these genes has well-established clinical utility fulfilling the ACCE principles. Multigene panel testing is widely available in current clinical practice. We are against indiscriminate large-scale commercial panel testing without well-established clinical benefit/utility in the population-testing context. The low incidence of moderate penetrance genes, poor precision, and wide confidence intervals around prevalence and penetrance estimates require more data on the clinical significance of pathogenic variants in multigene panels, and these are reasons against currently implementing large multigene panel testing in the general population [51,52]. The USPSTF currently recommends against population testing in the general population [51]. More data are needed on the 'E' (Ethical, legal, and social implications) of a population-based *BRCA* testing approach across different populations and health systems. There is an urgent need for multiple implementation studies across countries for evaluating general population *BRCA* testing and to develop local/regional and context-specific implementation pathways. These studies will need to provide prospective data on the impact of population testing on psychological well-being, quality of life, long-term health behaviour, socio-ethics, and lifestyle outcomes. A number of challenges and logistic hurdles will need to be overcome, including varying levels of workforce expansion/upskilling and the reorganisation of health services infrastructure. These include increasing public and health-professional awareness, establishing/expanding laboratory testing infrastructure, expanding downstream management pathways, and involving general practitioners, genetics services, gynaecologists, and breast clinicians/services. A framework/structure for data management and legal and regulatory protections will need to be established. These changes will need to be system/country and context-specific.

4. Materials and Methods

We developed a Markov model (Figure 3) (TreeAge-Pro-2018 Williamson, MA, USA) to compare the lifetime costs and effects of *BRCA1/BRCA2* testing all general population women ≥30 years compared with clinical-criteria/FH-based testing. We describe separate analyses for populations in the UK, USA, Netherlands, China, Brazil, and India using both payer and societal perspectives. While some countries only consider a payer perspective, a societal perspective is recommended by the WHO and other international bodies [53]. In the model, all women ≥30 years in the Population testing arm and only those fulfilling clinical/FH criteria in the Clinical-Criteria/FH-based testing arm undergo genetic testing for *BRCA* mutations. We include pre-test counselling for all and assume a 70% uptake of genetic testing (from the published literature) [22]. We include the cost of post-test counselling for mutation carriers as well as the cost of post-test counselling for those with variants of uncertain significance (VUS). We assume a VUS prevalence of 2% [54]. Model probabilities are described in Table 4, Appendix A, and costs are outlined in Appendix B. *BRCA* carriers identified are offered RRSO to reduce OC risk [4] and MRI/mammography screening, chemoprevention with SERM or RRM [8] to reduce their BC risk [10]. OC screening is excluded given the lack of mortality benefit. Women undergoing RRSO receive hormone replacement therapy (HRT) until 51 years. We include the costs of bone health monitoring and dual energy X-ray scans. We incorporate the excess risk and mortality from coronary heart disease (CHD) after premenopausal RRSO for women who do not take HRT (absolute mortality increase = 3.03%) [33]. Associated costs are modelled over an individual's lifetime. The Markov cycles' run depends on life expectancy and these are different across countries (starting from age 30): UK = 53 cycles, US = 52 cycles, Netherlands = 53 cycles, China = 48 cycles, Brazil = 49 cycles, and India = 38 cycles. Cancer incidence is estimated by summing the probabilities of pathways ending in OC or BC.

4.1. Probabilities

The model probabilities for different pathways are given in Table 4, and a detailed explanation is given in Appendix A. The age-specific incidence of BC and OC among general population women is obtained from Cancer Research UK [55,56], USA Cancer Statistics [57], and the International Agency for Research on Cancer (GLOBOCAN-2018) [58]. The BC/OC incidence for *BRCA1/BRCA2* carriers is obtained from the literature [3].

Figure 3 is a schematic diagram showing the Markov model structure for population and clinical-criteria/family-history (FH)-based *BRCA1/BRCA2* testing. In the Population testing arm, all women ≥30 years old are offered *BRCA1/BRCA2* testing and get classified as *BRCA*-positive and *BRCA*-negative. *BRCA* mutation carriers identified are offered options of risk-reducing mastectomy (RRM) and risk-reducing salpingo-oophorectomy (RRSO). Depending on the probability of *BRCA* women undertaking RRM and/or RRSO (+/− chemoprevention), they are placed into different health states and then progress to either *BRCA*-associated breast cancer (BC) or *BRCA*-associated ovarian cancer (OC). All women undergoing RRSO have an increased risk of fatal coronary heart disease (CHD). In addition, they have a probability of dying from the background all-cause mortality. Hence, patients in the model can go from intervention to death without ever developing breast cancer, ovarian cancer, or coronary artery disease. Patients can move from healthy state to death as they have a probability of dying from the background all-cause mortality. *BRCA*-positive women who do not progress or die would stay in the health states and undertake the next cycle. *BRCA1/BRCA2*-negative women progress to sporadic non-*BRCA* OC or non-*BRCA* BC based on the age-dependent probabilities. They also have a probability of dying from the background all-cause mortality. Women do not progress or die would stay in the health states to undertake the next cycle.

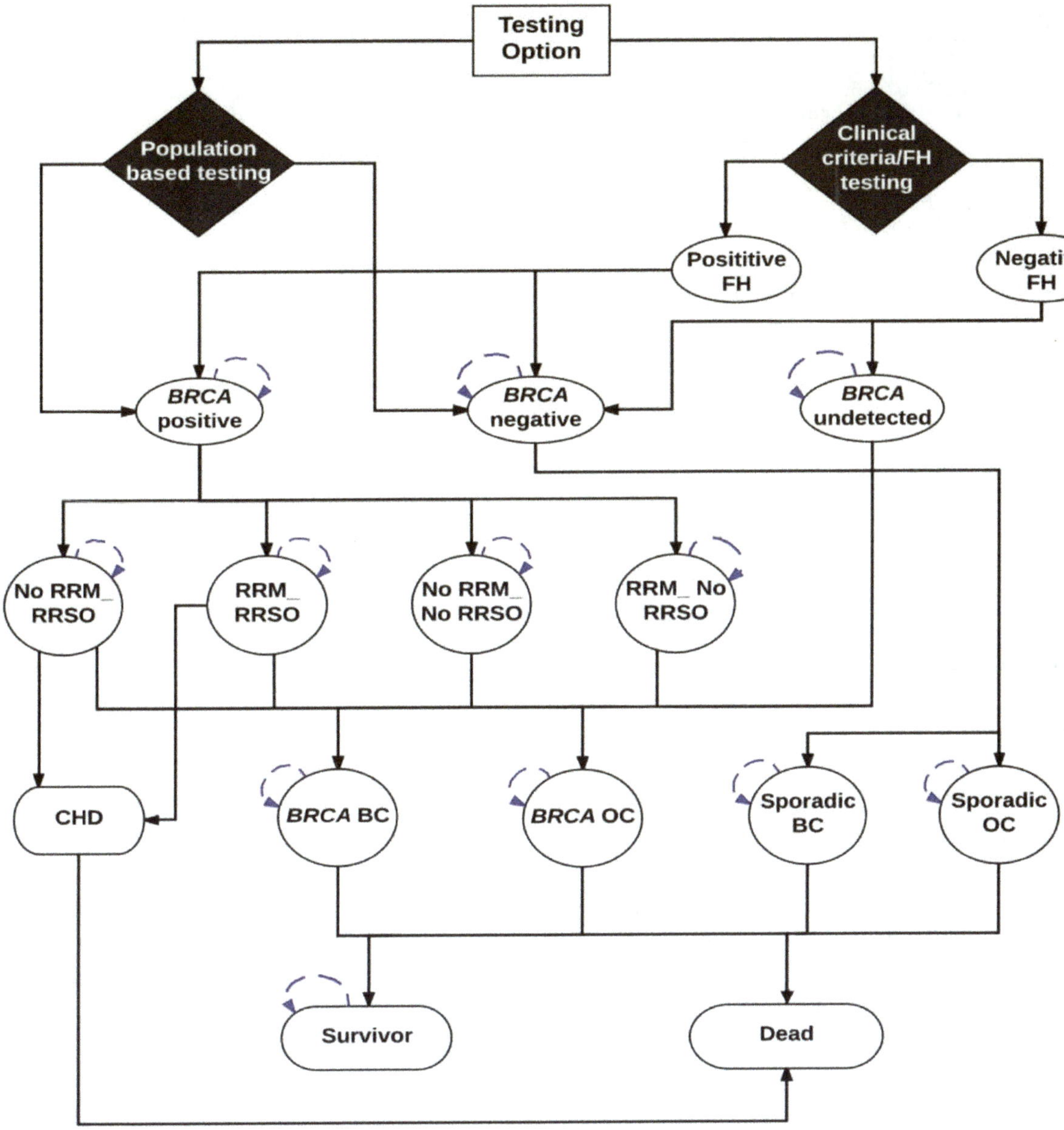

Figure 3. BC, breast cancer; CHD, coronary heart disease; FH, family history; OC, ovarian cancer; RRM, risk-reducing mastectomy; RRSO, risk-reducing salpingo-oophorectomy.

In the Clinical criteria/FH arm, only women whose FH fulfil current clinical criteria (based on current guidelines) undergo *BRCA1/BRCA2* genetic testing and get classified as *BRCA*-positive and *BRCA*-negative. Women with a negative FH are either *BRCA* negative or have an undetected *BRCA* mutation. Options of RRM and RRSO and disease progression for identified *BRCA* mutation carriers and disease progression for *BRCA* negative women are the same as those in the population testing arm and are described above. All women undergoing RRSO have an increased risk of fatal coronary heart disease (CHD). Undetected *BRCA* women are not offered RRM or RRSO. Depending on the baseline risk (no risk-reducing options), they progress to *BRCA*-associated BC or *BRCA*-associated OC. In addition, they have a probability of dying from the background all-cause mortality. Hence, patients in the model can go from intervention to death without developing breast cancer, ovarian cancer, or coronary artery disease. Patients can move from healthy state to death as they may die from the background all-cause mortality. Women who do not progress or die stay in the health state of *BRCA* undetected and undertake the next cycle.

Progression through the model is dependent on the probabilities provided in Table 4.

Table 4. Probability Values.

Probability	Description	Value	(95% CI) (Range)	Source
P1	BRCA1/2 mutation prevalence in general population	0.0067	(0.0059, 0.0077)	[59]
P2	Probability that carriers will undergo RRM	0.47	(0.34, 0.56)	[60]
P3	Reduction in ovarian cancer risk from RRSO	0.96	[0.8, 0.96]	[4,6]
P4	Probability of having a positive FH	0.0098	(0.0047, 0.0179)	ABCFS
P5	BRCA1/2 mutation prevalence in FH-positive individuals	0.1		[10]
P6	BRCA1/2 mutation prevalence in FH-negative individuals	0.0058	(0.0051, 0.0068)	[59], ABCFS
P7	Reduction in breast cancer risk from RRM without RRSO in BRCA1/2 carriers	0.91	(0.62, 0.98)	[8]
P8	Probability that carriers will undergo RRSO	0.55	(0.45, 0.64)	[61]
P9	Hazard ratio in breast cancer risk from RRSO alone	0.49	(0.37,0.65)	[4]
P10	Reduction in risk of breast cancer from RRM with RRSO	0.95	(0.78, 0.99)	[8]
P11	Excess CHD risk	0.0072	(0.0068, 0.0076)	[33]
P12	Fatal CHD risk	0.0303	(0.011, 0.043)	[33]
P13	Compliance with HRT	0.8	(0.76, 0.83)	[62]
P14	HR of breast cancer risk from breast cancer chemoprevention	0.71	(0.6, 0.83)	[63]
P15	Uptake of breast cancer chemoprevention	0.163	(0.136, 0.19)	[64]

95%CI—95% confidence interval, ABCFS—Australia Breast Cancer Family Study, CHD—coronary heart disease, FH—family history, RRM—risk-reducing mastectomy, RRSO—risk-reducing salpingo-oophorectomy. A detailed explanation of probabilities is given in Appendix A.

4.2. Costs

The analysis was conducted from both a payer perspective and societal perspective. All costs are reported at 2016 USA dollars, which was converted by purchasing power parity (PPP) factor [28]. PPP reflects the value of a country's currency required to purchase equivalent amounts of goods and services in the domestic market as the USA dollar would buy in the USA. Thus, it is used to translate and compare costs of goods/services between countries using the USA dollar as a common reference point. For comparison, we convert values in all other country currencies (£s, €s, ¥, ₹, R$) to $ (USA) using the purchasing power parity (PPP) factor [28]. In line with the National Institute of Health and Care Excellence (NICE) recommendations, future healthcare costs not associated with BC/OC/heart disease were not considered [25]. We collected primary data on relevant direct medical costs from the Urban Basic Medical Insurance Database in China [65]; the Dutch Healthcare Authority (NZA) in Netherlands; Management System of Procedures/Medical drugs/Orthotics/Prosthetics/Special Materials (SIGTAP) [66], the Health Price Bank (BPS) [67], and Chamber of Regulation of the Market of Medicines (CMED) [68] in Brazil; and an accredited cancer centre (Tata Medical Centre) in India (details in Appendix B). Costing data were obtained from published national health service (NHS) reference costs for the UK [69,70] and published literature for the USA (details in Appendix B). We adopted a standard internationally available *BRCA* testing cost (US $200) for our base case and explored the impact of change in testing costs on the overall results in the sensitivity analyses.

The retirement ages for females are 65 in the UK, 62 in the USA, 50–55 in China, 60 in Brazil, 68 in Netherlands, and 60–65 in India. We used the lower values of the retirement age ranges in China and India to get the conservative estimates of productivity loss. The female labour force participation rates are 56.77% in the UK, 55.99% in the USA, 62.03% in China, 53.32% in Brazil, 58.02% in the Netherlands, and 27.45% in India, which were obtained from the World Bank [71]. For the hourly wage rates across countries, see Appendix C. Additionally, we categorised costs due to productivity loss (for details: see Appendix C) as three subcomponents: (1) temporary disability due to short-term work absences following diagnosis, (2) permanent disability from reduced working hours following return to work or workforce departure; and (3) premature mortality due to death before retirement [72]. We estimated temporary disability as time absent from work multiplied by age-specific gross earnings. We calculated productivity costs due to permanent disability by applying age-specific gross earnings to the reduction in working hours, or the number of working hours in cases of permanent workforce departure, until retirement age. Regarding productivity loss from premature mortality, we assumed that without cancer, the productive capacity of an individual would continue from the age of diagnosis until the age of retirement. We multiplied the projected years of life lost by the age-specific gross earnings for the remainder of the working life to generate monetary estimates (see Appendix C). While we included productivity loss, we did not include all indirect costs in the analysis.

4.3. Life Years

Lifetime tables from each country were used to model the lifetime health outcomes, and these were obtained from the World Health Organisation (WHO) [73]. The median ages for RRM and RRSO in unaffected *BRCA* carriers were assumed to be 37 and 40 years [60]. BC and OC survival were modelled using five-year survival data from the CONCORD global surveillance of cancer survival [74]. No significant overall long-term survival differences between germ-line and sporadic BC/OC have been found [75–77]. After five years, the probability of death was assumed to be the same as that of the general population. Modelling estimated the number of BC cases, OC cases, BC deaths, OC deaths, and excess CHD deaths per million women aged 30 years in the six countries, and it calculated the number of cases prevented and deaths prevented. The actual numbers of cases prevented and deaths prevented were estimated based on the number of female population aged over 30 years in the six countries [29].

4.4. Quality-Adjusted Life Years (QALY)

QALYs are recommended by NICE as the appropriate summary measure of health effects for economic evaluation. Utility scores multiplied by life years provides QALYs. QALY = (survival in life years) x (utility score). Utility score is an adjustment for quality of life. It is an indication of individual preferences for specific health states where 1 = perfect health and 0 = death. The utility scores for early, advanced, recurrent, and end-stage breast cancer are 0.71, 0.65, 0.45, and 0.16 [78]. The utility scores used for early, advanced, recurrent, and end-stage OC are 0.81, 0.55, 0.61, and 0.16, respectively [79]. Additionally, utility scores used for RRM is 0.88 (SD = 0.22) and RRSO is 0.95 (SD = 0.10) [80].

4.5. Analysis

The Markov model is illustrated in Figure 3. Model outcomes include OC, BC, and excess deaths from CHD. Future costs and health effects are discounted at WHO-recommended 3% rate for the WHO analyses [81] and at country-recommended rates for country-specific analyses (see Table 1). The lifetime costs and QALYs were estimated in both population-testing and clinical-criteria/FH-testing arms. The incremental cost-effectiveness ratio (ICER) was calculated by dividing the difference in cost by the difference in health effects between these two strategies. ICER = $(\text{Cost}^{\text{Population-Testing}} - \text{Cost}^{\text{Criteria/FH-testing}})/(\text{Effect}^{\text{Population-Testing}} - \text{Effect}^{\text{Criteria/FH-testing}})$. The potential population impact was estimated by calculating the additional reduction in BC and OC incidence/deaths obtained through *BRCA* testing women aged >30 years. We present analyses using a range of cost-effectiveness thresholds. For all countries, we present the initial WHO recommendation of three times gross domestic product (GDP) per capita (threshold of being cost-effective) and one-time GDP per capita (threshold for being highly cost-effective) [82]. For countries (UK [25], USA [26], Netherlands [27]) with specific health economic willingness-to-pay (WTP) threshold guidelines, we also present analysis using those guidelines: UK = £20,000–30,000 [25]; USA = $50,000–100,000 [26]; Netherlands = €20,000–50,000. [27] Additionally, given the lack of a clear established threshold, we evaluate changes in ICER/QALY with *BRCA* testing costs for China, Brazil, and India to identify the *BRCA* testing cost threshold for a given economic cost-effectiveness threshold. We use $ (USA) conversion with PPP for comparison [28].

We also explored a number of scenario analyses, including: (1) no BC risk reduction from RRSO (p9 = 1); (2) no HRT uptake (p13 = 0); (3) 50% reduction in RRM uptake; (4) 50% reduction in RRSO uptake; (5) lower *BRCA*-testing costs of $100; and (6) the maximum genetic testing costs at which population *BRCA* testing remains cost-effective (see Table 3, Appendix D). In the one-way sensitivity analysis, each parameter is varied to evaluate their individual impact on results. Probabilities and utility scores were varied according to 95% confidence intervals or ranges where available or by +/−10%.

Costs were varied by +/−30%. Probabilistic sensitivity analysis (PSA) was undertaken, and parameters varied simultaneously across their distributions. Costs were specified as having a Gamma distribution, quality of life was specified as having a log-normal distribution, and probability was specified as having a beta distribution, as recommended [83]. A cost-effectiveness acceptability curve was used to plot the results of 1000 simulations for each country, showing the probability of population-based *BRCA* testing being cost-effective at different WTP thresholds. Different curves were generated for payer and societal perspectives.

5. Conclusions

The increasing societal awareness and acceptability of genetic testing, falling costs, computational advancements, and technological advancements provides the ability to implement large-scale population testing. We have demonstrated the potential cost-effectiveness of *BRCA* testing on a much broader scale in the general population and across a number of health systems. This is cost-effective for HIC and UMIC health systems and can prevent tens of thousands more BC and OC than the current clinical strategy. Such an approach can bring about a new paradigm for improving global cancer prevention. Context-specific implementation strategies and pathways for population testing need to be developed. A number of implementation studies providing data on the impact of population *BRCA* testing on real-world outcomes are needed. All this is essential for population genomics to achieve its potential for maximising early detection and cancer prevention.

Author Contributions: Conceptualisation, R.M.; methodology, L.S., S.P., R.M. and R.L. software, L.S.; validation, L.S., S.P., R.M., and R.L.; formal analysis, L.S., R.M., S.P., R.L., A.B., S.D., and Z.S.; data curation, J.W., H.B., A.M., Z.H., L.S., L.Y., B.C., P.C.D.S., J.H., F.G., and O.E.; writing—original draft preparation, R.M., L.S., and R.L.; writing—review and editing, all authors.; visualisation, L.S., R.M., R.L., F.G., and O.E.; All authors have read and agreed to the published version of the manuscript.

Acknowledgments: We are grateful to Melissa Southey (Monash University, Australia) for her support of this work. The study is supported by researchers at the Barts Cancer Research UK Centre for Excellence, Queen Mary University of London (C16420/A18066). This study/analysis received full ethics approval from the Institute of Child Health/ Great Ormond Street Hospital Research Ethics Committee on (REC Reference number 08/H0713/44, Substantial Amendment 3/7/2018).

Appendix A. Probability Values and Explanation

Table A1. Probability Values.

Probability	Description	Value	(95% CI) (Range)	Source
P1	BRCA1/2 mutation prevalence in general population	0.0067	(0.0059, 0.0077)	[59]
P2	Probability that carriers will undergo RRM	0.47	(0.34, 0.56)	[60]
P3	Reduction in ovarian cancer risk from RRSO	0.96	(0.8, 0.96)	[4,6]
P4	Probability of having a positive FH	0.0098	(0.0047, 0.0179)	ABCFS
P5	BRCA1/2 mutation prevalence in FH positive individuals	0.1		[84]
P6	BRCA1/2 mutation prevalence in FH negative individuals	0.0058	(0.0051, 0.0068)	[59], ABCFS
P7	Reduction in breast cancer risk from RRM without RRSO in BRCA1/2 carriers	0.91	(0.62, 0.98)	[8]
P8	Probability that carriers will undergo RRSO	0.55	(0.45, 0.64)	[61]
P9	Hazard ratio in breast cancer risk from RRSO alone	0.49	(0.37,0.65)	[4]

Table A1. *Cont.*

Probability	Description	Value	(95% CI) (Range)	Source
P10	Reduction in risk of breast cancer from RRM with RRSO	0.95	(0.78, 0.99)	[8]
P11	Excess CHD risk	0.0072	(0.0068, 0.0076)	[33]
P12	Fatal CHD risk	0.0303	(0.011, 0.043)	[33]
P13	Compliance with HRT	0.8	(0.76, 0.83)	[62]
P14	HR of breast cancer risk from breast cancer chemoprevention	0.71	(0.6, 0.83)	[63]
P15	Uptake of breast cancer chemoprevention	0.163	(0.136, 0.19)	[64]

95%CI—95% confidence interval, ABCFS—Australia Breast Cancer Family Study, CHD—coronary heart disease, FH—family history, RRM—risk-reducing mastectomy, RRSO—risk-reducing salpingo-oophorectomy.

Explanations

P1: *BRCA1/2* mutation prevalence in the general population is calculated based on Jervis 2015 [59].

P2: The probability that unaffected carriers will undergo RRM is taken from an analysis of UK *BRCA1/2* carriers by Evans et al. 2009 [60]. A composite uptake rate for *BRCA1* (60% RRM rate) and *BRCA2* (43% RRM rate) carriers weighted for the relative prevalence of *BRCA1* and *BRCA2* mutations was computed [60].

P3: The reduction in ovarian cancer risk obtained from RRSO is taken from previous studies which report a 4% residual risk of primary peritoneal cancer following RRSO [6].

P4: The probability of having a positive family history in general population is obtained from the Australia Breast Cancer Family Study (ABCFS).

P5: The overall *BRCA1/BRCA2* mutation prevalence (10%) among FH-positive breast cancer patients is based on the current testing guideline.

P6: The *BRCA1/2* mutation prevalence in FH negative individuals is calculated based on the *BRCA1/2* mutation prevalence in the general population, the BRCA1/2 mutation prevalence in FH-positive individuals, and the probability of having a positive FH.

P7: The reduction in breast cancer risk from RRM in *BRCA1/BRCA2* mutation carriers not undergoing RRSO is taken from the PROSE study data by Rebbeck et al. 2004 [8].

P8: The uptake of RRSO in unaffected *BRCA1/BRCA2* carriers is taken from a study among high-risk UK women [7].

P9: The hazard ratio for breast cancer in premenopausal unaffected *BRCA1/BRCA2* women undergoing RRSO alone is taken from a meta-analysis by Rebbeck et al. 2009 [4].

P10: The reduction in breast cancer risk in *BRCA1/BRCA2* mutation carriers undergoing RRM and RRSO is taken from the PROSE study data by Rebbeck et al. 2004 [8].

P11: Excess risk of CHD after RRSO is estimated using data from Parker 2013 [33]. The absolute excess CHD incidence is obtained by subtracting CHD incidence in women undergoing RRSO from those who have not.

P12: The risk of CHD mortality is obtained from the Nurses Health Study (Parker et al. 2013) [33]. Death from CHD is reported in 1 in 33 premenopausal women undergoing RRSO and not taking HRT [33].

P13: HRT compliance rate is obtained from a UK cohort (Read et al., 2010) [62].

P14: The Hazard Ratio for breast cancer risk from chemoprevention in high-risk women is obtained from the extended long-term follow-up of the IBIS-I breast cancer prevention trial (Cuzick et al. 2015) [63].

P15: The uptake of breast cancer chemoprevention is obtained from a recent meta-analysis by Smith et al. 2016 [64].

Appendix B. Medical Costs in 2016 Values (USA Dollars Converted by PPP)

Table A2. Medical costs in 2016 values (USA dollars converted by PPP).

Cost descriptions	UK		US	Netherlands		China		Brazil		India	
	GBP	USD	USD	EUR	USD	RMB	USD	BRL	USD	INR	USD
Cost of genetic testing		200	200		200		200		200		200
Cost of genetic counselling	29	42	42	55	67	0	0	135	68	733	42
Cost of prophylactic bilateral salpingo-oophorectomy	2799	3999	7904	3713	4584	4525	1308	957	483	82,368	4712
Cost of ovarian cancer diagnosis and treatment	14,268	20,383	133,121	23,238	28,689	12,991	3755	12,564	6345	613,662	35,107
Annual cost of ovarian cancer in years 1 to 2	5433	7761	14,635	10,865	13,413	48,495	14,016	4442	2244	290,086	16,595
Annual cost of ovarian cancer in years 3 to 5	5090	7271	14,635	10,480	12,939	48,021	13,879	4278	2161	280,720	16,059
Terminal care cost with ovarian cancer	16,452	23,503	93,005	11,325	13,981	10,060	2907	1358	686	80,623	4612
Cost of risk reducing mastectomy	4143	5919	13,101	2950	3642	2634	761	867	438	278,474	15,931
Annual cost of hormone replacement therapy	60	86	52	61	76	2148	621	217	110	15,595	892
Cost of mammography	60	85	156	95	117	82	24	42	21	2051	117
Cost of MRI	203	290	1477	215	265	605	175	252	127	7222	413
Cost of breast cancer diagnosis and treatment in general population	18,148	25,926	85,372	11,977	14,786	74,959	21,664	23,218	11,726	226,451	12,955
Annual cost of breast cancer in general population	1388	1982	8048	2718	3355	12,360	3572	2328	1176	55,519	3176
Cost of breast cancer diagnosis and treatment in BRCA1/2 carriers	16,499	23,570	78,964	10,780	13,309	68,476	19,791	20,861	10,536	200,902	11,493
Annual cost of breast cancer in BRCA1/2 carriers	1400	2000	8048	2656	3279	10,827	3129	1999	1009	53,959	3087
Terminal care cost with breast cancer	16,452	23,503	68,022	11,325	13,981	10,060	2907	1358	686	80,623	4612
Cost of fatal coronary heart disease	3387	4839	23,934	3008	3714	11,972	3460	2953	1491	47,673	2727
Annual cost of excess coronary heart disease	122	175	7277	109	134	526	152	124	63	3708	212
Annual cost of chemoprevention	19	27	899	36	45	93	27	499	252	62	4

CHD—coronary heart disease, HRT—hormone replacement therapy, MRI—magnetic resonance imaging, RRM—risk-reducing mastectomy, RRSO—risk-reducing salpingo-oophorectomy, PPP—purchasing power parity.

Appendix B.1. Explanations

All costs are adjusted for 2016 consumer price index.

For comparison, we convert values in all other country currencies (£s, €s, ¥, ₹, R$) to $ (USA) using purchasing power parity (PPP) factor [28].

We collected primary data on relevant direct medical costs from the Urban Basic Medical Insurance Database in China [65]; the Dutch Healthcare Authority (NZA) in Netherlands; Management System of Procedures/Medical drugs/Orthotics/Prosthetics/Special Materials (SIGTAP) [66], the Health Price Bank (BPS) [67] and Chamber of Regulation of the Market of Medicines (CMED) [68] in Brazil; and an accredited Cancer Centre (Tata Medical Centre) in India. UK costing data were obtained from published NHS reference costs for the UK [69,70].

Appendix B.2. Cost of Genetic Testing/Counselling

We use a standard international cost for genetic testing for all countries (US$ 200 in 2016). We assume a 71% uptake of genetic testing (based on our previous population based research studies) [22]. All participants have pre-test counselling and post-test counselling is received by those testing positive (pathogenic/likely pathogenic carriers). We assume a VUS prevalence of 2% and include the cost of post-test counselling for VUS in these 2% cases [54].

The cost of *BRCA1/BRCA2* testing is based on testing costs for these genes in our population testing research programme as well as confirmatory testing costs in an accredited national genetics laboratory for those testing positive. The UK national unit cost assumed for genetic counselling is £44 per hour of client contact from PSSRU Unit costs of Health and Social Care 2010 [22,85,86]. The US genetic counselling costs are obtained from Schwartz 2014 and include ancillary preparation (scheduling/administration), counsellor preparation, and counselling [87]. The genetic counselling costs in the Netherlands, Brazil, and India were obtained from primary data. There is no additional physician genetic counselling cost charged from patients in China; hence, this was not incorporated for Chinese analysis.

Appendix B.3. RRSO Costs

The UK RRSO costs are obtained from NHS reference costs [88], and the US costs are from Grann 2011 [89] inflated using the medical component of the USA consumer price index to 2016 US$. Costs of HRT for the UK are taken from BNF [90] and for the USA from William-Frame 2009 [91]. The costs of RRSO and HRT in Netherlands, China, Brazil, and India are obtained from primary data. Costs assume HRT is given from average age of RRSO to the average age of menopause (51 years). These costs are calculated for the 80% assumed to be compliant with HRT. Costs include the cost of three follow-up DEXA scans for monitoring bone health and calcium and vitamin-D3 for additional osteo-protection.

Appendix B.4. RRM

The UK RRM costs are obtained from NHS reference costs [88], and the USA costs are from Grann 2011 [89] inflated using the medical component of the US consumer price index to 2016 US$. The RRM costs in Netherlands, China, Brazil and India are obtained from primary data.

Appendix B.5. Costs of Ovarian Cancer

We assume that the costs of ovarian cancer diagnosis include a pelvic examination, ultrasound scan, CA125 test, CT scan, percutaneous biopsy, and peritoneal cytology. The costs of ovarian cancer treatment include the reference cost for a lower and upper genital tract very complex major procedure and administration of chemotherapy based on 6 cycles of carboplatin and paclitaxel treatment. It is assumed that in the first and second years, treated survivors would have a further three consultant visits, a CT scan, and four CA125 tests each year. In the third to fifth years post-surgery, it is assumed that survivors would have two consultant visits and two CA125 tests.

Costs for ovarian cancer diagnosis and treatment in the UK are derived from national reference costs and a recent ovarian cancer guideline developed by NICE [88,92]. Annual costs of ovarian cancer treatment in the USA are taken from Grann et al. 2011 [89] and inflated using the medical component of the USA consumer price index to 2016 US$. We include the costs of treatment of recurrence taken from Cancer Research UK [93] and Grann 2011 [89]. The costs of ovarian cancer diagnosis and treatment in Netherlands, China, Brazil, and India are obtained from primary data.

The costs of ovarian cancer terminal care are derived from end-of-life costs for cancer patients based on a report from the National Audit office UK [94]. For the USA, the terminal care costs for ovarian cancer are obtained from Grann 2011 [89], which were inflated using the medical component of the USA consumer price index to 2016 US$. The costs of ovarian cancer terminal care are obtained from primary data in the Netherlands, China, Brazil and India. In line with NICE recommendations, future healthcare costs not associated with ovarian cancer are not considered [95].

Appendix B.6. Costs of Breast Cancer

In the general population, 10% breast cancer is non-invasive DCIS and 90% is invasive. 95% of invasive breast cancer is early and locally advanced (stages 1–3), and 5% of invasive breast cancer is advanced breast cancer (stage 4) [96]. In *BRCA1/2* carriers, 20% of cancers are DCIS and 80% are invasive [9,97].

Seventy percent of invasive breast cancers are ER-positive [98,99], among which 49% are premenopausal; 15% of early/locally advanced breast cancers and 25% of advanced breast cancers are HER2-positive; 27% *BRCA1* and 67% *BRCA2* breast cancers are ER-positive; 5% *BRCA1* and 14% *BRCA2* breast cancers are HER2-positive [100–105]. All costs are adjusted for *BRCA1/BRCA2* breast cancers for differences in stage at presentation, the proportion of being non-invasive, and the proportion of being ER-positive or HER2-positive.

Annual breast cancer treatment costs in the USA are obtained from Grann et al. 2011 [89] and inflated using the medical component of the USA consumer price index to 2016 US$. In the UK, Netherlands, China, Brazil, and India, breast cancer treatment costs are estimated based on clinical guidelines and unit costs are detailed as below.

Diagnosis costs: Whether suspected at breast screening or through presentation to the GP, diagnosis in the breast clinic is made by triple assessment (clinical assessment, mammography, and ultrasound imaging with core biopsy and/or fine needle aspiration cytology) [98]. Clinical examination and mammography costs are from the paper by Robertson C et al. [106]. Breast ultrasound and biopsy costs are obtained from NHS reference costs [88] in the UK and from primary data in Netherlands, China, Brazil, and India. For all patients presented with suspected advanced breast cancer, MRI should be offered to assess for bone metastases [99].

Sentinel lymph node biopsy (SLNB) costs: SLNB is used for staging axilla for early invasive breast cancer and no evidence of lymph node involvement on ultrasound or a negative ultrasound-guided needle biopsy (73% of early and locally advanced invasive cancers). The SLNB costs in the UK are obtained from NHS reference costs including sentinel lymph node scan and unilateral intermediate breast procedures [88]. The SLNB costs in Netherlands, China, Brazil, and India are obtained from the primary data sources described above.

Pretreatment axilla ultrasound costs: Pretreatment ultrasound evaluation of the axilla should be performed for all patients being investigated for early invasive breast cancer and, if morphologically abnormal lymph nodes are identified, ultrasound-guided needle sampling should be offered [96]. The commissioning cost of pretreatment ultrasound evaluation of the breast and axilla is the same as that of the breast only [88]. The costing model considers the cost of ultrasound-guided needle sampling only, obtained from NHS reference costs (UK) [24] and primary data (Netherlands, China, Brazil, and India).

Axillary lymph node dissection (ALND) costs: ALNB is undertaken for lymph node positive cancers (approximately 31% early and locally advanced invasive cancers—NICE guideline and

BCCOM project [96,98,107]; 30% node positive for BRCA1/2 breast cancer—familial breast cancer screening studies, breast cancer case series and Early Breast Cancer Trialists' Collaborative Group data) [97,100–102,108]. The cost of ALND is assumed to be 25% of the cost of breast surgery as per NICE guideline development group recommendations [96].

Breast surgery costs include costs of breast-conserving surgery (assumed for all non-invasive cancers and 75% of early/locally advanced invasive cancers) and costs of mastectomy with reconstruction (for 25% early/locally advanced and all advanced cancers). Costs are obtained from the national NHS reference costs (UK) [88] and primary data (Netherlands, China, Brazil, and India).

Chemotherapy and radiotherapy costs: Invasive breast cancers who are not at low risk [107,109,110] receive adjuvant treatment in line with NICE guidelines. Costs include radiotherapy costs for 60% of early invasive/locally advanced, radiotherapy, and chemotherapy costs for 40% early invasive/locally advanced, and chemotherapy for all advanced cancers. Radiotherapy costs include planning and 40Gy in 15 fractions over 3 weeks [98] or palliative treatment; these were taken from national NHS reference costs [88]. Chemotherapy costs based on polychemotherapy [108] include administration costs, the costs of first and second-line therapy and toxicity from NICE guidelines [96,99]. In the Netherlands, China, Brazil, and India, radiotherapy costs and chemotherapy costs are obtained from the primary data sources described above.

Endocrine therapy costs: As per NICE guidelines [96,98], ER-positive invasive breast cancers receive Tamoxifen 20 mg/day (premenopausal) or Anastrazole 1mg/day (postmenopausal). Seventy percent of invasive breast cancers are ER-positive [98,99], among which 49% are premenopausal. We assume that the length of endocrine therapy is 5 years. The drug costs are obtained from the BNF [26] in the UK. ER testing costs are obtained from a local NHS trust and included for all invasive breast cancers. The costs of drugs and ER testing are obtained from primary data sources in the Netherlands, China, Brazil, and India described above.

Target therapy costs: HER2-positive breast cancer patients can be given at 3-week intervals for 1 year or until disease recurrence as per NICE guidelines. Breast cancer patients with positive HER2 are eligible for treatment with trastuzumab [98,99]. Ten percent of the eligible patients are intolerant of trastuzumab. Among women suitable for this treatment, 80% receive trastuzumab [96]. HER2 testing costs are obtained from a local NHS trust and included for all invasive breast cancers. The trastuzumab cost per patient including the administration of treatment and cardiac monitoring is £15080, which was obtained from the NICE costing report [96]. In the Netherlands, China, Brazil, and India, the costs of HER2 testing and trastuzumab are obtained from the primary data sources described above.

Follow-up costs: Breast cancer patients are offered mammographic surveillance and clinical follow up, with the screening cost of £141.45 per women in 2011 [106]. We assume that patients are followed up every four months in the first two years, every six months from the third to the fifth year, and every year from the sixth to the 10th year.

Bisphosphonate costs: Bisphosphonates is considered to be offered to patients newly diagnosed with bone metastases to prevent skeletal-related events and reduce pain [99]. Seventy-four percent of patients with advanced breast cancer will develop bone metastases, and 65% of patients with bone metastases are offered bisphosphonates [96,111]. Bisphosphonates that are currently offered include oral sodium clodronate, ibandronic acid, zoledronic acid, and pamidronate. The proportions of patients receiving the four drugs are 20%, 30%, 25%, and 25%, respectively. The annual costs including administration for the four drugs are £1971, £2541.96, £3208, and £3208 respectively, which were obtained from the NICE costing report [96]. We assume that the average length of bisphosphonates treatment is 2.7 years, which is the life expectancy of advanced breast cancers based on one-year survival rate (63.2%) [112]. The bisphosphonate costs in the Netherlands, China, Brazil, and India are obtained from the primary data sources described above.

Recurrence costs: For non-invasive breast cancers, the non-invasive and invasive relapse rates are both 12.5%. Thirty-five percent of early and locally advanced invasive breast cancers progress to advanced disease [96]. The recurrence rates for early and locally advanced breast cancer are 15.9% for node-positive [113] and 11% for node-negative disease [114]. Weighted for 31% node positive and 69% node negative, the composite recurrence rate for early and locally advanced breast cancer is 12.5%. The recurrence rate for the advanced disease is 66% (34% relapse-free five-year survival) [115].

Terminal care costs: The costs of terminal care for breast cancer are derived from end-of-life costs for cancer patients based on a report from the National Audit office UK [30]. For the US, the terminal care costs for breast cancer are obtained from Grann 2011 [89], and these were inflated using the medical component of the US consumer price index to 2016 US$. The costs of breast cancer terminal care are obtained from primary data sources in the Netherlands, China, Brazil, and India. In line with NICE recommendations, future healthcare costs not associated with breast cancer were not considered [95].

Appendix B.7. Cost of Breast Cancer Screening

For non-carriers, we assume routine triennial mammography between 50 and 70 years as per the UK NHS breast cancer screening programme [116] (seven mammograms on average). Breast screening in the USA assumes mammography every two years starting at 50 years [117]. In the Netherlands, the National Breast Cancer Screening Programme is designed for women between 50 and 75 years of age. Once every 2 years, women in this age group are invited for a mammogram. The guidelines from the Brazilian Ministry of Health is for all women aged 50–69 years to be screened with mammography only every 2 years. The coverage in the target age group remains low ranging from 27% to 51% [118]. To obtain a conservative estimate of the cost-effectiveness of population-based genetic testing, we adopted the highest value of uptake (51%) in Brazil. There is no national breast cancer screening programme in China or India.

For BRCA1/BRCA2 mutation carriers, we assume an annual mammogram from 40 to 69 years and annual MRI from 30–49 years as per NICE guidelines for familial breast cancer [119] (30 mammograms and 20 MRIs on average). We assume that breast cancer screening policies for BRCA1/2 carriers in the Netherlands, China, Brazil, and India, are the same as that in the UK. For the USA, it is based on annual mammography and MRI starting at 30 years, and annual mammography only from age 50 years [117].

Appendix B.8. Cost of Chemoprevention

BRCA1/BRCA2 mutation carriers are offered tamoxifen (premenopausal) or raloxifene (postmenopausal) for 5 years [119,120] to reduce breast cancer risk. The drug costs are obtained from the BNF (UK) [90], Grann 2011 (US) [89], and primary data (Netherlands, China, Brazil, and India). A 16.3% uptake is assumed for chemoprevention [64].

Appendix B.9. Cost of CHD

Cost of excess CHD: British Heart Foundation statistics reports costs per capita across four commissioning regions in England (London, Midlands and East, North, and South) [121].

The costs of CHD and stroke are averaged across the four regions. The prevalence of CHD is estimated at 12.0% in the UK [121] and 11.7% in the USA [122], with the onset of CHD estimated at 55 years of age [33,123].

The yearly cost of CHD in the UK is obtained by dividing the per capita cost by the population prevalence of CHD [121]. Using the report published by the American Heart Association [124], the total cost of CHD, CHF, and stroke were divided by the population with CHD [122,125], giving the yearly cost of CHD in the USA. This yearly cost is multiplied by the number of years between onset of CHD and average life expectancy to provide the cost attributed to excess CHD.

Cost of fatal CHD: This is costed on the basis of a fatal myocardial infarction using NHS reference costs [88]. USA costs are obtained from Afana et al. 2015 [126], and these are inflated using the medical component of the US consumer price index to 2016 US$.

We used the ratio of breast cancer treatment costs in the Netherlands, China, Brazil, and India compared to treatment costs in the UK to impute the costs of excess CHD and fatal CHD in each of these countries (Netherlands, China, Brazil, and India) based on the cost of CHD in the UK.

Appendix C. Estimation of Productivity Loss

The retirement ages for females are 65 in the UK, 62 in the USA, 50–55 in China, 60 in Brazil, 68 in Netherlands, and 60–65 in India. We used the lower values of the retirement age ranges in China and India to get the conservative estimates of productivity loss. The female labour force participation rates are 56.77% in the UK, 55.99% in the USA, 62.03% in China, 53.32% in Brazil, 58.02% in Netherlands, and 27.45% in India, which were obtained from the World Bank [71]. The hourly wage rage across countries are presented in Table A3.

Table A3. Hourly wage rage across countries (USA dollars in 2016).

Age	UK	USA	Netherlands	China	Brazil	India
30–34	19.47	13.08	16.85	5	5.54	4.77
35–39	19.47	14.75	22.37	5	5.54	4.58
40–44	19.33	14.75	22.37	5	5.54	4.58
45–49	19.33	14.97	24.11	5	5.54	6.56
50–54	17.42	14.97	24.11		5.54	6.56
55–59	17.42	15.10	24.19		5.54	3.71
60–64	15.08	15.10	24.19			
65–69			21.32			
Source	[127]	[128]	[129]	[130]	[131]	[132]

We categorised the productivity costs as three subcomponents: (1) temporary disability due to short-term work absences following diagnosis, (2) permanent disability due to reduced working hours following a return to work or workforce departure; and (3) premature mortality due to death before retirement [72], as detailed in Table A4.

Table A4. Descriptive statistics for productivity loss in breast and ovarian cancer patients.

Variables	Breast Cancer	Ovarian Cancer
(1) Temporary disability		
Percentage of temporary disability cases	94.0%	98% [1]
Average time taken off work following diagnosis (weeks)	44.9	47.22 [2]
(2) Permanent disability		
Percentage of permanent disability: reduced hours	26%	40% [3]
Reduced hours per week after returning to work (hours)	5.5	5.5
(3) Premature mortality (before retirement)		
Percentage of permanent disability: workforce departure	12.9%	30% [3]

Source: Hanly P, et al., 2012 [72]. [1] We assume 98% ovarian cancer patients have cancer-related short-term work absences after diagnosis. [2] We assume ovarian cancer patients experience four weeks for surgery, 24 weeks for chemotherapy, and 24 weeks for recurrence treatment with the recurrence rate of 80% [133]. [3] We assume the percentages of permanent disability for ovarian cancer are 40% for reduced working hours and 30% for workforce departure.

We estimated temporary disability as time absent from work multiplied by age-specific gross earnings.

We calculated productivity costs due to permanent disability by applying age-specific gross earnings to the reduction in working hours, or the number of working hours if permanent workforce departure, until retirement age. Regarding productivity loss from premature mortality, we assumed that without cancer, the productive capacity of an individual would continue from the age of diagnosis until age of retirement. We multiplied the projected years of life lost by the age-specific gross earnings for the remainder of the working life to generate monetary estimates.

Appendix D. Maximum Values of Genetic Testing Costs at Which Offering Genetic Testing for the Population Remains Cost-Effective.

Table A5. Maximum values of genetic testing costs at which offering genetic testing for the population remains cost-effective.

	Payer Perspective		Societal Perspective	
	Lower WTP #	**Higher WTP ##**	**Lower WTP #**	**Higher WTP ##**
Thresholds based on GDP				
UK	$412 ($42,648/QALY)	$1254 ($127,869/QALY)	$677 ($42,639/QALY)	$1520 ($127,960/QALY)
USA	$519 ($57,490/QALY)	$1417 ($172,735/QALY)	$680 ($57,582/QALY)	$1577 ($172,698/QALY)
Netherlands	$442 ($50,539/QALY)	$1407 ($151,520/QALY)	$792 ($50,517/QALY)	$1758 ($151,603/QALY)
China	$146 ($15,402/QALY)	$354 ($46,536/QALY)	$183 ($15,522/QALY)	$390 ($46,506/QALY)
Brazil	$130 ($15,143/QALY)	$493 ($45,490/QALY)	$219 ($15,168/QALY)	$582 ($45,515/QALY)
India	Not cost-effective	$95 ($19,670/QALY)	$62 ($6,540/QALY)	$172 ($19,685/QALY)
Thresholds based on local economic evaluation guidelines				
UK	$238 ($28,386/QALY)	$365 ($42,826/QALY)	$481 ($28,406/QALY)	$608 ($42,845/QALY)
USA	$460 ($49,919/QALY)	$850 ($99,969/QALY)	$620 ($49,882/QALY)	$1010 ($99,933/QALY)
Netherlands∫	$293 ($24,364/QALY)	$800 ($60,934/QALY)	$582 ($24,369/QALY)	$1089 ($60,939/QALY)

1*GDP per capita, ## 3*GDP per capita, WTP—willingness to pay (threshold), GDP—gross domestic product.

The appendix describes the maximum genetic testing costs and corresponding ICER/QALY (in brackets) at which offering *BRCA* testing for the population will remain cost-effective. Results are presented for both the payer and societal perspectives.

For GDP-based thresholds: This is cost-effective at the standard 3*GDP per capita WTP threshold and highly cost-effective at the 1*GDP per capita WTP threshold [82]. The discount rate is 3% for costs and health effects (LYs and QALYs) [81].

For country-specific thresholds:

For the UK, this is £20,000 to £30,000 [25,134]; for the USA, this is $50,000 to $100,000 [26,135]; for the Netherlands, this is: €20,000 to €50,000 [27]. Values in £s and €s have been converted to $ using PPP (purchasing power parity) [28].

For country-specific thresholds:

For the UK, the discount rate is 3.5% discount for costs and QALYs [25,134]; for the USA, this is 3% discount for costs and QALYs [53]; for the Netherlands, this is 4% discount for costs and 1.5% discount for QALYs [136].

Perspective:

WHO guidelines recommend a societal perspective [81,82].

Dutch guidelines recommend a societal perspective [136]. UK NICE guidelines recommend a payer perspective [25]. US guidelines recommend presentation of both societal and payer perspectives [53].

Appendix E. One-Way Sensitivity Analyses

One-way sensitivity analysis for all probabilities, costs, and utilities in terms of ICER of population-based BRCA testing compared to a clinical-criteria/FH-based approach in the UK, USA, Netherlands, China, Brazil, and India from both the payer perspective and the societal perspective.

X-axis: Incremental cost-effectiveness ratio (ICER): cost (£s or $s) per quality-adjusted life year (QALY) (discounted).

Y-axis: Probability, cost, and utility parameters in the model. The model is run at both lower and upper values/limits of the 95% confidence interval or range of all probability parameters described in Table 1, and both lower and upper values/limits of the cost and utility-score parameters given in the methods and Table 2.

'Upper value' represents outcomes for the upper limit of the parameter, and 'Lower value' represents outcomes for lower limit of the parameter.

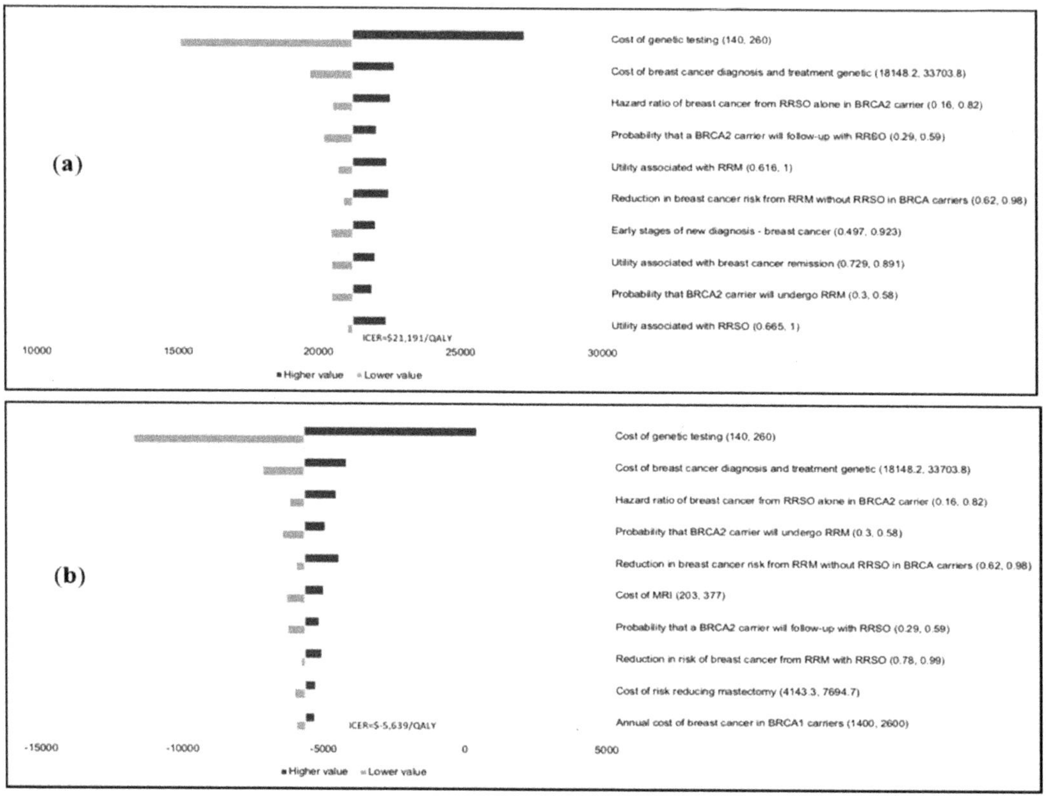

Figure A1. Tornado Diagram in the UK (**a**) from the healthcare payer perspective. (**b**) from the societal perspective.

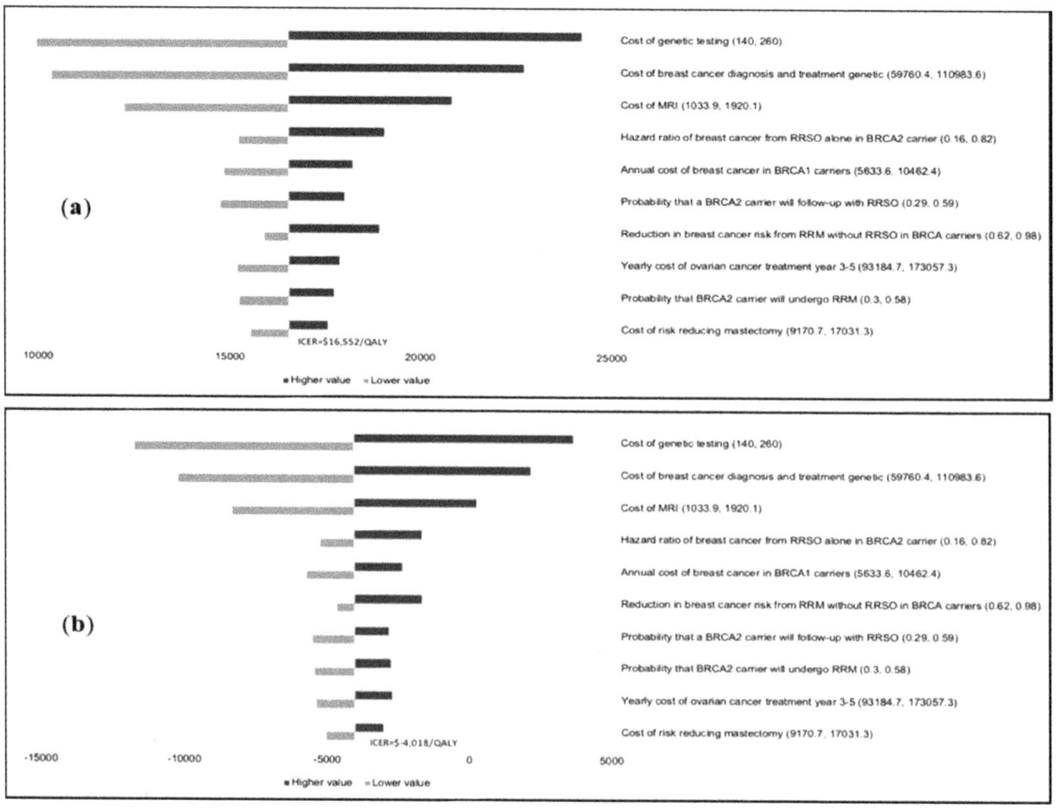

Figure A2. Tornado Diagram in the USA (**a**) from the healthcare payer perspective. (**b**) from the societal perspective.

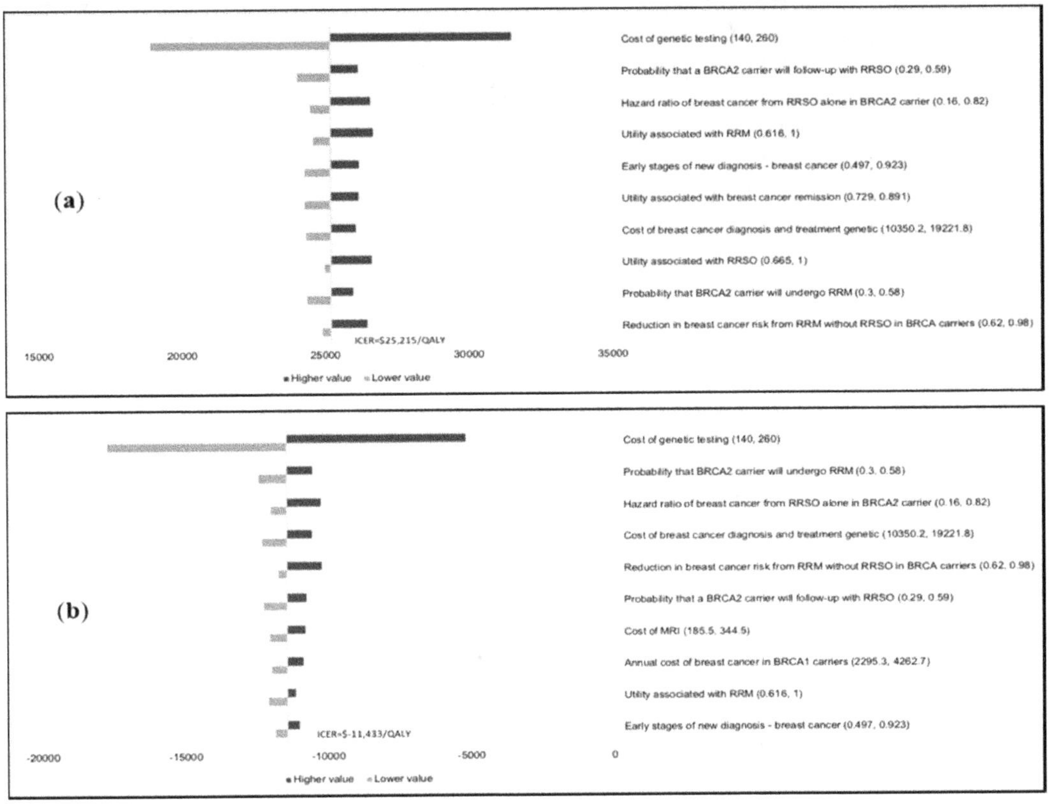

Figure A3. Tornado Diagram in the Netherlands (**a**) from the healthcare payer perspective. (**b**) from the societal perspective.

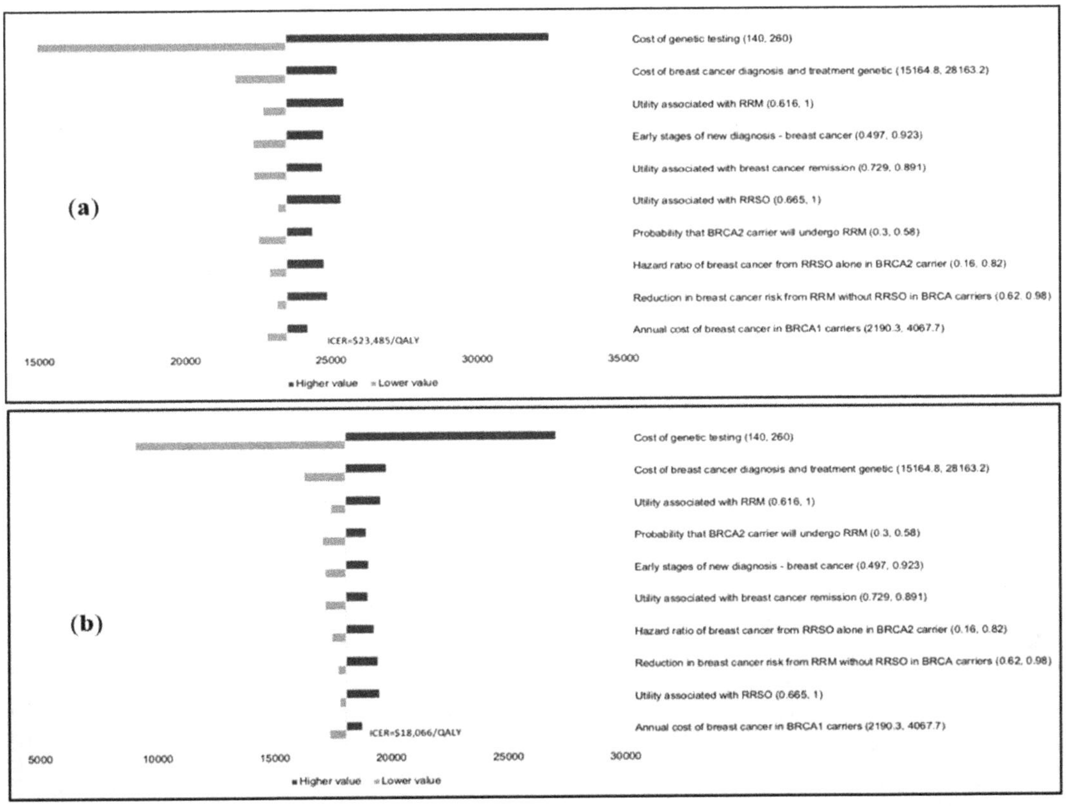

Figure A4. Tornado Diagram in China (**a**) from the healthcare payer perspective. (**b**) from the societal perspective.

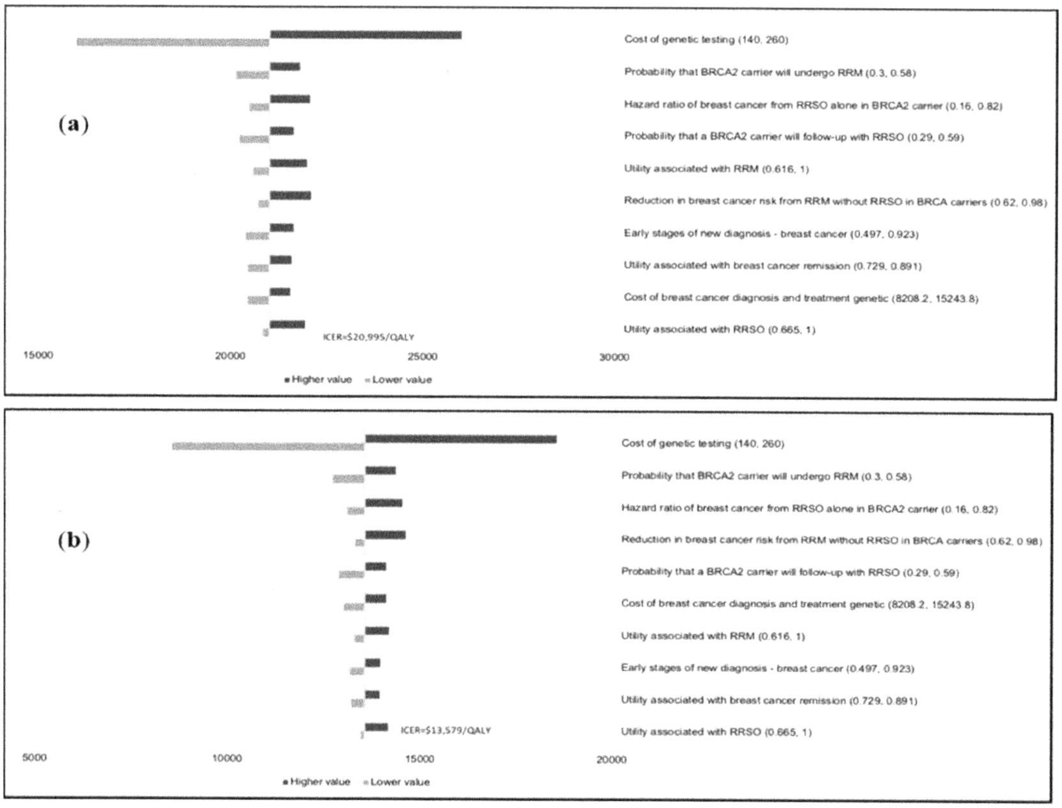

Figure A5. Tornado Diagram in Brazil (**a**) from the healthcare payer perspective. (**b**) from the societal perspective.

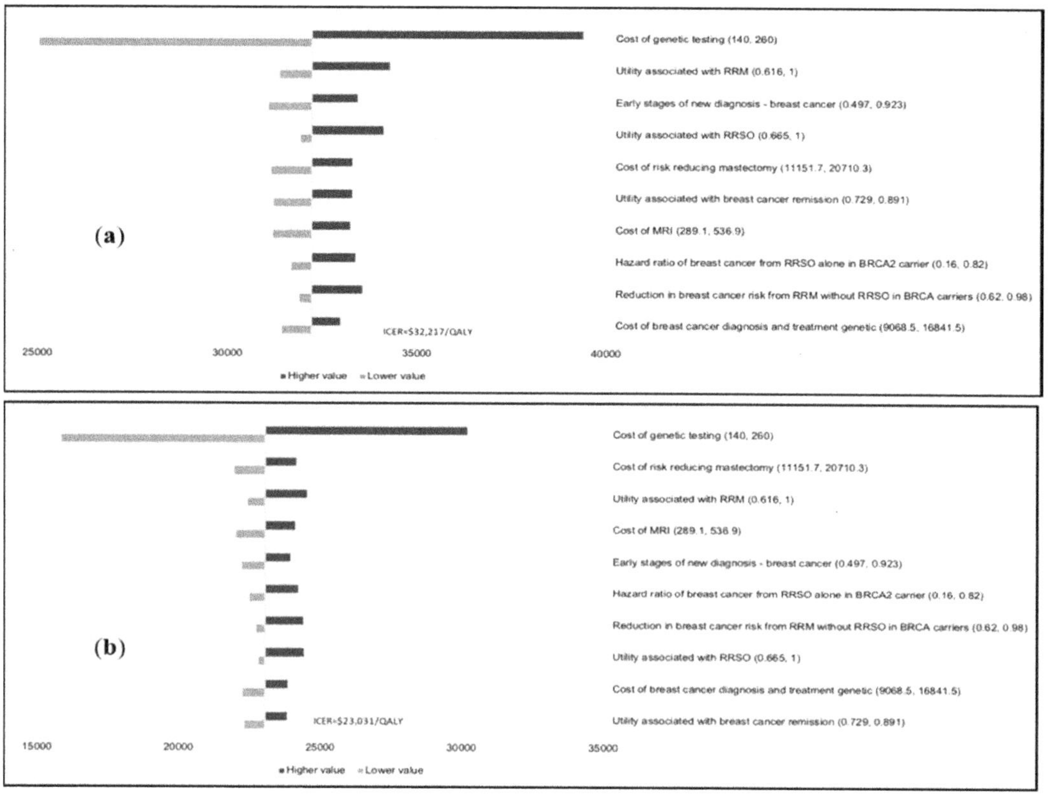

Figure A6. Tornado Diagram in India (**a**) from the healthcare payer perspective. (**b**) from the societal perspective.

References

1. Harter, P.; Hauke, J.; Heitz, F.; Reuss, A.; Kommoss, S.; Marme, F.; Heimbach, A.; Prieske, K.; Richters, L.; Burges, A.; et al. Prevalence of deleterious germline variants in risk genes including BRCA1/2 in consecutive ovarian cancer patients (AGO-TR-1). *PLoS ONE* **2017**, *12*, e0186043. [CrossRef]
2. Buys, S.S.; Sandbach, J.F.; Gammon, A.; Patel, G.; Kidd, J.; Brown, K.L.; Sharma, L.; Saam, J.; Lancaster, J.; Daly, M.B. A study of over 35,000 women with breast cancer tested with a 25-gene panel of hereditary cancer genes. *Cancer* **2017**, *123*, 1721–1730. [CrossRef] [PubMed]
3. Kuchenbaecker, K.B.; Hopper, J.L.; Barnes, D.R.; Phillips, K.A.; Mooij, T.M.; Roos-Blom, M.J.; Jervis, S.; Van Leeuwen, F.E.; Milne, R.L.; Andrieu, N.; et al. Risks of Breast, Ovarian, and Contralateral Breast Cancer for BRCA1 and BRCA2 Mutation Carriers. *JAMA* **2017**, *317*, 2402–2416. [CrossRef] [PubMed]
4. Rebbeck, T.R.; Kauff, N.D.; Domchek, S.M. Meta-analysis of risk reduction estimates associated with risk-reducing salpingo-oophorectomy in BRCA1 or BRCA2 mutation carriers. *J. Natl. Cancer Inst.* **2009**, *101*, 80–87. [CrossRef] [PubMed]
5. Kauff, N.D.; Domchek, S.M.; Friebel, T.M.; Robson, M.E.; Lee, J.; Garber, J.E.; Isaacs, C.; Evans, D.G.; Lynch, H.; Eeles, R.A.; et al. Risk-reducing salpingo-oophorectomy for the prevention of BRCA1- and BRCA2-associated breast and gynecologic cancer: A multicenter, prospective study. *J. Clin. Oncol.* **2008**, *26*, 1331–1337. [CrossRef]
6. Finch, A.; Beiner, M.; Lubinski, J.; Lynch, H.T.; Moller, P.; Rosen, B.; Murphy, J.; Ghadirian, P.; Friedman, E.; Foulkes, W.D.; et al. Salpingo-oophorectomy and the risk of ovarian, fallopian tube, and peritoneal cancers in women with a BRCA1 or BRCA2 Mutation. *JAMA* **2006**, *296*, 185–192. [CrossRef]
7. Nelson, H.D.; Fu, R.; Zakher, B.; Pappas, M.; McDonagh, M. Medication Use for the Risk Reduction of Primary Breast Cancer in Women: Updated Evidence Report and Systematic Review for the US Preventive Services Task Force. *JAMA* **2019**, *322*, 868–886. [CrossRef]
8. Rebbeck, T.R.; Friebel, T.; Lynch, H.T.; Neuhausen, S.L.; Van't Veer, L.; Garber, J.E.; Evans, G.R.; Narod, S.A.; Isaacs, C.; Matloff, E.; et al. Bilateral prophylactic mastectomy reduces breast cancer risk in BRCA1 and BRCA2 mutation carriers: The PROSE Study Group. *J. Clin. Oncol.* **2004**, *22*, 1055–1062. [CrossRef] [PubMed]
9. Nelson, H.D.; Pappas, M.; Zakher, B.; Mitchell, J.P.; Okinaka-Hu, L.; Fu, R. Risk assessment, genetic counseling, and genetic testing for BRCA-related cancer in women: A systematic review to update the U.S. Preventive Services Task Force recommendation. *Ann. Intern. Med.* **2014**, *160*, 255–266. [CrossRef] [PubMed]
10. NICE. Familial Breast Cancer: Classification and Care of People at Risk of Familial Breast Cancer and Management of Breast Cancer and Related Risks in People with a Family History of Breast Cancer. In *NICE Clinical Guideline CG164*; National Institute for Health and Care Excellence: London, UK, 2013.
11. Childers, C.P.; Childers, K.K.; Maggard-Gibbons, M.; Macinko, J. National Estimates of Genetic Testing in Women With a History of Breast or Ovarian Cancer. *J. Clin. Oncol.* **2017**, *35*, 3800–3806. [CrossRef] [PubMed]
12. Manchanda, R.; Blyuss, O.; Gaba, F.; Gordeev, V.S.; Jacobs, C.; Burnell, M.; Gan, C.; Taylor, R.; Turnbull, C.; Legood, R.; et al. Current detection rates and time-to-detection of all identifiable BRCA carriers in the Greater London population. *J. Med. Genet.* **2018**, *55*. [CrossRef] [PubMed]
13. NHS England. *Clinical Commissioning Policy: Genetic Testing for BRCA1 and BRCA2 Mutations*; NHS England Specialised Services Clinical Reference Group for Medical Genetics: London, UK, 2015.
14. Manchanda, R.; Lieberman, S.; Gaba, F.; Lahad, A.; Levy-Lahad, E. Population Screening for Inherited Predisposition to Breast and Ovarian Cancer. *Annu. Rev. Genom. Hum. Genet.* **2020**. [CrossRef] [PubMed]
15. Gabai-Kapara, E.; Lahad, A.; Kaufman, B.; Friedman, E.; Segev, S.; Renbaum, P.; Beeri, R.; Gal, M.; Grinshpun-Cohen, J.; Djemal, K.; et al. Population-based screening for breast and ovarian cancer risk due to BRCA1 and BRCA2. *Proc. Natl. Acad. Sci. USA* **2014**, *111*, 14205–14210. [CrossRef] [PubMed]
16. Manchanda, R.; Burnell, M.; Gaba, F.; Desai, R.; Wardle, J.; Gessler, S.; Side, L.; Sanderson, S.; Loggenberg, K.; Brady, A.F.; et al. Randomised trial of population-based BRCA testing in Ashkenazi Jews: Long-term outcomes. *BJOG* **2020**, *127*, 364–375. [CrossRef]
17. George, A.; Riddell, D.; Seal, S.; Talukdar, S.; Mahamdallie, S.; Ruark, E.; Cloke, V.; Slade, I.; Kemp, Z.; Gore, M.; et al. Implementing rapid, robust, cost-effective, patient-centred, routine genetic testing in ovarian cancer patients. *Sci. Rep.* **2016**, *6*, 29506. [CrossRef]

18. Moller, P.; Hagen, A.I.; Apold, J.; Maehle, L.; Clark, N.; Fiane, B.; Lovslett, K.; Hovig, E.; Vabo, A. Genetic epidemiology of BRCA mutations—Family history detects less than 50% of the mutation carriers. *Eur. J. Cancer* **2007**, *43*, 1713–1717. [CrossRef] [PubMed]
19. Norum, J.; Grindedal, E.M.; Heramb, C.; Karsrud, I.; Ariansen, S.L.; Undlien, D.E.; Schlichting, E.; Maehle, L. BRCA mutation carrier detection. A model-based cost-effectiveness analysis comparing the traditional family history approach and the testing of all patients with breast cancer. *ESMO Open* **2018**, *3*, e000328. [CrossRef]
20. Beitsch, P.D.; Whitworth, P.W.; Hughes, K.; Patel, R.; Rosen, B.; Compagnoni, G.; Baron, P.; Simmons, R.; Smith, L.A.; Grady, I.; et al. Underdiagnosis of Hereditary Breast Cancer: Are Genetic Testing Guidelines a Tool or an Obstacle? *J. Clin. Oncol.* **2018**, *37*. [CrossRef]
21. Manchanda, R.; Legood, R.; Burnell, M.; McGuire, A.; Raikou, M.; Loggenberg, K.; Wardle, J.; Sanderson, S.; Gessler, S.; Side, L.; et al. Cost-effectiveness of population screening for BRCA mutations in Ashkenazi jewish women compared with family history-based testing. *J. Natl. Cancer Inst.* **2015**, *107*, 380. [CrossRef]
22. Manchanda, R.; Loggenberg, K.; Sanderson, S.; Burnell, M.; Wardle, J.; Gessler, S.; Side, L.; Balogun, N.; Desai, R.; Kumar, A.; et al. Population testing for cancer predisposing BRCA1/BRCA2 mutations in the Ashkenazi-Jewish community: A randomized controlled trial. *J. Natl. Cancer Inst.* **2015**, *107*, 379. [CrossRef]
23. Manchanda, R.; Gaba, F. Population Based Testing for Primary Prevention: A Systematic Review. *Cancers* **2018**, *10*, 424. [CrossRef]
24. Griffiths, U.K.; Legood, R.; Pitt, C. Comparison of Economic Evaluation Methods Across Low-income, Middle-income and High-income Countries: What are the Differences and Why? *Health Econ.* **2016**, *25* (Suppl. 1), 29–41. [CrossRef] [PubMed]
25. NICE. *Guide to the Methods of Technology Appraisal*; National Institute of Health and Care Excellence: London, UK, 2013.
26. Neumann, P.J.; Cohen, J.T.; Weinstein, M.C. Updating cost-effectiveness—The curious resilience of the $50,000-per-QALY threshold. *N. Engl. J. Med.* **2014**, *371*, 796–797. [CrossRef]
27. *Kosteneffectiviteit in de Praktijk*; Zorginstituut Nederland (National Health Care Institute, Netherlands): Diemen, The Netherlands, 2015.
28. The World Bank. PPP Conversion Factor, GDP. Available online: http://data.worldbank.org/indicator/PA.NUS.PPP (accessed on 9 August 2019).
29. World Bank. Population, Female. Available online: https://data.worldbank.org/indicator/SP.POP.TOTL.FE.IN?year_high_desc=true (accessed on 29 January 2019).
30. Woods, B.; Revill, P.; Sculpher, M.; Claxton, K. Country-Level Cost-Effectiveness Thresholds: Initial Estimates and the Need for Further Research. *Value Health* **2016**, *19*, 929–935. [CrossRef] [PubMed]
31. Bertram, M.Y.; Lauer, J.A.; De Joncheere, K.; Edejer, T.; Hutubessy, R.; Kieny, M.P.; Hill, S.R. Cost-effectiveness thresholds: Pros and cons. *Bull. World Health Organ.* **2016**, *94*, 925–930. [CrossRef]
32. Ottersen, T.; Forde, R.; Kakad, M.; Kjellevold, A.; Melberg, H.O.; Moen, A.; Ringard, A.; Norheim, O.F. A new proposal for priority setting in Norway: Open and fair. *Health Policy* **2016**, *120*, 246–251. [CrossRef]
33. Parker, W.H.; Feskanich, D.; Broder, M.S.; Chang, E.; Shoupe, D.; Farquhar, C.M.; Berek, J.S.; Manson, J.E. Long-term mortality associated with oophorectomy compared with ovarian conservation in the nurses' health study. *Obstet. Gynecol.* **2013**, *121*, 709–716. [CrossRef]
34. Metcalfe, K.; Eisen, A.; Senter, L.; Armel, S.; Bordeleau, L.; Meschino, W.S.; Pal, T.; Lynch, H.T.; Tung, N.M.; Kwong, A.; et al. International trends in the uptake of cancer risk reduction strategies in women with a BRCA1 or BRCA2 mutation. *Br. J. Cancer* **2019**, *121*. [CrossRef] [PubMed]
35. Manchanda, R.; Abdelraheim, A.; Johnson, M.; Rosenthal, A.N.; Benjamin, E.; Brunell, C.; Burnell, M.; Side, L.; Gessler, S.; Saridogan, E.; et al. Outcome of risk-reducing salpingo-oophorectomy in BRCA carriers and women of unknown mutation status. *BJOG* **2011**, *118*, 814–824. [CrossRef]
36. Miller, M.E.; Czechura, T.; Martz, B.; Hall, M.E.; Pesce, C.; Jaskowiak, N.; Winchester, D.J.; Yao, K. Operative risks associated with contralateral prophylactic mastectomy: A single institution experience. *Ann. Surg. Oncol.* **2013**, *20*, 4113–4120. [CrossRef] [PubMed]
37. Gaba, F.; Manchanda, R. Systematic review of acceptability, cardiovascular, neurological, bone health and HRT outcomes following risk reducing surgery in BRCA carriers. *Best Pract. Res. Clin. Obstet. Gynaecol.* **2020**, *65*. [CrossRef] [PubMed]

38. Metcalfe, K.A.; Poll, A.; Royer, R.; Llacuachaqui, M.; Tulman, A.; Sun, P.; Narod, S.A. Screening for founder mutations in BRCA1 and BRCA2 in unselected Jewish women. *J. Clin. Oncol.* **2010**, *28*, 387–391. [CrossRef] [PubMed]
39. Lieberman, S.; Tomer, A.; Ben-Chetrit, A.; Olsha, O.; Strano, S.; Beeri, R.; Koka, S.; Fridman, H.; Djemal, K.; Glick, I.; et al. Population screening for BRCA1/BRCA2 founder mutations in Ashkenazi Jews: Proactive recruitment compared with self-referral. *Genet. Med.* **2016**, *19*. [CrossRef]
40. Metcalfe, K.A.; Poll, A.; Llacuachaqui, M.; Nanda, S.; Tulman, A.; Mian, N.; Sun, P.; Narod, S.A. Patient satisfaction and cancer-related distress among unselected Jewish women undergoing genetic testing for BRCA1 and BRCA2. *Clin. Genet.* **2010**, *78*, 411–417. [CrossRef] [PubMed]
41. Yuen, J.; Cousens, N.; Barlow-Stewart, K.; O'Shea, R.; Andrews, L. Online BRCA1/2 screening in the Australian Jewish community: A qualitative study. *J. Community Genet.* **2019**, *11*. [CrossRef] [PubMed]
42. Manchanda, R. Predicting risk of ovarian malignancy improved screening and early detection feasibility study. In *ISRCTN Registry: ISRCTN54246466*; BioMed Central: London, UK, 2017.
43. Plon, S.E.; Eccles, D.M.; Easton, D.; Foulkes, W.D.; Genuardi, M.; Greenblatt, M.S.; Hogervorst, F.B.; Hoogerbrugge, N.; Spurdle, A.B.; Tavtigian, S.V.; et al. Sequence variant classification and reporting: Recommendations for improving the interpretation of cancer susceptibility genetic test results. *Hum. Mutat.* **2008**, *29*, 1282–1291. [CrossRef] [PubMed]
44. Global Burden of Disease Cancer, C.; Fitzmaurice, C.; Akinyemiju, T.F.; Al Lami, F.H.; Alam, T.; Alizadeh-Navaei, R.; Allen, C.; Alsharif, U.; Alvis-Guzman, N.; Amini, E.; et al. Global, Regional, and National Cancer Incidence, Mortality, Years of Life Lost, Years Lived With Disability, and Disability-Adjusted Life-Years for 29 Cancer Groups, 1990 to 2016: A Systematic Analysis for the Global Burden of Disease Study. *JAMA Oncol.* **2018**, *4*, 1553–1568. [CrossRef]
45. International Agency for Research on Cancer. Cancer Tomorrow. In *A Tool That Predicts the Future Cancer Incidence and Mortality Burden Worldwide from the Current Estimates in 2018 up until 2040*; International Agency for Research on Cancer (IARC): Lyon, France, 2018.
46. Wilson, J.; Jungner, G. *Principles and Practice of Screening for Disease*; 34; World Health Organisation: Geneva, Switzerland, 1968.
47. UK, N.S.C. Criteria for Appraising the Viability, Effectiveness and Appropriateness of a Screening Programme. Available online: https://www.gov.uk/government/publications/evidence-review-criteria-national-screening-programmes/criteria-for-appraising-the-viability-effectiveness-and-appropriateness-of-a-screening-programme (accessed on 1 December 2019).
48. Khoury, M.J.; McCabe, L.L.; McCabe, E.R. Population screening in the age of genomic medicine. *N. Engl. J. Med.* **2003**, *348*, 50–58. [CrossRef]
49. CDC. ACCE Model Process for Evaluating Genetic Tests. In *Genomic Testing*; The Office of Public Health Genomics (OPHG), Centers for Disease Control and Prevention (CDC): Atlanta, GA, USA, 2010.
50. Burke, W.; Zimmerman, R. *Moving Beyond ACCE: An Expanded Framework for Genetic Test Evaluation*; PHG Foundation: London, UK, 2007.
51. Force, U.S.P.S.T.; Owens, D.K.; Davidson, K.W.; Krist, A.H.; Barry, M.J.; Cabana, M.; Caughey, A.B.; Doubeni, C.A.; Epling, J.W., Jr.; Kubik, M.; et al. Risk Assessment, Genetic Counseling, and Genetic Testing for BRCA-Related Cancer: US Preventive Services Task Force Recommendation Statement. *JAMA* **2019**, *322*, 652–665. [CrossRef]
52. Nelson, H.D.; Pappas, M.; Cantor, A.; Haney, E.; Holmes, R. Risk Assessment, Genetic Counseling, and Genetic Testing for BRCA-Related Cancer in Women: Updated Evidence Report and Systematic Review for the US Preventive Services Task Force. *JAMA* **2019**, *322*, 666–685. [CrossRef]
53. Sanders, G.D.; Neumann, P.J.; Basu, A.; Brock, D.W.; Feeny, D.; Krahn, M.; Kuntz, K.M.; Meltzer, D.O.; Owens, D.K.; Prosser, L.A.; et al. Recommendations for Conduct, Methodological Practices, and Reporting of Cost-effectiveness Analyses: Second Panel on Cost-Effectiveness in Health and Medicine. *JAMA* **2016**, *316*, 1093–1103. [CrossRef] [PubMed]
54. Eggington, J.M.; Bowles, K.R.; Moyes, K.; Manley, S.; Esterling, L.; Sizemore, S.; Rosenthal, E.; Theisen, A.; Saam, J.; Arnell, C.; et al. A comprehensive laboratory-based program for classification of variants of uncertain significance in hereditary cancer genes. *Clin. Genet.* **2014**, *86*, 229–237. [CrossRef] [PubMed]

55. Cancer Research UK. Breast Cancer Incidence (Invasive) Statistics. Available online: http://www.cancerresearchuk.org/health-professional/cancer-statistics/statistics-by-cancer-type/breast-cancer/incidence-invasive#collapseOne (accessed on 14 March 2019).
56. Cancer Research UK. Ovarian Cancer Incidence Statistics. Available online: http://www.cancerresearchuk.org/health-professional/cancer-statistics/statistics-by-cancer-type/ovarian-cancer/incidence#heading-One (accessed on 14 March 2019).
57. United States Cancer Statistics. Rate of New Cancers by Age Group, All Races, Female. Available online: https://gis.cdc.gov/Cancer/USCS/DataViz.html (accessed on 19 November 2019).
58. International Agency for Research on Cancer. Estimated Number of New Cases in 2018, Worldwide, Females, All Ages. Available online: http://gco.iarc.fr/today/online-analysis-table (accessed on 21 November 2019).
59. Jervis, S.; Song, H.; Lee, A.; Dicks, E.; Harrington, P.; Baynes, C.; Manchanda, R.; Easton, D.F.; Jacobs, I.; Pharoah, P.P.; et al. A risk prediction algorithm for ovarian cancer incorporating BRCA1, BRCA2, common alleles and other familial effects. *J. Med. Genet.* **2015**, *52*, 465–475. [CrossRef] [PubMed]
60. Evans, D.G.; Lalloo, F.; Ashcroft, L.; Shenton, A.; Clancy, T.; Baildam, A.D.; Brain, A.; Hopwood, P.; Howell, A. Uptake of risk-reducing surgery in unaffected women at high risk of breast and ovarian cancer is risk, age, and time dependent. *Cancer Epidemiol. Biomark. Prev.* **2009**, *18*, 2318–2324. [CrossRef]
61. Manchanda, R.; Burnell, M.; Abdelraheim, A.; Johnson, M.; Sharma, A.; Benjamin, E.; Brunell, C.; Saridogan, E.; Gessler, S.; Oram, D.; et al. Factors influencing uptake and timing of risk reducing salpingo-oophorectomy in women at risk of familial ovarian cancer: A competing risk time to event analysis. *BJOG* **2012**, *119*, 527–536. [CrossRef] [PubMed]
62. Read, M.D.; Edey, K.A.; Hapeshi, J.; Foy, C. Compliance with estrogen hormone replacement therapy after oophorectomy: A prospective study. *Menopause Int.* **2010**, *16*, 60–64. [CrossRef]
63. Cuzick, J.; Sestak, I.; Cawthorn, S.; Hamed, H.; Holli, K.; Howell, A.; Forbes, J.F.; Investigators, I.-I. Tamoxifen for prevention of breast cancer: Extended long-term follow-up of the IBIS-I breast cancer prevention trial. *Lancet Oncol.* **2015**, *16*, 67–75. [CrossRef]
64. Smith, S.G.; Sestak, I.; Forster, A.; Partridge, A.; Side, L.; Wolf, M.S.; Horne, R.; Wardle, J.; Cuzick, J. Factors affecting uptake and adherence to breast cancer chemoprevention: A systematic review and meta-analysis. *Ann. Oncol.* **2016**, *27*, 575–590. [CrossRef]
65. Chen, H.; Chen, Y.; Cui, B. The association of multimorbidity with healthcare expenditure among the elderly patients in Beijing, China. *Arch. Gerontol. Geriatr.* **2018**, *79*, 32–38. [CrossRef] [PubMed]
66. SIGTAP. *Sistema de Gerenciamento da Tabela de Procedimentos, Medicamentos e OPM do SUS*; Ministry of Health, Brazil: Brasilia, Brazil, 2020.
67. BPS. *Banco de Preços em Saúde*; Health Price Bank; Ministry of Health, Brazil: Brasilia, Brazil, 2019.
68. CMED. *Câmara de Regulação do Mercado de Medicamentos*; ANVISA, Barzilian Health Regulatory Agency: Brasilia, Brazil, 2016.
69. Curtis, L.; Burns, A. *Unit Costs of Health and Social Care 2016*; Personal Social Services Research Unit (PSSRU): Canterbury, Kent, UK, 2016.
70. NHS Improvement. *NHS Reference Costs 2016/17*; NHS Improvement: London, UK, 2017.
71. The World Bank. Labor Force Participation Rate, Female (% of Female Population Ages 15+) (Modeled ILO Estimate). Available online: https://data.worldbank.org/indicator/SL.TLF.CACT.FE.ZS (accessed on 7 November 2019).
72. Hanly, P.; Timmons, A.; Walsh, P.M.; Sharp, L. Breast and prostate cancer productivity costs: A comparison of the human capital approach and the friction cost approach. *Value Health* **2012**, *15*, 429–436. [CrossRef]
73. World Health Organisation. Life Tables. Available online: http://apps.who.int/gho/data/node.main.687?lang=en (accessed on 27 January 2020).
74. Allemani, C.; Matsuda, T.; Di Carlo, V.; Harewood, R.; Matz, M.; Niksic, M.; Bonaventure, A.; Valkov, M.; Johnson, C.J.; Esteve, J.; et al. Global surveillance of trends in cancer survival 2000-14 (CONCORD-3): Analysis of individual records for 37,513,025 patients diagnosed with one of 18 cancers from 322 population-based registries in 71 countries. *Lancet* **2018**, *391*, 1023–1075. [CrossRef]
75. Bordeleau, L.; Panchal, S.; Goodwin, P. Prognosis of BRCA-associated breast cancer: A summary of evidence. *Breast Cancer Res. Treat.* **2010**, *119*, 13–24. [CrossRef] [PubMed]

76. Rennert, G.; Bisland-Naggan, S.; Barnett-Griness, O.; Bar-Joseph, N.; Zhang, S.; Rennert, H.S.; Narod, S.A. Clinical outcomes of breast cancer in carriers of BRCA1 and BRCA2 mutations. *N. Engl. J. Med.* **2007**, *357*, 115–123. [CrossRef] [PubMed]

77. McLaughlin, J.R.; Rosen, B.; Moody, J.; Pal, T.; Fan, I.; Shaw, P.A.; Risch, H.A.; Sellers, T.A.; Sun, P.; Narod, S.A. Long-term ovarian cancer survival associated with mutation in BRCA1 or BRCA2. *J. Natl. Cancer Inst.* **2013**, *105*, 141–148. [CrossRef] [PubMed]

78. National Institue for Health and Care Excellence (NICE). *Clinical Guideline (CG81)—Advanced Breast Cancer: Diagnosis and Treatment*; National Collaborating Centre for Cancer, National Institute for Health and Clinical Excellence: Cardiff, UK, 2009.

79. Havrilesky, L.J.; Broadwater, G.; Davis, D.M.; Nolte, K.C.; Barnett, J.C.; Myers, E.R.; Kulasingam, S. Determination of quality of life-related utilities for health states relevant to ovarian cancer diagnosis and treatment. *Gynecol. Oncol.* **2009**, *113*, 216–220. [CrossRef]

80. Grann, V.R.; Patel, P.; Bharthuar, A.; Jacobson, J.S.; Warner, E.; Anderson, K.; Tsai, W.Y.; Hill, K.A.; Neugut, A.I.; Hershman, D. Breast cancer-related preferences among women with and without BRCA mutations. *Breast Cancer Res. Treat.* **2010**, *119*, 177–184. [CrossRef]

81. Edejer, T.; Baltussen, R.; Adam, T.; Hutubessy, R.; Acharya, A.; Evans, D.; Murray, C. *WHO Guide to Cost-Effectiveness Analysis*; World Health Organisation: Geneva, Switzerland, 2003.

82. Hutubessy, R.; Chisholm, D.; Edejer, T.T. Generalized cost-effectiveness analysis for national-level priority-setting in the health sector. *Cost Eff. Resour. Alloc.* **2003**, *1*, 8. [CrossRef]

83. Briggs, A. Probabilistic analysis of cost-effectiveness models: Statistical representation of parameter uncertainty. *Value Health* **2005**, *8*, 1–2. [CrossRef]

84. National Institute for Health and Care Excellence (NICE). *Familial Breast Cancer: Classification, Care and Managing Breast Cancer and Related Risks in People with a Family History of Breast Cancer*; National Institute for Health and Clinical Excellence: Cardiff, UK, 2013.

85. Manchanda, R.; Burnell, M.; Loggenberg, K.; Desai, R.; Wardle, J.; Sanderson, S.C.; Gessler, S.; Side, L.; Balogun, N.; Kumar, A.; et al. Cluster-randomised non-inferiority trial comparing DVD-assisted and traditional genetic counselling in systematic population testing for BRCA1/2 mutations. *J. Med. Genet.* **2016**, *53*, 472–480. [CrossRef]

86. Curtis, L. *Unit Costs of Health and Social Care 2011*; Personal Social Services Research Unit (PSSRU): Canterbury, UK, 2011.

87. Schwartz, M.D.; Valdimarsdottir, H.B.; Peshkin, B.N.; Mandelblatt, J.; Nusbaum, R.; Huang, A.T.; Chang, Y.; Graves, K.; Isaacs, C.; Wood, M.; et al. Randomized noninferiority trial of telephone versus in-person genetic counseling for hereditary breast and ovarian cancer. *J. Clin. Oncol.* **2014**, *32*, 618–626. [CrossRef]

88. NHS Reference Costs 2015 to 2016. Available online: https://assets.publishing.service.gov.uk/government/uploads/system/uploads/attachment_data/file/577083/Reference_Costs_2015-16.pdf (accessed on 1 March 2019).

89. Grann, V.R.; Patel, P.R.; Jacobson, J.S.; Warner, E.; Heitjan, D.F.; Ashby-Thompson, M.; Hershman, D.L.; Neugut, A.I. Comparative effectiveness of screening and prevention strategies among BRCA1/2-affected mutation carriers. *Breast Cancer Res. Treat.* **2011**, *125*, 837–847. [CrossRef] [PubMed]

90. British National Formulary. *British National Formulary*; BMJ Group and Pharmaceutical Press (Royal Pharmaceutical Society of Great Britain): London, UK, 2018.

91. Williams-Frame, A.; Carpenter, J.S. Costs of hormonal and nonhormonal prescription medications for hot flashes. *Womens Health (Lond)* **2009**, *5*, 497–502. [CrossRef]

92. National Institue for Health and Care Excellence (NICE). *Ovarian Cancer: The Recognition and initial Management of Ovarian Cancer*; National Institute for Health and Clinical Excellence (NICE): Cardiff, UK, 2011.

93. Cancer Research UK. *Saving Lives, Averting Costs. an Analysis of the Financial Implications of Achieving Earlier Diagnosis of Colorectal, Lung and Ovarian Cancer*; CRUK: London, UK, 2014.

94. National Audit Office. *End of Life Care*; National Audit Office (NAO), House of Commons: London, UK, 2008.

95. National Institute of Health and Clinical Excellence. *Guide to the Methods of Technology Appraisal*; National Institute for Health and Clinical Excellence (NICE): London, UK, 2013.

96. National Institute for Health and Clinical Excellence. *National Costing Report: Early and Locally Advanced Breast Cancer/Advanced Breast Cancer*; National Institute for Health and Clinical Excellence: London, UK, 2009.

97. Heijnsdijk, E.A.; Warner, E.; Gilbert, F.J.; Tilanus-Linthorst, M.M.; Evans, G.; Causer, P.A.; Eeles, R.A.; Kaas, R.; Draisma, G.; Ramsay, E.A.; et al. Differences in natural history between breast cancers in BRCA1 and BRCA2 mutation carriers and effects of MRI screening-MRISC, MARIBS, and Canadian studies combined. *Cancer Epidemiol. Biomarkers Prev.* **2012**, *21*, 1458–1468. [CrossRef] [PubMed]

98. National Institue for Health and Care Excellence (NICE). *Early and Locally Advanced Breast Cancer: Diagnosis and Treatment*; National Collaborating Centre for Cancer, National Institute for Health and Clinical Excellence: Cardiff, UK, 2009.

99. National Institute for Health and Care Excellence (NICE). *Advanced Breast Cancer: Diagnosis and Treatment*; National Institute for Health and Clinical Excellence: London, UK, 2009.

100. Cortesi, L.; Turchetti, D.; Marchi, I.; Fracca, A.; Canossi, B.; Battista, R.; Ruscelli, S.; Pecchi, A.R.; Torricelli, P.; Federico, M. Breast cancer screening in women at increased risk according to different family histories: An update of the Modena Study Group experience. *BMC Cancer* **2006**, *6*, 210. [CrossRef] [PubMed]

101. MARIBS Study Group. Screening with magnetic resonance imaging and mammography of a UK population at high familial risk of breast cancer: A prospective multicentre cohort study (MARIBS). *Lancet* **2005**, *365*, 1769–1778. [CrossRef]

102. Robson, M.E.; Chappuis, P.O.; Satagopan, J.; Wong, N.; Boyd, J.; Goffin, J.R.; Hudis, C.; Roberge, D.; Norton, L.; Begin, L.R.; et al. A combined analysis of outcome following breast cancer: Differences in survival based on BRCA1/BRCA2 mutation status and administration of adjuvant treatment. *Breast Cancer Res.* **2003**, *6*, R8–R17. [CrossRef]

103. Comen, E.; Davids, M.; Kirchhoff, T.; Hudis, C.; Offit, K.; Robson, M. Relative contributions of BRCA1 and BRCA2 mutations to "triple-negative" breast cancer in Ashkenazi Women. *Breast Cancer Res. Treat.* **2011**, *129*, 185–190. [CrossRef] [PubMed]

104. Tung, N.; Garber, J.E.; Lincoln, A.; Domchek, S.M. Frequency of triple-negative breast cancer in BRCA1 mutation carriers: Comparison between common Ashkenazi Jewish and other mutations. *J. Clin. Oncol.* **2012**, *30*, 4447–4448. [CrossRef]

105. Chappuis, P.O.; Nethercot, V.; Foulkes, W.D. Clinico-pathological characteristics of BRCA1- and BRCA2-related breast cancer. In *Seminars in Surgical Oncology*; John Wiley & Sons: Hoboken, NJ, USA, 2000; Volume 18, pp. 287–295.

106. Robertson, C.; Arcot Ragupathy, S.K.; Boachie, C.; Dixon, J.M.; Fraser, C.; Hernandez, R.; Heys, S.; Jack, W.; Kerr, G.R.; Lawrence, G.; et al. The clinical effectiveness and cost-effectiveness of different surveillance mammography regimens after the treatment for primary breast cancer: Systematic reviews registry database analyses and economic evaluation. *Health Technol. Assess* **2011**, *15*, i–vi. [CrossRef]

107. Bates, T.; Kearins, O.; Monypenny, I.; Lagord, C.; Lawrence, G. Clinical outcome data for symptomatic breast cancer: The Breast Cancer Clinical Outcome Measures (BCCOM) Project. *Br. J. Cancer* **2009**, *101*, 395–402. [CrossRef]

108. Breast, E.; Trialist, C. Group C. Effects of chemotherapy and hormonal therapy for early breast cancer on recurrence and 15-year survival: An overview of the randomised trials. *Lancet* **2005**, *365*, 1687–1717. [CrossRef]

109. Blamey, R.W.; Ellis, I.O.; Pinder, S.E.; Lee, A.H.; Macmillan, R.D.; Morgan, D.A.L.; Robertson, J.F.R.; Mitchell, M.J.; Ball, G.R.; Haybittle, J.L.; et al. Survival of invasive breast cancer according to the Nottingham Prognostic Index in cases diagnosed in 1990–1999. *Eur. J. Cancer* **2007**, *43*, 1548–1555. [CrossRef] [PubMed]

110. Gribbin, J.; Dewis, R. *Adjuvant! Online: Review of Evidence Concerning Its Validity, and Other Considerations Relating to Its Use in the NHS*; National Institute for Health and Clinical Excellence: Cardiff, UK, 2009.

111. Kozlow, W.; Guise, T.A. Breast cancer metastasis to bone: Mechanisms of osteolysis and implications for therapy. *J. Mammary Gland Biol.* **2005**, *10*, 169–180. [CrossRef] [PubMed]

112. Breast cancer survival statistics. Available online: https://www.cancerresearchuk.org/health-professional/cancer-statistics/statistics-by-cancer-type/breast-cancer/survival (accessed on 1 April 2018).

113. Wapnir, I.L.; Anderson, S.J.; Mamounas, E.P.; Geyer, C.E., Jr.; Jeong, J.H.; Tan-Chiu, E.; Fisher, B.; Wolmark, N. Prognosis after ipsilateral breast tumor recurrence and locoregional recurrences in five National Surgical Adjuvant Breast and Bowel Project node-positive adjuvant breast cancer trials. *J. Clin. Oncol.* **2006**, *24*, 2028–2037. [CrossRef] [PubMed]
114. Anderson, S.J.; Wapnir, I.; Dignam, J.J.; Fisher, B.; Mamounas, E.P.; Jeong, J.H.; Geyer Jr, C.E.; Wickerham, D.L.; Costantino, J.P.; Wolmark, N. Prognosis after ipsilateral breast tumor recurrence and locoregional recurrences in patients treated by breast-conserving therapy in five National Surgical Adjuvant Breast and Bowel Project protocols of node-negative breast cancer. *J. Clin. Oncol.* **2009**, *27*, 2466–2473. [CrossRef]
115. Gennari, A.; Conte, P.; Rosso, R.; Orlandini, C.; Bruzzi, P. Survival of metastatic breast carcinoma patients over a 20-year period: A retrospective analysis based on individual patient data from six consecutive studies. *Cancer* **2005**, *104*, 1742–1750. [CrossRef]
116. Waldron, J. *Breast Screening Programme, England 2008-09*; NHS Digital: Leeds, UK, 2010.
117. CDC. Breast Cancer Screening Guidelines for Women. Available online: https://www.cdc.gov/cancer/breast/pdf/breastcancerscreeningguidelines.pdf (accessed on 1 April 2018).
118. Dos-Santos-Silva, I. Breast cancer control policies in Brazil: Where to go from here? *Cadernos De Saude Publica* **2018**, *34*. [CrossRef]
119. National Institute for Health and Care Excellence. *Familial Breast Cancer: Classification and Care of People at Risk of Familial Breast Cancer and Management of Breast Cancer and Related Risks in People with a Family History of Breast Cancer*; National Institute for Health and Care Excellence: London, UK, 2013.
120. Cuzick, J.; Sestak, I.; Bonanni, B.; Costantino, J.P.; Cummings, S.; DeCensi, A.; Dowsett, M.; Forbes, J.F.; Ford, L.; LaCroix, A.Z.; et al. Selective oestrogen receptor modulators in prevention of breast cancer: An updated meta-analysis of individual participant data. *Lancet* **2013**, *381*, 1827–1834. [CrossRef]
121. Townsend, N.; Bhatnagar, P.; Wilkins, E. *Cardiovascular Disease Statistics*; British Heart Foundation: London, UK, 2015.
122. CDC. Heart Disease. Available online: https://www.cdc.gov/nchs/fastats/heart-disease.htm (accessed on 17 March 2018).
123. Who Is at Risk for Coronary Heart Disease? Available online: https://www.nhlbi.nih.gov/health-topics/coronary-heart-disease#Risk-Factors (accessed on 17 March 2018).
124. American Heart Association. Cardiovascular Disease: A Costly Burden for America—Projections through 2035. Available online: http://www.heart.org/idc/groups/heart-public/@wcm/@adv/documents/downloadable/ucm_491543.pdf (accessed on 17 March 2018).
125. Population, total. Available online: https://data.worldbank.org/indicator/SP.POP.TOTL?view=chart (accessed on 7 November 2019).
126. Afana, M.; Brinjikji, W.; Cloft, H.; Salka, S. Hospitalization costs for acute myocardial infarction patients treated with percutaneous coronary intervention in the United States are substantially higher than Medicare payments. *Clin. Cardiol.* **2015**, *38*, 13–19. [CrossRef]
127. Office for National Statistics. Employee earnings in the UK: 2018. Available online: https://www.ons.gov.uk/employmentandlabourmarket/peopleinwork/earningsandworkinghours/bulletins/annualsurveyofhoursandearnings/2018 (accessed on 7 November 2019).
128. Bureau of Labor Statistics. Labor Force Statistics from the Current Population Survey. Available online: https://www.bls.gov/cps/earnings.htm#demographics (accessed on 7 November 2019).
129. Statistics Netherlands. Available online: www.cbs.nl (accessed on 7 November 2019).
130. World Economic Forum. The Global Gender Gap Report 2016. Available online: http://reports.weforum.org/global-gender-gap-report-2016/economies/#economy=CHN (accessed on 7 November 2019).
131. Brazilian Institute of Geography and Statistics. Estatísticas de Gênero - Indicadores sociais das mulheres no Brasil. Available online: https://www.ibge.gov.br/estatisticas-novoportal/multidominio/genero/20163-estatisticas-de-genero-indicadores-sociais-das-mulheres-no-brasil.html?=&t=o-que-e (accessed on 7 November 2019).
132. National Sample Survey Office. *Employment and Unemployment Survey, 68th Round, 2012-13, Government of India, Ministry of Statistics & Programme Implementation*; National Sample Survey Office (NSSO): New Delhi, India, 2013.
133. National Ovarian Cancer Coalition. Ovarian Cancer Recurrence: Discussion With an Expert. Available online: http://ovarian.org/component/content/article/33/385 (accessed on 7 November 2019).

134. National Institue for Health and Care Excellence (NICE). *Social Value Judgements: Principles for the Development of NICE Guidance*; National Institute for Health and Clinical Excellence: Cardiff, UK, 2008.
135. Ubel, P.A.; Hirth, R.A.; Chernew, M.E.; Fendrick, A.M. What is the price of life and why doesn't it increase at the rate of inflation? *Arch. Intern. Med.* **2003**, *163*, 1637–1641. [CrossRef]
136. *Richtlijn Voor Het Uitvoeren van Economische Evaluaties in de Gezondheidszorg*; Zorginstituut Nederland (National Health Care Institute, Netherlands): Diemen, The Netherlands, 2016. Available online: https://www.zorginstituutnederland.nl/publicaties/publicatie/2016/02/29/richtlijn-voor-het-uitvoeren-van-economische-evaluaties-in-de-gezondheidszorg (accessed on 21 March 2019).

11

Worldwide Review and Meta-Analysis of Cohort Studies Measuring the Effect of Mammography Screening Programmes on Incidence-Based Breast Cancer Mortality

Amanda Dibden [1], Judith Offman [2], Stephen W. Duffy [1,*] and Rhian Gabe [1]

1 Centre for Cancer Prevention, Wolfson Institute of Preventive Medicine, Queen Mary University of London, Charterhouse Square, London EC1M 6BQ, UK; a.dibden@qmul.ac.uk (A.D.); r.gabe@qmul.ac.uk (R.G.)

2 Comprehensive Cancer Centre, School of Cancer & Pharmaceutical Sciences, Faculty of Life Sciences & Medicine, King's College London, Innovation Hub, Guys Cancer Centre, Guys Hospital, Great Maze Pond, London SE1 9RT, UK; judith.offman@kcl.ac.uk

* Correspondence: s.w.duffy@qmul.ac.uk

Abstract: In 2012, the Euroscreen project published a review of incidence-based mortality evaluations of breast cancer screening programmes. In this paper, we update this review to October 2019 and expand its scope from Europe to worldwide. We carried out a systematic review of incidence-based mortality studies of breast cancer screening programmes, and a meta-analysis of the estimated effects of both invitation to screening and attendance at screening, with adjustment for self-selection bias, on incidence-based mortality from breast cancer. We found 27 valid studies. The results of the meta-analysis showed a significant 22% reduction in breast cancer mortality with invitation to screening, with a relative risk of 0.78 (95% CI 0.75–0.82), and a significant 33% reduction with actual attendance at screening (RR 0.67, 95% CI 0.61–0.75). Breast cancer screening in the routine healthcare setting continues to confer a substantial reduction in mortality from breast cancer.

Keywords: breast cancer; screening; mammography; incidence-based mortality

---

1. Introduction

Reviews of randomised controlled trials (RCTs) of mammography screening estimate that invitation to screening reduces risk of death from breast cancer by around 20% [1,2]. However, as the majority of RCTs were carried out over 30 years ago, they do not take account of changes in breast cancer incidence [3], mortality [4], screening techniques and treatments that have occurred over time. Furthermore, the results may not be representative of the effectiveness of individual population mammography screening programmes [5], which are affected by factors such as varying round lengths, radiographer skill and technology [6]. While RCTs provide reliable evidence and proof of principle that mammography screening is likely to be beneficial, once population screening programmes have been introduced, randomisation to a non-interventional control is no longer ethical and it is necessary to measure the effectiveness of screening in practice through observational studies.

Cohort studies have been used to achieve this objective but there can be important, subtle differences in methods of analysis used. One method is to use incidence-based mortality (IBM) [7], where deaths from breast cancer are only included in women diagnosed after screening has been introduced [8]. This avoids contamination of deaths in the screening period of women who were diagnosed prior to the start of screening, which would bias results against screening [9]. The aim of this review is to provide an overview of all IBM studies evaluating the impact of mammography screening on breast cancer mortality and to establish an up to date estimate of the long term benefit of breast screening.

2. Materials and Methods

2.1. Search Strategy

A systematic search of PubMed was performed in October 2019 with search terms based on those used by Njor et al. in their review of European IBM studies (Euroscreen project) [8]. Inclusion criteria were that (i) the study used IBM in the analysis, (ii) the study outcome was breast cancer mortality and (iii) the paper was in English. No restrictions were placed on age of study participants included to enable the inclusion of as many studies, and hence women, as possible.

2.2. Selection of Sources of Evidence

The titles and abstracts were initially assessed for relevance. A random selection of 100 papers were independently assessed by three reviewers (A.D., S.W.D. and J.O.) for accuracy. Following observation of more than 90% agreement among reviewers, the remainder of the papers were assessed by one reviewer (A.D.). The main text of the potentially eligible papers was then assessed by two reviewers (A.D. and S.W.D.) in order to make a final decision regarding inclusion in the review. We prepared a list of variables to extract from each paper (if available). These included programme characteristics, person years accrued and relative risks associated with invitation and/or exposure to screening as well as the proportion participating in screening (the latter to assist in correction for self-selection bias).

2.3. Statistical Methods

Random effects meta-analyses were undertaken to obtain overall estimates of the effects of (i) invitation to screening and (ii) attendance to screening on risk of breast cancer mortality [10]. It is important to note that when assessing the effect of invitation on mortality, it pertains to populations offered screening and the effect of attendance pertains to women who actually take up the offer of screening and is thus effected by the participation rate. Analyses were repeated stratified by age group (i) 50 and over, (ii) under 50. We chose age 50 to stratify the data as the majority of studies reported on the effects of screening in women aged 50–69, reflecting many national screening programmes, and in order to provide separate evidence in women under 50 years where possible as there has been uncertainty about whether screening younger women is effective and hence, cost-effective. Heterogeneity between studies was assessed using the χ^2 test. Where studies used overlapping data, the largest study was chosen on the basis of better precision with a smaller variance.

Statistical analyses were conducted using Stata Version 13 (StataCorp, College Station, TX, USA) [11].

Adjustment for Self-Selection Bias

Studies have shown that women who do not comply with an invitation to screening usually, but not invariably, have a higher risk of breast cancer mortality than those who choose to attend, resulting in a bias in favour of screening [12]. In order to account for such self-selection bias in studies reporting the effect of attending, we used the statistical adjustment proposed by Duffy et al. [13]. This uses the relative risk of attenders versus non-attenders from the current study, the participation rate, and the risk of death in non-attenders versus uninvited from an appropriate external source (Table 1). The relative risk of non-attenders versus uninvited women of 1.17 (95% CI 1.08–1.26) reported in the Swedish Organised Service Screening Evaluation Group (SOSSEG) study was used in this review as it was a large population based service screening study investigating IBM [14].

Table 1. Statistical adjustments to estimate effect of invitation and attendance to screening.

RR_1: Effect of Invitation to Screening	RR_2: Effect of Attendance Adjusted for Self-Selection
$RR_1 = D_r(pRR_A + 1 - p)$	$RR_2 = \frac{pRR_A D_r}{1-(1-p)D_r}$

RR_A = the relative risk of breast cancer death associated with attending screening versus not attending; p = the proportion of women who attend screening; D_r = the relative risk of breast cancer death for non-attenders versus uninvited = 1.17; Formulae for the variance, and thus the 95% confidence intervals, of these estimates can be found elsewhere [13].

3. Results

3.1. Literature Selection

The literature search identified a total of 5232 titles from three searches performed in PubMed (see Appendix A for details of searches 1, 2 and 3), and 43 were deemed relevant for our review after assessment of abstracts and full text (Figure 1). Of these, four studies assessed the effectiveness of screening programmes outside Europe, one each from Canada [15] and the USA [16], and two from New Zealand [17,18]. The remaining 39 studies were European with twelve from Sweden [14,19–29], nine from Finland [30–38], five from Norway [39–43], four from both Italy [44–47] and Denmark [48–51], two from the Netherlands [52,53] and the UK [54,55] and one from Spain [56].

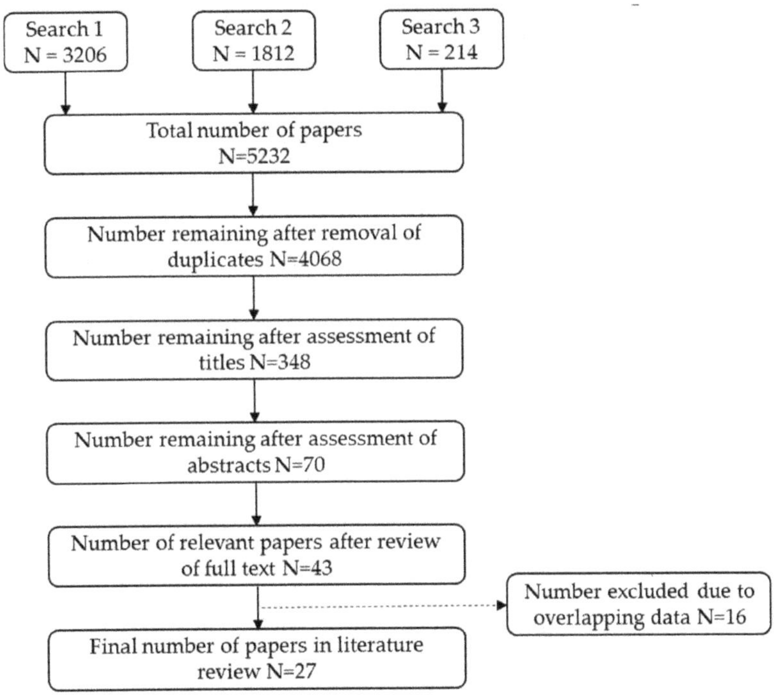

Figure 1. Literature search flow diagram.

There was overlap between some papers, whereby authors used the same data to estimate the effect of different outcomes or updated results with longer follow-up. This resulted in sixteen exclusions (one paper from Denmark [51], four from Finland [31,34,35,37], two from Italy [44,46], three from Norway [39,42,43] and six from Sweden [19,21,22,26,27,29]). The remaining twenty-seven papers included in this review, representing independent populations, are summarized in Table 2.

Table 2. Overview of Studies.

Reference (by Country and Date)	Region	Age Range of Screening	Screening Interval	Comparison Group(s)	Accrual/follow up Period in Screening Group	Accrual/follow up Period in Comparison Group	Person-Years Study/Comparison Groups(Average Population)
Coldman, 2014 [15]	7 provinces, Canada	40–79 depending on province	2 years [1]	Contemporaneous	1990–2009	Same	20,155,000
Beau, 2018 [48]	Copenhagen, Denmark	50–69	2 years	Regional and historical	1991–2007	1977–1991 (pre-screening) 1991–2007 (screening)	976,743/17,804,549
Njor, 2015 [49]	Funen, Denmark	50–69	2 years	Regional and historical	1993–2007/09	1979–1993/95 (pre-screening) 1993–2007/09 (screening)	870,465/ 7,096,056; 828,508; 6,151,011
Olsen, 2005 [50]	Copenhagen, Denmark	50–69	2 years	Regional and historical	1991–2001	1981–1991 (pre-screening) 1991–2001 (screening)	430,823/ 534,224; 4,396,417; 4,055,004
Parvinen, 2015 [30]	Turku, Finland	40–74	2 years [2]	Regional and historical	1987–2009	1976–1986 (pre-screening) 1987–2009 (screening)	853,297/ Helsinki: 2,700,574; Rest of Finland: 21,761,900
Sarkeala, 2008 [33]	8 municipalities, Finland	50–69	2 years	Historical	1992–2003	1974–1985 (pre-screening) 1992–2003 (screening)	228,527
Sarkeala, 2008 [32]	260 municipalities, Finland	50–69	2 years	Historical	1992–2003	1974–1985 (pre-screening) 1992–2003 (screening)	2,731,268
Anttila, 2002 [36]	Helsinki, Finland	50–59	2 years	Contemporaneous [3]	1986–1997	Same	161,400/155,400
Hakama, 1997 [38]	Finland	50–64	2 years	Contemporaneous	1987–1989/1992	Same	400,804/299,228
Puliti, 2012 [45]	Florence, Italy	50–69	2 years	Contemporaneous	1991–2007/08	Same	50–59: 270,399/113,409 60–69: 233,543/151,615
Paci, 2002 [47]	Florence, Italy	50–69	2 years	Contemporaneous	1990–1996/99	Same	254,890
Van Dijck, 1997 [52]	Nijmegen, Netherlands	68–83	2 years	Regional	1977–1990	1978–1990	60,313/ 61,832
Peer, 1995 [53]	Nijmegen, Netherlands	35–49	2 years	Regional	1975–1990	1976–1990	166,307/ 154,103
Taylor, 2019 [18]	New Zealand	50–64 45–49/ 65–69	2 years	Historical	2001–03/ 2009–11 2006–08/ 2009–11	1996–98/ 2004–06 2001–03/ 2004–06	930,000/766,000 480,000/409,000 249,000/205,000 [4]

Table 2. *Cont.*

Morrell, 2017 [17]	New Zealand	45–69	2 years	Contemporaneous	1999–2011/ 2000–2011	Same	3,707,483/ 5,405,518
Weedon-Fekjær, 2014 [41]	Norway	50–69	2 years	Contemporaneous	1986–2009	Same	2,407,709/ 12,785,325
Hofvind, 2013 [40]	Norway	50–69	2 years	Contemporaneous [5]	1996–2009/10	Same	4,814,060/ 988,641
Ascunce, 2007 [56]	Navarre, Spain	50–69	2 years	Historical	1991–2001/ 1997–2001	1980–1990/ 1986–1990	293,000/ 289,000 [6]
Hellquist, 2011 [20]	Sweden	40–49	1.5–2 years	Regional	1986–2005	Same	7,261,415/ 8,843,852
SOSSEG, 2006 [14]	13 counties, Sweden	40–69 depending on county	2 years	Historical	1980–2001 depending on county	1958–1989 depending on county	7,542,833/ 7,265,841
Tabar, 2003 [23]	Östergötland and Dalarna, Sweden	40–69	1.5–2 years	Historical	1978–1997	1958–1977	2,399,000/ 2,416,000
Jonsson, 2003 [25]	10 counties, Sweden	70–74	2 years	Regional and historical	1986–1998	1976–1988 (pre-screening) 1986–1998 (screening)	1,251,300/ 580,100; 533,400; 1,162,800
Jonsson, 2003 [24]	Gävleborg, Sweden	40–64	2 years [7]	Regional and historical	1974–1986/1998	1964–1973/1985 (pre-screening) 1974–1986/1998 (screening)	855,000/ 2,581,000; 12,619,000
Jonsson, 2001 [28]	7 counties, Sweden	50–69	2 years	Regional and historical	1986–1994/97	1979–1987/1990 (pre-screening) 1987–1993/97 (screening)	2,0360,00/ 1,265,000; 2,046,000; 1,296,000
Johns, 2017 [54]	England and Wales, UK	49–64	3 years	Contemporaneous	1991–2005 [8]	Same	1,675,356/ 4,719,228
UK Trial of Early Detection of Breast Cancer Group, 1999 [55]	Guildford and Edinburgh, UK	45–64	2 years	Regional	1979–1995	Same	(45,607/ 127,123)
Thompson [16]	Washington, USA	40+ if high risk/50+ if low risk	3 years	Contemporaneous	1982–1988	Same	(94,656)

[1] Two Provinces, British Columbia and Nova Scotia, invited women aged 40–49 annually; [2] Women aged 40–49 were invited yearly for women born in even years, triennially for women born in odd years; [3] Invited women born 1935–1939 were compared with uninvited women born in 1930–1934; [4] Estimated from data in the paper; [5] All women followed from 1986 but screening began in 1995; [6] Estimated from data in the paper; [7] The average interval between the first and second, and second and third round was 38 months (range 22–65), but was 23 months between rounds 3 and 4; [8] The 15-year period 1991–2005 was partitioned into observation periods of two years accrual and up to nine years follow-up.

3.2. *Study Findings*

Whilst the majority of studies included women in the age range 50–64 years, the youngest age of invitation was 35 years and the oldest 83 years. Most countries invite women every two years, with the range between 18 months and three years. Table 3 shows the unadjusted relative risk for the effect of invitation and attendance on the outcome of incidence-based breast cancer mortality as reported in the studies, and corresponding relative risks adjusted for self-selection bias as described above. The effect sizes and the participation rates reported in the studies suggest differences in risk of breast cancer mortality within countries as well as between countries. Participation rates ranged from 44% in Canada to above 90% in Finland.

The studies reviewed used one or more of three types of comparison groups used to estimate breast cancer mortality in an uninvited population: contemporaneous, regional and historical. (i) The contemporaneous comparison group compared women not yet invited, during the same time period and in the same region, as the women invited. (ii) The regional comparison group is often concurrent to the invited women, but in a region not yet invited. (iii) The historical comparison group compares women invited with women from an epoch not yet invited.

Ten studies compared the screening population with a contemporaneous comparison group, five of which estimated the effect of invitation to screening and seven the effect of attending screening. The effect of invitation fell within a narrow range from 0.72 (95% CI 0.64–0.79) [41] to 0.81 (95% CI 0.64–1.01) [47] and the effect of attendance was 0.38 (95% CI 0.30–0.49) [17] to 0.67 (95% CI 0.49–0.97) [38].

A further six studies used a historical comparison group to compare the impact of introducing screening in a particular region or country, the majority of which reported both the effect of invitation and attendance. The range of the respective effect sizes was wider for invitation than the studies that used a contemporaneous comparison group but narrower for attendance at 0.58 (95% CI 0.44–0.75) [56] to 0.83 (95% CI 0.73–0.95) [18] and 0.52 (95% CI 0.46–0.59) [23] to 0.66 (95% CI 0.58–0.75) [32] respectively.

Only four studies used a regional comparison group without any adjustment for differences in underlying cancer incidence between regions. All studies estimated the effect of invitation, with the results ranging from 0.73 (95% CI 0.63–0.84) [55] to 0.94 (95% CI 0.68–1.29) [53]. Just one study reported the effect of attending screening and found a 29% reduction in breast cancer mortality (95% CI 0.62–0.80) [20] in women who attended screening compared to those who did not.

The remaining seven studies used a combination of regional and historical data, and again, all studies estimated the effect of invitation, with effect estimates ranging between 0.75 (95% CI 0.63–0.89) [50] to 0.97 (95% CI 0.73–1.28) [25], which is almost identical to the results of those studies that used a regional control group alone. The two studies that estimated the effect of attendance reported relative risks of 0.60 (95% CI 0.49–0.74) [50] and 0.68 (95% CI 0.59–0.79) [49] respectively.

Table 3. Unadjusted and adjusted relative risks.

Reference (by Country and Date)	Country	Age at Screening	Attendance	RR: Unadjusted Effect on Incidence-Based Breast Cancer Mortality		RR Calculated from Effect of Attendance	RR Adjusted for Self-Selection
				Invited Versus not Invited [1]	Screened Versus not Screened [1]	Invited Versus not Invited(RR_1) [1]	Screened Versus not Screened (RR_2) [1]
Coldman, 2014 [15]	7 provinces, Canada	40–79	0.437	NR	0.60 (0.52–0.67)	0.97 (0.88–1.06)	0.90 (0.68–1.18)
		40–49			0.56 (0.45–0.67) [2]	0.95 (0.85–1.05)	0.84 (0.61–1.16)
		50–59			0.60 (0.49–0.70)	0.97 (0.87–1.07)	0.90 (0.66–1.23)
		60–69			0.58 (0.50–0.67)	0.96 (0.87–1.05)	0.87 (0.69–1.10)
		70–79			0.65 (0.56–0.74) [3]	0.99 (0.90–1.09)	0.97 (0.74–1.29)
Beau, 2018 [48]	Copenhagen, Denmark	50–69	0.71 [4]	0.89 (0.82–0.98)	NR	NA	NA
Njor,2015 [49]	Funen, Denmark	50–69	0.84	0.78 (0.68–0.89)	0.68 (0.59–0.79)	0.86 (0.75–0.98)	0.82 (0.69–0.98)
Olsen, 2005 [50]	Copenhagen, Denmark	50–69	0.71	0.75 (0.63–0.89) [5]	0.60 (0.49–0.74)	0.84 (0.72–0.97)	0.75 (0.60–0.96)
Parvinen, 2015 [30]	Turku, Finland	40–49	0.867	0.73 (0.50–1.06)	NR	NA	NA
		50–59		0.98 (0.71–1.35)			
		60–74		0.85 (0.66–1.10)			
Sarkeala, 2008 [33]	8 municipalities, Finland	50–69	0.905	0.72 (0.51–0.97)	0.62 (0.43–0.85)	0.77 (0.56–1.06)	0.74 (0.51–1.08)
Sarkeala, 2008 [32]	260 municipalities, Finland	50–69	0.924	0.78 (0.70–0.87)	0.66 (0.58–0.75)	0.80 (0.70–0.92)	0.78 (0.67–0.92)
Anttila, 2002 [36]	Helsinki, Finland	50–59	0.82	0.81 (0.62–1.05)	NR	NA	NA
Hakama, 1997 [38]	Finland	50–64	0.85	0.76 (0.53–1.09)	0.67 (0.46–0.97) [6]	0.84 (0.62–1.15)	0.81 (0.55–1.19)
Puliti, 2012 [45]	Florence, Italy	50–69	0.64	NR	0.44 (0.36–0.54) [7]	0.75 (0.67–0.85)	0.57 (0.45–0.73)
		50–59			0.55 (0.41–0.75)	0.83 (0.71–0.98)	0.71 (0.51–0.98)
		60–69			0.49 (0.38–0.64)	0.79 (0.68–0.91)	0.63 (0.47–0.85)
Paci, 2002 [47]	Florence, Italy	50–69	0.60	0.81 (0.64–1.01)	NR	0.75 (0.67–0.85)	0.57 (0.45–0.73)
Van Dijck, 1997 [52]	Nijmegen, Netherlands	68–83	0.46	0.80 (0.53–1.22)	NR	NA	NA
Peer,1995 [53]	Nijmegen, Netherlands	35–49	0.65	0.94 (0.68–1.29)	NR	NA	NA
Taylor, 2019 [18]	New Zealand	45–49	0.72	1.00 (0.71–1.42) [8]	NR	NA	NA
		50–64		0.83 (0.73–0.95)			
		65–69		0.81 (0.57–1.16)			
Morrell, 2017 [17]	New Zealand	45–69	0.64	NR	0.38 (0.30–0.49)	0.71 (0.62–0.80)	0.49 (0.37–0.65)
Weedon-Fekjær, 2014 [41]	Norway	50–69	0.76	0.72 (0.64–0.79)	NR	NA	NA
Hofvind, 2013 [40]	Norway	50–69	0.84	NR	0.39 (0.35–0.44)	0.57 (0.51–0.64)	0.47 (0.41–0.55)
Ascunce, 2007 [56]	Navarre, Spain	50–69	0.85	0.58 (0.44–0.75) [9]	NR	NA	NA
Hellquist, 2011 [20]	Sweden	40–49	0.80	0.79 (0.72–0.86)	NR	0.74 (0.66–0.83) [10]	0.71 (0.62–0.80)
SOSSEG, 2006 [14]	13 counties, Sweden	40–69	0.80 [11]	0.73 (0.69–0.77)	0.55 (0.51–0.59)	0.75 (0.68–0.82)	0.66 (0.58–0.74)
Tabar, 2003 [23]	Östergötland and Dalarna, Sweden	40–69	0.85	0.59 (0.53–0.66)	0.52 (0.46–0.59)	0.69 (0.61–0.78)	0.63 (0.54–0.73)
Jonsson, 2003 [25]	10 counties, Sweden	70–74	0.84 [12]	0.97 (0.73–1.28)	NR	NA	NA
Jonsson, 2003 [24]	Gävleborg, Sweden	40–64	0.84	0.86 (0.71–1.05)	NR	NA	NA
Jonsson, 2001 [28]	7 counties, Sweden	50–69	0.80 [11]	0.90 (0.74–1.10)	NR	NA	NA

Table 3. *Cont.*

Johns, 2017 [54]	England and Wales, UK	49–64	0.74	0.79 (0.73–0.84)	0.54 (0.51–0.57)	0.77 (0.71–0.84)	0.67 (0.59–0.76)
UK Trial of Early Detection of Breast Cancer Group, 1999 [55]	Guildford and Edinburgh, UK	45–64	0.654	0.73 (0.63–0.84)	NR	NA	NA
Thompson, 1994 [16]	Washington, USA	≥50	NR	NR	0.61 (0.23–1.62)	NA	NA
Pooled RR from all studies		Random effects		0.78 (0.75–0.82)	0.54 (0.49–0.59)	0.76 (0.71–0.83)	0.67 (0.61–0.75)
		Heterogeneity p-value		<0.001	<0.001	<0.001	<0.001
Pooled RR from studies inviting women aged 50 and over		Random effects		0.80 (0.77–0.84)	0.57 (0.51–0.64)	0.82 (0.74–0.92)	0.74 (0.64–0.85)
		Heterogeneity p-value		0.175	<0.001	<0.001	<0.001
Pooled RR from studies inviting women under 50 years		Random effects		0.81 (0.74–0.87)	0.56 (0.45–0.67) [13] –	0.84 (0.66–1.06)	0.73 (0.65–0.82)
		Heterogeneity p-value		0.418		0.002	0.343

[1] RR, relative risk (95% confidence interval), NR, not reported, NA, not applicable; [2] Pooled RR of three provinces; [3] Pooled RR of four provinces; [4] Participation rate not reported so taken from Olsen AH, Njor SH, Vejborg I, Schwartz W, Dalgaard P, Jensen, M.B.; et al. Breast cancer mortality in Copenhagen after introduction of mammography screening: cohort study. *BMJ* **2005**, *330*, 220. [50]; [5] Not included in meta-analysis due to later paper by Beau et al.; [6] Calculated from data in the paper; [7] Unadjusted RR calculated from data in the paper; [8] RR calculated from data in the paper. The accrual period for women aged 50–64 was 2001–2003 and for women aged 45–49 and 65–69 was 2006–2008; [9] Excludes prevalent cases; [10] RR1 and RR2 are as reported by authors in the paper; [11] Attendance rate not reported so taken from Giordano L, von Karsa L, Tomatis M, Majek O, de Wolf C, Lancucki L, et al. Mammographic screening programmes in Europe: organization, coverage and participation. *J. Med Screen.* **2012**, *19*, 72–82. [57] as region reported invites women until the age of 74; [12] Attendance rate not reported so taken from Swedish Organised Service Screening Evaluation Group. Reduction in breast cancer mortality from the organised service screening with mammography: 2. Validation with alternative analytic methods. *Cancer Epidemiol Biomark. Prev.* **2006**, *15*, 52–56. [58]; [13] One study only.

3.3. *Meta-Analysis by Age-Group of Women*

There were twenty-two studies that assessed the effect of invitation to screening (Table 3 and Figure 2). All studies had a relative risk of less than or equal to 1, with the largest studies achieving statistical significance. The largest studies were those by SOSSEG [14] and Johns et al. [54] who found a 20–30% reduction in breast cancer mortality. The pooled rate ratio was 0.78 (95% CI 0.75–0.82) with significant heterogeneity ($p < 0.001$).

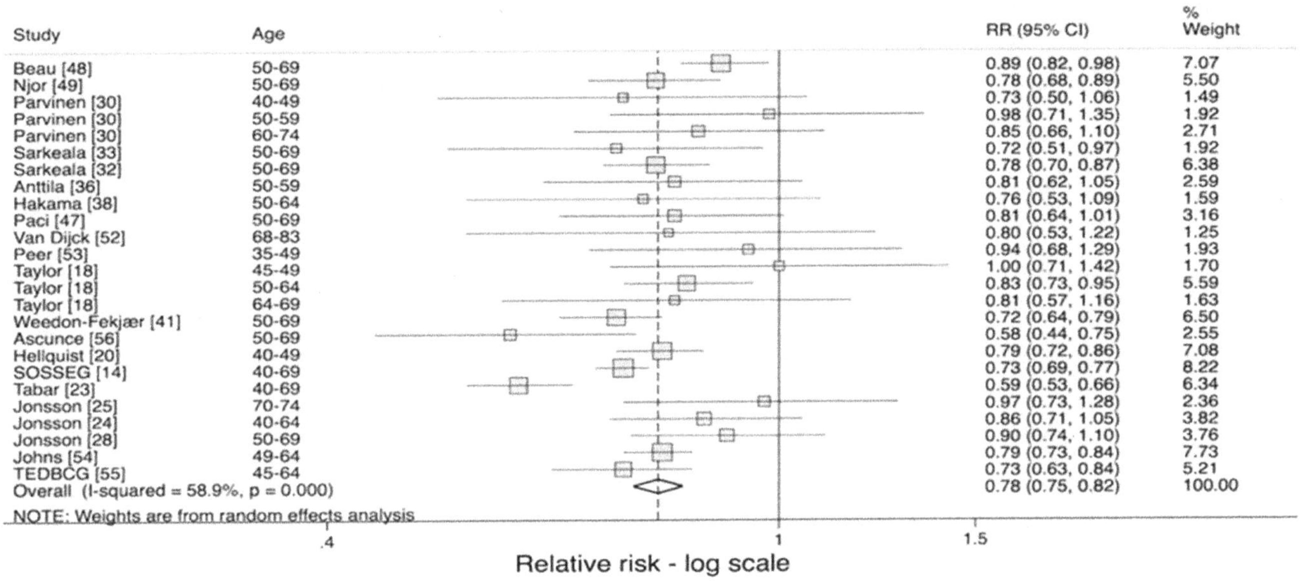

Figure 2. Effect of invitation on risk of breast cancer mortality [14,18,20,23–25,28,30,32,33,36,38,41,47–49,52–56].

Fourteen studies reported on the effect of being screened, eight of which also reported on the effect of being invited. All but one study reported a statistically significant result with the largest studies again by SOSSEG [14] and Johns et al. [54] with relative risks of 0.54 and 0.55 respectively. This therefore led to a pooled estimate of 0.54 (95% CI 0.49–0.59) with significant heterogeneity at $p < 0.001$. However, as discussed previously, the effect estimate of being screened is likely to be subject to self-selection bias. Therefore, an adjustment was made to account for this.

To be able to calculate the adjustments for self-selection suggested by Duffy et al. [13], it is necessary to know the proportion of women attending screening. This is not reported in the paper by Thompson et al. [16] and so the adjusted relative risks cannot be estimated. However, this study is small and therefore omission of this study in the calculation of the pooled relative risk would not have a substantial effect.

The intention to treat estimate, RR_1, was 0.76 (95% CI 0.71–0.83) with significant heterogeneity ($p < 0.001$). This estimate is almost identical to the effect size presented in Figure 2 (RR 0.78). The adjusted pooled relative risk for the effect of being screened, RR_2, was 0.67 (95% CI 0.61–0.75) and again there was significant heterogeneity between studies with $p < 0.001$ (Figure 3).

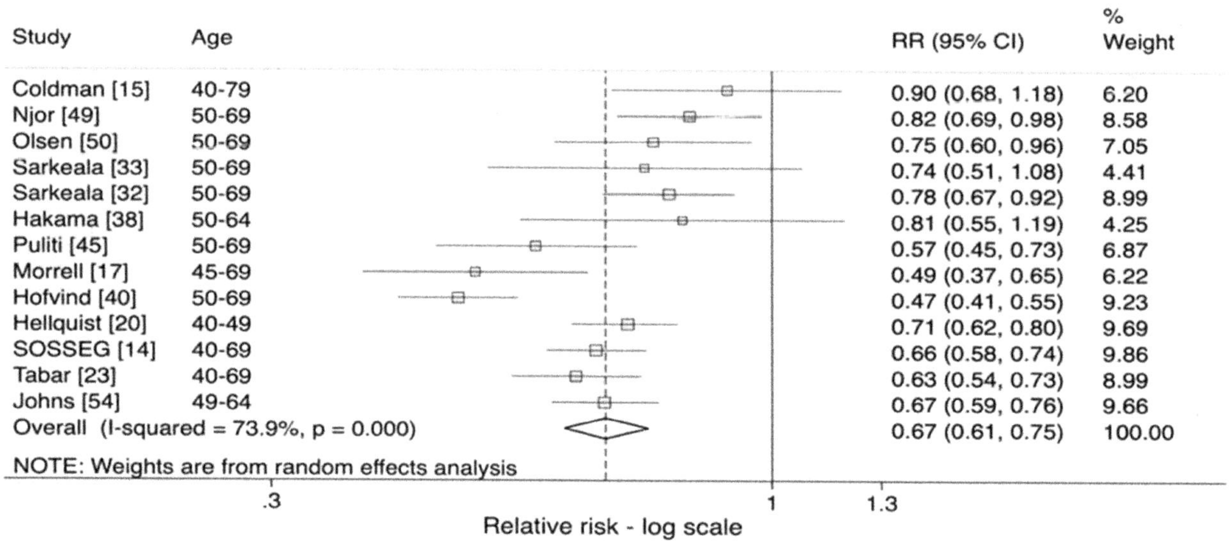

Figure 3. Estimated effect of attendance adjusted for self-selection on risk of breast cancer mortality (RR_2) [14,15,17,20,23,32,33,38,40,45,49,50,54].

When assessing the effect of invitation in women aged 50 and over (Figure 4), whilst the pooled relative risk was similar to that in women of all ages, the p-value was 0.175, suggesting no heterogeneity between studies. However, there was still evidence of heterogeneity when assessing the effect of attendance with a relative risk, adjusted for self-selection, of 0.74 (95% CI 0.64–0.85) and a p-value of <0.001 (Figure 5).

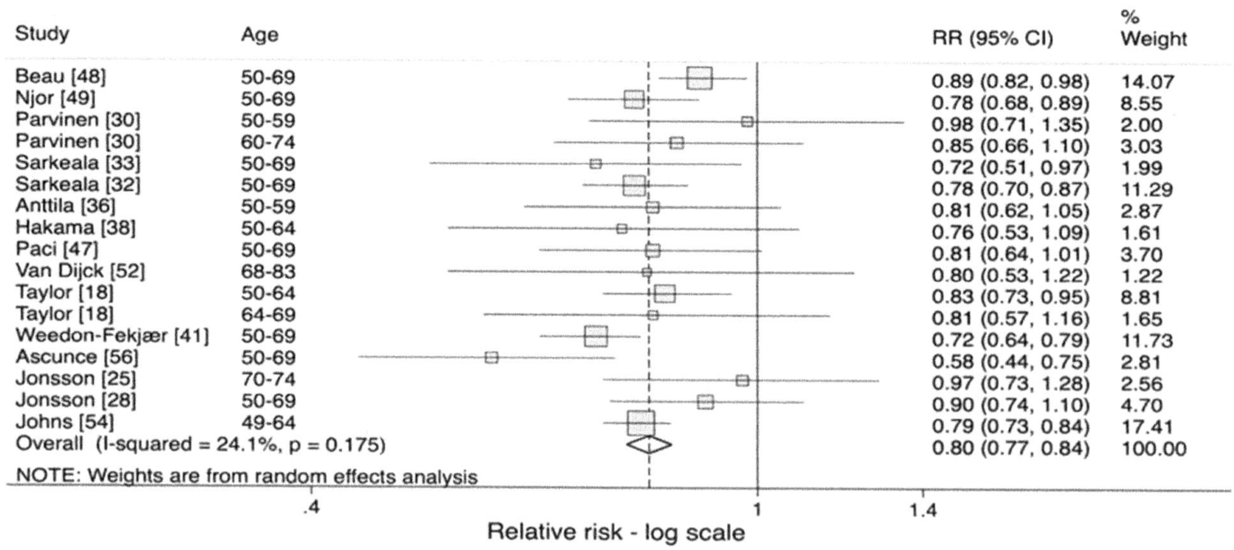

Figure 4. Effect of invitation on risk of breast cancer mortality in women aged 50 and over [18,25,28,30,32,33,36,38,41,47–49,52,54,56].

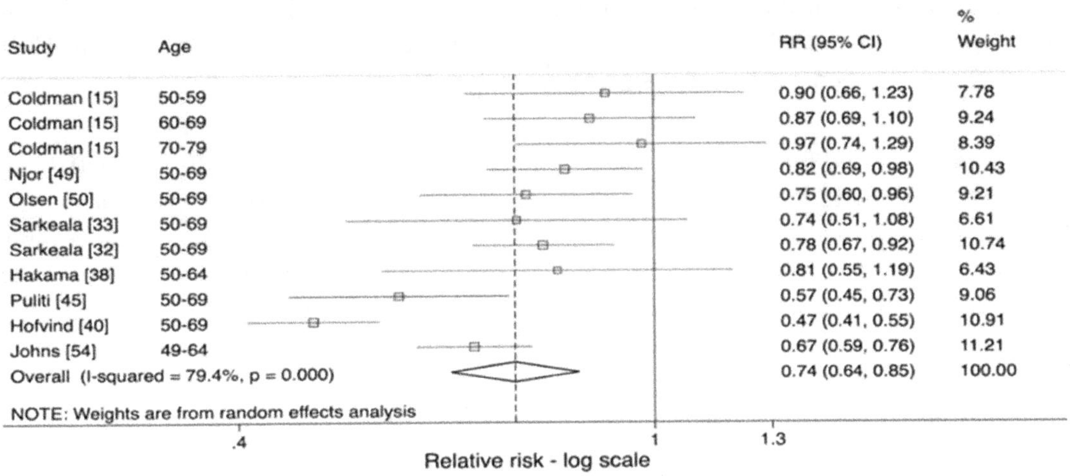

Figure 5. Estimated effect of attendance adjusted for self-selection on risk of breast cancer mortality (RR_2) in women aged 50 and over [15,32,33,38,40,45,49,50,54].

There were five studies that reported on the effect of screening in women under 50 years. Four studies [18,20,30,53] report the effect of invitation with a pooled relative risk of 0.81 (95% CI 0.74–0.87) and no evidence of heterogeneity ($p = 0.418$). Two studies [15,20] reported the effect of attendance to screening and the adjusted relative risk was 0.73 (95% CI 0.65–0.82).

4. Discussion

This systematic review and meta-analysis of IBM studies estimates that the risk of death from breast cancer in women invited for screening is reduced by 22% compared to women not invited (RR 0.78, 95% CI 0.75–0.82), with similar results across age groups. This result is consistent with earlier overviews of cohort studies [5,6] and from the RCTs in breast cancer screening, which suggest invitation to screening reduces mortality by approximately 20% [1].

The studies with contemporaneous control groups are likely to be least biased, with the regional and historical comparison groups potentially affected by differences in the underlying risk of breast cancer mortality between regions or across time periods respectively. When assessing the effect of invitation, the results of studies with contemporaneous control groups ranged from 0.72 (95% CI 0.64–0.79) in the Norwegian study by Weedon-Fekjær [41] to 0.81 (95% CI 0.64–1.01) in the Italian study by Paci [47].

The relative risk, RR_2, estimates the effect of attendance adjusted for self-selection bias. Using population specific attendance rates and $D_r = 1.17$ from the SOSSEG study [14] results in a mortality decrease of 33% (RR: 0.67, 95% CI 0.61–0.75). This is slightly more conservative than the relative risk estimated by Broeders et al. [5] although it is unclear whether their result is adjusted for self-selection bias.

The relative risk, RR_1, estimating the effect of invitation to screening from the relative risk of attendance adjusting for potential self-selection bias, is almost identical to the pooled effect estimated directly. The agreement between the two measures suggests that the adjustment method is valid.

There appears to be significant heterogeneity of the effect of invitation in the meta-analysis of all studies, which disappears when the analysis is stratified by the age. This suggests that there is a difference in the effect of invitation in differing age groups, and that the varying distributions by age among studies is contributing to the heterogeneity of the effect for all ages combined. The heterogeneity of the effect of attendance adjusted for self-selection bias (RR_2), however, is present for women screened at any age and in women screened over the age of 50 years, suggesting that variation in age distributions is not entirely responsible for heterogeneity among studies. It is likely that this is partly due to differing screening regimens and practices.

Attendance rates varied between studies, from 0.44 in the Canadian study [15] to 0.92 in the study by Sarkeala et al. [32]. Canada differs from other countries in respect of protocol for call and recall, requiring women to self-refer in some provinces. When this opportunistic screening is taken into account, the attendance rate is estimated to be 63.1% [59]. Additionally, the screening programme has a high retention rate, with nearly 80% of previous participants attending a subsequent screen within 36 months.

IBM studies have been the focus of this review but they are not without their limitations. The main limitation is the identification of an appropriate comparison group in the absence of screening [8]. In addition, they are prospective studies and require a long follow-up period to accumulate enough deaths to achieve statistical power [60] and to see the full benefit of screening. Results from the Swedish Two-County Trial suggest that the full benefit of screening requires follow-up of at least 20 years [61]. The majority of studies included in this review had at least 10 years follow-up, with some having over 20 years. In addition, the length of the accrual period should be equal in comparison groups and should be equal to the length of the follow-up period. The effect of screening will be underestimated if the accrual period is shorter than the follow-up period, as more cases will accrue in the screened population than the non-screened population. Seventeen studies in this review had equal accrual and follow-up periods, with ten studies having a shorter accrual period.

Our results update and confirm those of the Euroscreen project for IBM studies [5,8]. Case-control studies reviewed in the Euroscreen project tended to find rather stronger effects than the IBM studies with the effect of invitation 0.69 (95% CI 0.57–0.83) and the effect of attendance adjusted for self-selection bias 0.52 (95% CI 0.42–0.65). This may be due to ascertainment biases in the case-control approach [12]. In addition, the Euroscreen project estimated the effect from trend studies to be between 28–36%, which is comparable to the results in this review [62].

There have been suggestions of alternative analysis methods using the IBM approach. Tabar et al. [63] suggest using as the endpoint the incidence of breast cancers subsequently proving fatal, within ten or twenty years. This method links exposure to endpoint more accurately, but requires a long follow-up period. Sasieni et al. [64] propose a method for estimating the expected number of deaths in the population without screening, which can be used when there is no contemporaneous comparison group. Neither of these methods have been used extensively up to now.

5. Conclusions

IBM studies yield estimates uncontaminated by pre-screening cancers. Results from these international studies indicate that inviting women to screening results in a 22% reduction in breast cancer mortality and that the effect of attending screening reduces the risk of death by around 30%. Breast cancer screening in the routine healthcare setting continues to confer a substantial reduction in mortality from breast cancer.

Author Contributions: Conceptualization, S.D. and A.D.; methodology, A.D., J.O., S.W.D. and R.G.; data extraction A.D.; writing—original draft preparation, A.D., S.W.D. and R.G.; writing—review and editing, A.D., J.O., S.W.D. and R.G. All authors have read and agree to the published version of the manuscript.

Appendix A

Search Strategy

The following search terms were used to conduct the review of the literature in PubMed. These search terms were taken from previous review by Njor et al. [8], however our search was restricted to three out of the four searches performed by Njor et al. and papers in English only.

(1) ("breast neoplasms/mortality*" [MeSH Terms] OR breast cancer mortality OR "mortality" [MeSH Terms]) AND (("mass screening" [MeSH Terms] OR screening) AND ("mammography" [MeSH Terms] OR mammography) AND English [lang] [8]
(2) (effect* OR evaluation OR impact OR trend) AND (service screening OR programme screening OR mass screening) AND breast cancer AND (mortality OR survival) AND English [lang]
(3) "Breast neoplasm/mortality*" [MeSH Terms] AND "mass screening" [MeSH Terms] AND ("mortality/trends" [MeSH Terms] OR "survival analysis" [MeSH Terms] OR "survival rate/trends" [MeSH Terms]) AND English [lang]

References

1. Independent UK Panel on Breast Cancer Screening. The benefits and harms of breast cancer screening: An independent review. *Lancet (Lond. Engl.)* **2012**, *380*, 1778–1786. [CrossRef]
2. Gotzsche, P.C.; Jorgensen, K.J. Screening for breast cancer with mammography. *Cochrane Database Syst. Rev.* **2013**. [CrossRef] [PubMed]
3. Cancer Research UK. Breast Cancer Incidence Statistics. Available online: https://www.cancerresearchuk.org/health-professional/cancer-statistics/statistics-by-cancer-type/breast-cancer/incidence-invasive#heading-Two (accessed on 24 April 2019).
4. Cancer Research UK. Breast Cancer Mortality Statistics. Available online: https://www.cancerresearchuk.org/health-professional/cancer-statistics/statistics-by-cancer-type/breast-cancer/mortality#heading-Two (accessed on 24 April 2019).
5. Broeders, M.; Moss, S.; Nystrom, L.; Njor, S.; Jonsson, H.; Paap, E.; Massat, N.; Duffy, S.; Lynge, E.; Paci, E. The impact of mammographic screening on breast cancer mortality in Europe: A review of observational studies. *J. Med. Screen.* **2012**, *19*, 14–25. [CrossRef] [PubMed]
6. Gabe, R.; Duffy, S.W. Evaluation of service screening mammography in practice: The impact on breast cancer mortality. *Ann. Oncol. Off. J. Eur. Soc. Med. Oncol.* **2005**, *16*, ii153–ii162. [CrossRef]
7. Chu, K.C.; Miller, B.A.; Feuer, E.J.; Hankey, B.F. A method for partitioning cancer mortality trends by factors associated with diagnosis: An application to female breast cancer. *J. Clin. Epidemiol.* **1994**, *47*, 1451–1461. [CrossRef]
8. Njor, S.; Nystrom, L.; Moss, S.; Paci, E.; Broeders, M.; Segnan, N.; Lynge, E. Breast cancer mortality in mammographic screening in Europe: A review of incidence-based mortality studies. *J. Med. Screen.* **2012**, *19*, 33–41. [CrossRef]
9. Duffy, S.W.; Chen, T.H.H.; Yen, A.M.F.; Tabar, L.; Gabe, R.; Smith, R.A. Methodologic Issues in the Evaluation of Service Screening. *Semin. Breast Dis.* **2007**, *10*, 68–71. [CrossRef]
10. Egger, M.; Davey Smith, G.; Schneider, M. *Systematic Reviews in Health Care: Meta-Analysis in Context*, 2nd ed.; BMJ Publishing Group: London, UK, 2008; Volume 2, pp. 211–227.
11. StataCorp. *Stata Statistical Software: Release 13*; StataCorp LP: College Station, TX, USA, 2013.
12. Duffy, S.W. Case-Control Studies to Evaluate the Effect of Mammographic Service Screening on Mortality from Breast Cancer. *Semin. Breast Dis.* **2007**, *10*, 61–63. [CrossRef]
13. Duffy, S.W.; Cuzick, J.; Tabar, L.; Vitak, B.; Hsiu-Hsi Chen, T.; Yen, M.-F.; Smith, R.A. Correcting for non-compliance bias in case–control studies to evaluate cancer screening programmes. *J. R. Stat. Soc. Ser. C (Appl. Stat.)* **2002**, *51*, 235–243. [CrossRef]
14. Swedish Organised Service Screening Evaluation Group. Reduction in breast cancer mortality from organized service screening with mammography: 1. Further confirmation with extended data. *Cancer Epidemiol. Biomark. Prev.* **2006**, *15*, 45–51. [CrossRef]

15. Coldman, A.; Phillips, N.; Wilson, C.; Decker, K.; Chiarelli, A.M.; Brisson, J.; Zhang, B.; Payne, J.; Doyle, G.; Ahmad, R. Pan-Canadian study of mammography screening and mortality from breast cancer. *J. Natl. Cancer Inst.* **2014**, *106*. [CrossRef] [PubMed]
16. Thompson, R.S.; Barlow, W.E.; Taplin, S.H.; Grothaus, L.; Immanuel, V.; Salazar, A.; Wagner, E.H. A population-based case-cohort evaluation of the efficacy of mammographic screening for breast cancer. *Am. J. Epidemiol.* **1994**, *140*, 889–901. [CrossRef] [PubMed]
17. Morrell, S.; Taylor, R.; Roder, D.; Robson, B.; Gregory, M.; Craig, K. Mammography service screening and breast cancer mortality in New Zealand: A National Cohort Study 1999–2011. *Br. J. Cancer* **2017**, *116*, 828–839. [CrossRef] [PubMed]
18. Taylor, R.; Gregory, M.; Sexton, K.; Wharton, J.; Sharma, N.; Amoyal, G.; Morrell, S. Breast cancer mortality and screening mammography in New Zealand: Incidence-based and aggregate analyses. *J. Med. Screen.* **2019**, *26*, 35–43. [CrossRef]
19. Hellquist, B.N.; Czene, K.; Hjalm, A.; Nystrom, L.; Jonsson, H. Effectiveness of population-based service screening with mammography for women ages 40 to 49 years with a high or low risk of breast cancer: Socioeconomic status, parity, and age at birth of first child. *Cancer* **2015**, *121*, 251–258. [CrossRef]
20. Hellquist, B.N.; Duffy, S.W.; Abdsaleh, S.; Bjorneld, L.; Bordas, P.; Tabar, L.; Vitak, B.; Zackrisson, S.; Nystrom, L.; Jonsson, H. Effectiveness of population-based service screening with mammography for women ages 40 to 49 years: Evaluation of the Swedish Mammography Screening in Young Women (SCRY) cohort. *Cancer* **2011**, *117*, 714–722. [CrossRef]
21. Jonsson, H.; Bordas, P.; Wallin, H.; Nystrom, L.; Lenner, P. Service screening with mammography in Northern Sweden: Effects on breast cancer mortality—An update. *J. Med. Screen.* **2007**, *14*, 87–93. [CrossRef]
22. Baker, S.G.; Kramer, B.S.; Prorok, P.C. Comparing breast cancer mortality rates before-and-after a change in availability of screening in different regions: Extension of the paired availability design. *BMC Med. Res. Methodol.* **2004**, *4*, 12. [CrossRef]
23. Tabar, L.; Yen, M.F.; Vitak, B.; Chen, H.H.; Smith, R.A.; Duffy, S.W. Mammography service screening and mortality in breast cancer patients: 20-year follow-up before and after introduction of screening. *Lancet (Lond. Engl.)* **2003**, *361*, 1405–1410. [CrossRef]
24. Jonsson, H.; Nystrom, L.; Tornberg, S.; Lundgren, B.; Lenner, P. Service screening with mammography. Long-term effects on breast cancer mortality in the county of Gavleborg, Sweden. *Breast (Edinb. Scotl.)* **2003**, *12*, 183–193. [CrossRef]
25. Jonsson, H.; Tornberg, S.; Nystrom, L.; Lenner, P. Service screening with mammography of women aged 70-74 years in Sweden. Effects on breast cancer mortality. *Cancer Detect. Prev.* **2003**, *27*, 360–369. [CrossRef]
26. Duffy, S.W.; Tabar, L.; Chen, H.H.; Holmqvist, M.; Yen, M.F.; Abdsalah, S.; Epstein, B.; Frodis, E.; Ljungberg, E.; Hedborg-Melander, C.; et al. The impact of organized mammography service screening on breast carcinoma mortality in seven Swedish counties. *Cancer* **2002**, *95*, 458–469. [CrossRef] [PubMed]
27. Tabar, L.; Vitak, B.; Chen, H.H.; Yen, M.F.; Duffy, S.W.; Smith, R.A. Beyond randomized controlled trials: Organized mammographic screening substantially reduces breast carcinoma mortality. *Cancer* **2001**, *91*, 1724–1731. [CrossRef]
28. Jonsson, H.; Nystrom, L.; Tornberg, S.; Lenner, P. Service screening with mammography of women aged 50-69 years in Sweden: Effects on mortality from breast cancer. *J. Med. Screen.* **2001**, *8*, 152–160. [CrossRef]
29. Jonsson, H.; Tornberg, S.; Nystrom, L.; Lenner, P. Service screening with mammography in Sweden–evaluation of effects of screening on breast cancer mortality in age group 40–49 years. *Acta Oncol. (Stockh. Swed.)* **2000**, *39*, 617–623.
30. Parvinen, I.; Heinavaara, S.; Anttila, A.; Helenius, H.; Klemi, P.; Pylkkanen, L. Mammography screening in three Finnish residential areas: Comprehensive population-based study of breast cancer incidence and incidence-based mortality 1976–2009. *Br. J. Cancer* **2015**, *112*, 918–924. [CrossRef]
31. Wu, J.C.-Y.; Anttila, A.; Yen, A.M.-F.; Hakama, M.; Saarenmaa, I.; Sarkeala, T.; Malila, N.; Auvinen, A.; Chiu, S.Y.-H.; Chen, T.H.-H. Evaluation of breast cancer service screening programme with a Bayesian approach: Mortality analysis in a Finnish region. *Breast Cancer Res. Treat.* **2010**, *121*, 671–678. [CrossRef]
32. Sarkeala, T.; Heinavaara, S.; Anttila, A. Organised mammography screening reduces breast cancer mortality: A cohort study from Finland. *Int. J. Cancer* **2008**, *122*, 614–619. [CrossRef]
33. Sarkeala, T.; Heinavaara, S.; Anttila, A. Breast cancer mortality with varying invitational policies in organised mammography. *Br. J. Cancer* **2008**, *98*, 641–645. [CrossRef]

34. Anttila, A.; Sarkeala, T.; Hakulinen, T.; Heinavaara, S. Impacts of the Finnish service screening programme on breast cancer rates. *BMC Public Health* **2008**, *8*, 38. [CrossRef]
35. Parvinen, I.; Helenius, H.; Pylkkanen, L.; Anttila, A.; Immonen-Raiha, P.; Kauhava, L.; Rasanen, O.; Klemi, P.J. Service screening mammography reduces breast cancer mortality among elderly women in Turku. *J. Med. Screen.* **2006**, *13*, 34–40. [CrossRef] [PubMed]
36. Anttila, A.; Koskela, J.; Hakama, M. Programme sensitivity and effectiveness of mammography service screening in Helsinki, Finland. *J. Med. Screen.* **2002**, *9*, 153–158. [CrossRef] [PubMed]
37. Hakama, M.; Pukkala, E.; Soderman, B.; Day, N. Implementation of screening as a public health policy: Issues in design and evaluation. *J. Med. Screen.* **1999**, *6*, 209–216. [CrossRef] [PubMed]
38. Hakama, M.; Pukkala, E.; Heikkila, M.; Kallio, M. Effectiveness of the public health policy for breast cancer screening in Finland: Population based cohort study. *BMJ (Clin. Res. Ed.)* **1997**, *314*, 864–867. [CrossRef]
39. Moller, M.H.; Lousdal, M.L.; Kristiansen, I.S.; Stovring, H. Effect of organized mammography screening on breast cancer mortality: A population-based cohort study in Norway. *Int. J. Cancer* **2019**, *144*, 697–706. [CrossRef]
40. Hofvind, S.; Ursin, G.; Tretli, S.; Sebuodegard, S.; Moller, B. Breast cancer mortality in participants of the Norwegian Breast Cancer Screening Program. *Cancer* **2013**, *119*, 3106–3112. [CrossRef]
41. Weedon-Fekjaer, H.; Romundstad, P.R.; Vatten, L.J. Modern mammography screening and breast cancer mortality: Population study. *BMJ (Clin. Res. Ed.)* **2014**, *348*, g3701. [CrossRef]
42. Olsen, A.H.; Lynge, E.; Njor, S.H.; Kumle, M.; Waaseth, M.; Braaten, T.; Lund, E. Breast cancer mortality in Norway after the introduction of mammography screening. *Int. J. Cancer* **2013**, *132*, 208–214. [CrossRef]
43. Kalager, M.; Zelen, M.; Langmark, F.; Adami, H.O. Effect of screening mammography on breast-cancer mortality in Norway. *N. Engl. J. Med.* **2010**, *363*, 1203–1210. [CrossRef]
44. Capodaglio, G.; Zorzi, M.; Tognazzo, S.; Greco, A.; Michieletto, F.; Fedato, C.; Montaguti, A.; Turrin, A.; Ferro, A.; Cinquetti, S.; et al. Impact of breast cancer screening in a population with high spontaneous coverage with mammography. *Tumori* **2018**, *104*, 258–265. [CrossRef]
45. Puliti, D.; Miccinesi, G.; Zappa, M.; Manneschi, G.; Crocetti, E.; Paci, E. Balancing harms and benefits of service mammography screening programs: A cohort study. *Breast Cancer Res. BCR* **2012**, *14*, R9. [CrossRef] [PubMed]
46. Paci, E.; Duffy, S.W.; Giorgi, D.; Zappa, M.; Crocetti, E.; Vezzosi, V.; Bianchi, S.; del Turco, M.R. Quantification of the effect of mammographic screening on fatal breast cancers: The Florence Programme 1990–1996. *Br. J. Cancer* **2002**, *87*, 65–69. [CrossRef] [PubMed]
47. Paci, E.; Giorgi, D.; Bianchi, S.; Vezzosi, V.; Zappa, M.; Crocetti, E.; Rosselli del Turco, M. Assessment of the early impact of the population-based breast cancer screening programme in Florence (Italy) using mortality and surrogate measures. *Eur. J. Cancer (Oxf. Engl. 1990)* **2002**, *38*, 568–573. [CrossRef]
48. Beau, A.B.; Andersen, P.K.; Vejborg, I.; Lynge, E. Limitations in the Effect of Screening on Breast Cancer Mortality. *J. Clin. Oncol. Off. J. Am. Soc. Clin. Oncol.* **2018**, *36*, 2988–2994. [CrossRef] [PubMed]
49. Njor, S.H.; Schwartz, W.; Blichert-Toft, M.; Lynge, E. Decline in breast cancer mortality: How much is attributable to screening? *J. Med. Screen.* **2015**, *22*, 20–27. [CrossRef] [PubMed]
50. Olsen, A.H.; Njor, S.H.; Vejborg, I.; Schwartz, W.; Dalgaard, P.; Jensen, M.B.; Tange, U.B.; Blichert-Toft, M.; Rank, F.; Mouridsen, H.; et al. Breast cancer mortality in Copenhagen after introduction of mammography screening: Cohort study. *BMJ (Clin. Res. Ed.)* **2005**, *330*, 220. [CrossRef]
51. Olsen, A.H.; Njor, S.H.; Lynge, E. Estimating the benefits of mammography screening: The impact of study design. *Epidemiology (Camb. Mass.)* **2007**, *18*, 487–492. [CrossRef]
52. Van Dijck, J.A.; Verbeek, A.L.; Beex, L.V.; Hendriks, J.H.; Holland, R.; Mravunac, M.; Straatman, H.; Werre, J.M. Breast-cancer mortality in a non-randomized trial on mammographic screening in women over age 65. *Int. J. Cancer* **1997**, *70*, 164–168. [CrossRef]
53. Peer, P.G.; Werre, J.M.; Mravunac, M.; Hendriks, J.H.; Holland, R.; Verbeek, A.L. Effect on breast cancer mortality of biennial mammographic screening of women under age 50. *Int. J. Cancer* **1995**, *60*, 808–811. [CrossRef]
54. Johns, L.E.; Coleman, D.A.; Swerdlow, A.J.; Moss, S.M. Effect of population breast screening on breast cancer mortality up to 2005 in England and Wales: An individual-level cohort study. *Br. J. Cancer* **2017**, *116*, 246–252. [CrossRef]

55. UK Trial of Early Detection of Breast Cancer Group. 16-year mortality from breast cancer in the UK Trial of Early Detection of Breast Cancer. *Lancet (Lond. Engl.)* **1999**, *353*, 1909–1914. [CrossRef]
56. Ascunce, E.N.; Moreno-Iribas, C.; Barcos Urtiaga, A.; Ardanaz, E.; Ederra Sanz, M.; Castilla, J.; Egues, N. Changes in breast cancer mortality in Navarre (Spain) after introduction of a screening programme. *J. Med. Screen.* **2007**, *14*, 14–20. [CrossRef] [PubMed]
57. Giordano, L.; von Karsa, L.; Tomatis, M.; Majek, O.; de Wolf, C.; Lancucki, L.; Hofvind, S.; Nyström, L.; Segnan, N.; Ponti, A. Mammographic screening programmes in Europe: Organization, coverage and participation. *J. Med. Screen.* **2012**, *19*, 72–82. [CrossRef] [PubMed]
58. Swedish Organised Service Screening Evaluation Group. Reduction in breast cancer mortality from the organised service screening with mammography: 2. Validation with alternative analytic methods. *Cancer Epidemiol. Biomark. Prev.* **2006**, *15*, 52–56. [CrossRef]
59. Doyle, G.P.; Major, D.; Chu, C.; Stankiewicz, A.; Harrison, M.L.; Pogany, L.; Mai, V.M.; Onysko, J. A review of screening mammography participation and utilization in Canada. *Chronic Dis. Inj. Can.* **2011**, *31*, 152–156.
60. Breslow, N.E.; Day, N.E. *Statistical Methods in Cancer Research. Vol II. The Deisgn and Analysis of Cohort Studies*; International Agency for Cancer Research: Lyon, France, 1987.
61. Tabár, L.; Vitak, B.; Chen, T.H.-H.; Yen, A.M.-F.; Cohen, A.; Tot, T.; Chiu, S.Y.-H.; Chen, S.L.-S.; Fann, J.C.-Y.; Rosell, J.; et al. Swedish Two-County Trial: Impact of Mammographic Screening on Breast Cancer Mortality during 3 Decades. *Radiology* **2011**, *260*, 658–663. [CrossRef]
62. Moss, S.M.; Nystrom, L.; Jonsson, H.; Paci, E.; Lynge, E.; Njor, S.; Broeders, M. The impact of mammographic screening on breast cancer mortality in Europe: A review of trend studies. *J. Med. Screen.* **2012**, *19*, 26–32. [CrossRef]
63. Tabar, L.; Dean, P.B.; Chen, T.H.; Yen, A.M.; Chen, S.L.; Fann, J.C.; Chiu, S.Y.; Ku, M.M.; Wu, W.Y.; Hsu, C.Y.; et al. The incidence of fatal breast cancer measures the increased effectiveness of therapy in women participating in mammography screening. *Cancer* **2019**, *125*, 515–523. [CrossRef]
64. Sasieni, P. On the expected number of cancer deaths during follow-up of an initially cancer-free cohort. *Epidemiology (Camb. Mass.)* **2003**, *14*, 108–110. [CrossRef]

12

Multi-Marker Longitudinal Algorithms Incorporating HE4 and CA125 in Ovarian Cancer Screening of Postmenopausal Women

Aleksandra Gentry-Maharaj [1,†], Oleg Blyuss [2,3,†], Andy Ryan [1], Matthew Burnell [1], Chloe Karpinskyj [1], Richard Gunu [4], Jatinderpal K. Kalsi [4], Anne Dawnay [5], Ines P. Marino [6], Ranjit Manchanda [1,7,8], Karen Lu [9], Wei-Lei Yang [9], John F. Timms [4], Mahesh Parmar [1], Steven J. Skates [10], Robert C. Bast Jr. [9,‡], Ian J. Jacobs [4,11,‡], Alexey Zaikin [3,4,12,13,‡] and Usha Menon [1,‡,*]

1 MRC Clinical Trials Unit at UCL, Institute of Clinical Trials & Methodology, London WC1V 6LJ, UK; a.gentry-maharaj@ucl.ac.uk (A.G.-M.); a.ryan@ucl.ac.uk (A.R.); m.burnell@ucl.ac.uk (M.B.); c.karpinskyj@ucl.ac.uk (C.K.); r.manchanda@qmul.ac.uk (R.M.); m.parmar@ucl.ac.uk (M.P.)

2 School of Physics, Astronomy and Mathematics, University of Hertfordshire, Hatfield AL10 9AB, UK; o.blyuss@qmul.ac.uk

3 Department of Paediatrics and Paediatric Infectious Diseases, Sechenov First Moscow State Medical University, Moscow 119991, Russia; alexey.zaikin@ucl.ac.uk

4 Department of Women's Cancer, Institute for Women's Health, University College London, London WC1E 6BT, UK; r.gunu@ucl.ac.uk (R.G.); j.k.kalsi@ucl.ac.uk (J.K.K.); john.timms@ucl.ac.uk (J.F.T.); i.jacobs@unsw.edu.au (I.J.J.)

5 Clinical Biochemistry, Barts Health NHS Trust, London E1 8PR, UK; anne.dawnay@bartshealth.nhs.uk

6 Department of Biology and Geology, Physics and Inorganic Chemistry, Universidad Rey Juan Carlos, 28933 Madrid, Spain; ines.perez@urjc.es

7 Wolfson Institute of Preventive Medicine, Barts CRUK Cancer Centre, Queen Mary University of London, London EC1M 6BQ, UK

8 Department of Gynaecological Oncology, St Bartholomew's Hospital, Barts Health NHS Trust, London EC1A 7BE, UK

9 University of Texas M.D. Anderson Cancer Center, Houston, TX 77030, USA; khlu@mdanderson.org (K.L.); wlyang@mdanderson.org (W.-L.Y.); rbast@mdanderson.org (R.C.B.J.)

10 Massachusetts General Hospital and Harvard Medical School, Boston, MA 02114, USA; sskates@mgh.harvard.edu

11 University of New South Wales, Sydney 2052, Australia

12 Department of Applied Mathematics, Lobachevsky University of Nyzhniy Novgorod, Nizhniy Novgorod 603105, Russia

13 Department of Mathematics, University College London, London WC1H 0AY, UK

* Correspondence: u.menon@ucl.ac.uk

† These authors contributed equally to this paper.

‡ Joint last author.

Abstract: Longitudinal CA125 algorithms are the current basis of ovarian cancer screening. We report on longitudinal algorithms incorporating multiple markers. In the multimodal arm of United Kingdom Collaborative Trial of Ovarian Cancer Screening (UKCTOCS), 50,640 postmenopausal women underwent annual screening using a serum CA125 longitudinal algorithm. Women (cases) with invasive tubo-ovarian cancer (WHO 2014) following outcome review with stored annual serum samples donated in the 5 years preceding diagnosis were matched 1:1 to controls (no invasive tubo-ovarian cancer) in terms of the number of annual samples and age at randomisation. Blinded samples were assayed for serum human epididymis protein 4 (HE4), CA72-4 and anti-TP53 autoantibodies. Multimarker method of mean trends (MMT) longitudinal algorithms were developed using the assay results and trial CA125 values on the training set and evaluated in the blinded validation set. The study set comprised of 1363 (2–5 per woman) serial samples from 179 cases and 181 controls. In the validation set, area under the curve (AUC) and sensitivity of longitudinal CA125-MMT algorithm were 0.911 (0.871–0.952) and 90.5% (82.5–98.6%). None of the longitudinal multi-marker algorithms (CA125-HE4, CA125-HE4-CA72-4, CA125-HE4-CA72-4-anti-TP53) performed better or improved on lead-time. Our population study suggests that longitudinal HE4, CA72-4, anti-TP53 autoantibodies adds little value to longitudinal serum CA125 as a first-line test in ovarian cancer screening of postmenopausal women.

Keywords: ovarian cancer; CA125; HE4; UKCTOCS; MMT; screening; postmenopausal women

1. Introduction

Ovarian cancer is the most fatal of all gynaecological malignancies [1]. Despite significant advances in treatment, the impact on mortality over the past three decades has been modest [2–5]. A key contributing factor is diagnosis at advanced stages when survival is poor (5-year survival rates for stage III/IV disease 35% versus 90% for stage I) [6]. Efforts over the past four decades have therefore focused on early detection. Advances in understanding the natural history has meanwhile clarified the need to focus on detecting invasive tubo-ovarian cancer (WHO 2014), especially Type II (high-grade serous) cancers as they account for most of the mortality.

Since its discovery in 1981, CA125 remains the best performing marker for ovarian cancer. It forms an integral part of differential diagnosis and has been studied extensively in the context of screening [7–10]. In screening, performance has been improved by the use of the Risk of Ovarian Cancer Algorithm (ROCA), which assesses serial changes in CA125 over time. As a first-line test for ovarian cancer screening, ROCA had a sensitivity of 85.8% in the United Kingdom Collaborative Trial of Ovarian Cancer Screening (UKCTOCS) during incidence screening [11]. Moreover, screening using the multimodal strategy (ROCA as the first-line test with transvaginal ultrasound as the second-line test) resulted for the first time in a stage shift in women diagnosed with invasive tubo-ovarian cancer compared with no screening, on an "intention to screen" analysis. The mortality benefit was however not definitive at the first analysis and further follow-up is underway [5]. Retrospective analysis using data from the trial suggests that other longitudinal CA125 algorithms such as parametric empirical Bayes (PEB) [12,13], parenclitic networks [14], deep learning [15] and method of mean trends (MMT) [16,17] are likely to perform similarly.

Over the years, data from small case–control studies [18,19] have suggested that markers like human epididymis protein 4 (HE4) and TP53 autoantibodies might complement CA125 in ovarian cancer screening. HE4 was the second best marker for invasive tubo-ovarian cancer after CA125 (sensitivity CA125 86%; HE4 73%) in a nested case–control study within the Prostate, Lung, Colorectal and Ovarian cancer screening (PLCO) trial using a single preclinical sample taken within 6 months of diagnosis [20]. Data from the Carotene and Retinol Efficacy Trial suggested that a panel including CA125, HE4 and mesothelin may provide a signal for ovarian cancer 3 years before diagnosis [21]. More recently, elevated anti-TP53 autoantibody levels were detected in 16% of cases not detected by ROCA in the UKCTOCS sample set, providing in these cases a lead time of 22 months [19]. Other studies have explored the performance of multi-marker (CA125, IGFBP2, LCAT, SHBG, GRP78 and calprotectin) [22] panels. All have used cut-offs for interpreting results. Longitudinal algorithms incorporating multiple markers have not been previously investigated.

We report on the performance of longitudinal multi-marker algorithms incorporating CA125, HE4, CA72-4 and anti-TP53 autoantibodies as a first-line test in ovarian cancer screening using the prospective specimen collection and the retrospective blinded evaluation (PRoBe) design [23] within the general population UKCTOCS trial.

2. Results

During a median follow-up of 11.1 (IQR 10.0–12.0) years, of the 46,237 women randomised to the multimodal screening (MMS) arm of UKCTOCS who had two or more annual screens, 238 were diagnosed with invasive tubo-ovarian cancer [24]. At the time of sample selection, 179 (75.2%) of the latter had adequate (>2 mL) serum in the biorepository. The final set comprised of 179 cases and 181 controls. Training and validation sets comprised of 181 women (90 invasive tubo-ovarian cancer cases, 91 controls; 676 annual samples) and 179 women (89 invasive tubo-ovarian cancer cases, 90 controls; 677 annual samples), respectively (Table 1), with 2–5 serial samples per woman.

Table 1. Details of cases (invasive tubo-ovarian cancer) and controls in training and validation sets.

Group	Overall		Annual Samples Available in Year Preceding Diagnosis	
	No. of Women	No. of Annual Samples	No. of Women	No. of Annual Samples
		Training Set		
Cases	90	317	68	68
Controls	91	359	113/167 *	608
		Validation Set		
Cases	89	332	74	74
Controls	90	355	105/173 *	613

* a case is included as a control until the screen is within a year of diagnosis for the purposes of this analysis—the first number is unique controls and the second number includes those who will become cases.

Of the cases, 68 and 74 were diagnosed within 1 year of sample in the training and validation set, respectively (Table 1). There was no difference in age between the cases and controls. Baseline and clinical characteristics of the women in the training and validation sets were well balanced (Table 2). There were 13 Type I, 74 Type II, and 3 Type uncertain tubo-ovarian cancers in the training set, and 11 Type I, 72 Type II, and 6 Type uncertain in the validation set. In the training set, four longitudinal multi-marker algorithms (CA125-HE4-MMT1, CA125-HE4-MMT2, CA125-HE4-CA72-4-MMT, CA125-HE4-CA72-4-anti-TP53-MMT) were derived and then applied to the validation set, which comprised of 670 annual samples from 179 women (Table 1).

For the detection of invasive tubo-ovarian cancers diagnosed within 1 year of last annual sample, at a fixed specificity of 87.6% (similar to ROCA as a first-line test in UKCTOCS), CA125, HE4 or CA72-4 alone had a sensitivity of 73%, 58.1%, and 37.8%, respectively (Table 3). Figure 1 shows the Receiver Operating Curve (ROC) for the performance of CA125-MMT versus the four newly developed models, CA125-HE4-MMT1, CA125-HE4-MMT2, CA125-HE4-CA72-4-MMT, CA125-HE4-CA72-4-anti-TP53-MMT, in the validation set. CA125-MMT provided a higher area under the curve (AUC) compared with any other model (0.911 versus 0.897–0.902) (Table 3). At a specificity of 87.6%, CA125-MMT outperformed all other multimarker models (sensitivity of 90.5% versus 81–86.5%) with CA125-HE4-MMT1 being the next best model.

Of the 74 invasive tubo-ovarian cancers in the validation set, 67 (90.5%) were detected by the CA125-MMT model, of whom 53 (79.1%) were Type II cancers (Table S1). Of the other models, the CA125-HE4-MMT1 detected 64 cancers with one additional woman with Type I cancer not detected by the CA125-MMT model.

In the lead time analysis, no multimarker algorithm outperformed CA125-MMT. The lead time from marker elevation/change point to diagnosis was on average 140–148 days (multimarker algorithms) compared with 152 days (CA125-MMT algorithm) (Table 4).

Table 2. Characteristics of cases and controls in training and validation sets.

Baseline Characteristics	Training Set	Validation Set
No. of women	181	179
Median age at recruitment (years)	63.54	63.68
BMI	26.46	25.99
OCP use	90 (49.7%)	88 (49.2%)
Median Duration of OCP use (years)	5 (*n* = 89)	5 (*n* = 86)
Hysterectomy	35 (19.3%)	34 (19.0%)
% White ethnicity	177 (97.8%)	174 (97.6%)
HRT use	25 (13.8%)	33 (18.4%)
Personal history of breast cancer	3 (1.66%)	7 (3.91%)
Morphology of Cases		
Invasive tubo-ovarian cancer	90	89
Histological Type of Invasive Tubo-Ovarian Cancer		
Type I	***13***	***11***
Endometrioid (low grade)	6	5
Serous (low grade)	1	2
Clear cell	6	4
Type II	***68***	***63***
High grade serous ovarian	57	62
Carcinoma, NOS	10	3
Endometrioid (high grade)	6	5
Carcinosarcoma	1	2
Type uncertain	***3***	***6***
Carcinoma, NOS	2	4
Serous (grade unknown)	1	2
Stage of Invasive Tubo-Ovarian Cancer		
I	21	20
II	12	10
III	47	53
IV	10	6

BMI, body mass index; OCP, oral contraceptive pill; HRT, hormone replacement therapy.

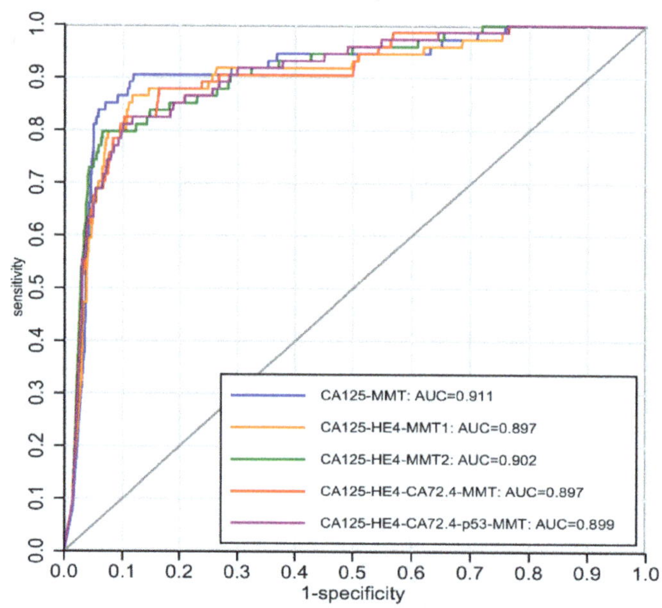

Figure 1. ROC curves with the AUC for each of the longitudinal algorithms.

Table 3. Sensitivity and area under the ROC curve (AUC) of algorithms for the detection of invasive tubo-ovarian cancer diagnosed within one year of sample in the validation set.

Algorithms	AUC (95%CI)	Sensitivity (95%CI) at 87.6% SPECIFICITY
CA125-MMT	91.1	90.5
	(87.1 to 95.2)	(82.5 to 98.6)
CA125-HE4-MMT1	89.7	86.5
	(85.6 to 93.8)	(77.7 to 95.2)
CA125-HE4-MMT2	90.2	81
	(86.4 to 94)	(71.8 to 90.4)
CA125-HE4-CA72-4-MMT	89.7	82.4
	(85.8 to 93.7)	(73.5 to 91.4)
CA125-HE4-CA72-4-anti-TP53-MMT	90	82.4
	(86.2 to 93.6)	(73.5 to 91.4)
CA125	86.5	73
	(81.1 to 91.9)	(61.1 to 84.8)
HE4	80.4	58.1
	(74.8 to 86)	(45.4 to 70.8)
CA72-4	71.7	37.8
	(65 to 78.5)	(22.9 to 49.8)

AUC, area under ROC curve; CI, confidence interval.

Table 4. Lead time of algorithms for the detection of invasive tubo-ovarian cancer in the validation set.

Algorithm	No. of Cases Detected by Algorithm	Mean Lead Time	SD
CA125-MMT	67	152	95
CA125-HE4-MMT1	64	148	95
CA125-HE4-MMT2	60	140	91
CA125-HE4-CA72-4-MMT	61	144	92
CA125-HE4-CA72-4-anti-TP53-MMT	61	144	92

The newer models offered no benefit in detecting poor prognostic cases (who died within 5 years of the last sample taken), with 12 of 67 (18.0%) women detected by the CA125-MMT model. The CA125-HE4-MMT2 model was able to detect 11 cases who died but at a cost of only detecting 60 cases. None of the other models were able to improve on this.

3. Discussion

3.1. Principal Findings

This is the first study to explore the added value of longitudinal multi-marker profiles to longitudinal CA125 for ovarian cancer screening. In this population-based case–control study, the addition of longitudinal HE4 or other markers such as CA72-4 and anti-TP53 did not improve on the performance of the longitudinal single marker CA125 algorithm in postmenopausal women [16]. There was also no improvement in lead time over longitudinal CA125. It would therefore be hard to justify the higher costs of including HE4 alongside CA125 in this population.

3.2. Results in Context

The current sensitivity of multimodal ovarian cancer screening is 87%. The MMS strategy consists of first-line screening using the longitudinal CA125 algorithm (ROCA) followed by repeat CA125 profiling and transvaginal ultrasound in women with intermediate or elevated test results. There has been longstanding interest in the possibility of increasing sensitivity by adding other markers that might help detect the 15% of the cases that are currently missed using the MMS strategy, which is probably due to the tumours not expressing CA125. HE4 has been the fore runner among potential markers ever since being highlighted in the study by Cramer and colleagues [20] using samples from the ovarian cancer screening arm of the PLCO trial. This study showed that out of 35 markers evaluated in a single sample taken 6 months prior to diagnosis in 118 women with ovarian cancer, HE4 (sensitivity 73%) was the second best marker to CA125 (sensitivity 86%). A previous exploratory study nested within the UKCTOCS cohort which was enriched for the missed cases also seemed to suggest that longitudinal HE4 and CA72-4 might improve sensitivity [25]. In the same UKCTOCS nested case–control study, p53 autoantibody profile was shown to complement CA125 in that it was able to detect 20.7% of those not detected by ROCA [19]. This was however not borne out in our rigorous study that used all available samples from the multimodal cohort. Our results using a cut-off as used in the PLCO analysis resulted in similar results (HE4 sensitivity 58.1% vs. 73% in PLCO; CA125 73% versus 86% in PLCO).

3.3. *Clinical and Research Implications*

There are now a number of longitudinal CA125 algorithms [16,26]. The advantage of the MMT methodologies presented here is that they incorporate longitudinal profiling of multiple biomarkers in a single algorithm. This sets the stage for future work incorporating novel markers as they gain recognition in ovarian cancer screening. Moreover, the longitudinal algorithms framework described here is applicable to other cancers and diseases where a serial profile of multiple markers is available.

3.4. *Strengths and Limitations*

The major strength is the decrease in bias through the use of a population-based nested case–control as per the PRoBE study design [23]. All samples were prospectively collected before outcome ascertainment. Linkage to electronic health records and independent outcome review of cases ensured complete and accurate data. The study has involved the largest dataset of serial samples up to 5 years prior to diagnosis of tubo-ovarian cancer in postmenopausal women from the general population that we are aware of. While the number of cases may seem small, the set consisted of 75% of all women who had two or more annual screens and were diagnosed with invasive tubo-ovarian cancer in the course of 343,156 screens. CA125, HE4 and CA72-4 assays were assayed by ELISA (enzyme-linked immunosorbent assay), the gold standard [27] in assaying markers. When applying the algorithm in the validation set, the statistician was blinded to the outcome. The algorithms described have a flexible modelling framework and hence can be used more widely. HE4 levels are known to increase with age in healthy people [28]. To address this in our design we have used age-matched controls. Moreover, as our models are based on trend indices rather than raw HE4 levels, the variation in age is unlikely to affect our results. While all women donated annual samples, it needs to be noted that the available serial repeat samples were influenced by the use of CA125 and ROCA in the trial. The results cannot be extrapolated to high-risk screening strategies where the frequency of screening is 6-monthly or less. In these high risk populations, ovarian cancer screening, if undertaken, usually starts at age 35 and in these premenopausal women HE4 may be helpful in ruling out endometriosis. We only used one control per case due to limited funds. Including a larger number of controls would have shed more light on the biological variation of HE4 in postmenopausal women.

4. Materials and Methods

4.1. *Subjects*

Between April 2001 and September 2005, 202,638 postmenopausal women aged 50–74 were recruited to UKCTOCS through 13 trial centres based in England, Wales and Northern Ireland (NI). The women were randomised to annual screening: (1) MMS using serum CA125 interpreted with the

ROCA followed by transvaginal ultrasound (TVS) as a second-line test ($n = 50,640$); (2) ultrasound (USS) screening using TVS alone ($n = 50,639$); or (3) no screening (control) group ($n = 101,359$) in a 1:1:2 ratio, as described previously [29,30]. In the MMS group, based on ROCA, women were triaged to (1) annual screening if normal; (2) repeat CA125 in 6 weeks if intermediate; (3) repeat CA125 and TVS if the risk was elevated. Women with abnormal ultrasound or persistent elevated risk (irrespective of scan findings) had clinical assessment by a trial clinician and additional investigations within the NHS. Women who had surgery or biopsy for suspected tubo-ovarian cancer after clinical assessment were considered trial-screen positive. Blood samples were taken at the trial centres in gel tubes (8 mL gel separation serum tubes; Greiner Bio-One 455071, Stonehouse, UK) and transported at room temperature overnight to the central UKCTOCS laboratory using the standard protocol [11,29,31]. The samples received within 56 h of venepuncture were processed by centrifuging at 1500× g for 10 min. The serum was separated and assayed for CA125. The excess serum was pre-cooled at −80 °C and stored in 500 μL straws in liquid nitrogen at an off-site cryorepository until the sample was retrieved and thawed for the current analysis.

UKCTOCS was approved by the UK North West Multicentre Research Ethics Committees (North West MREC 00/8/34) on 21 June 2000 with site-specific approval from the local regional ethics committees and the Caldicott guardians (data controllers) of the primary care trusts. The current study was approved by the NRES (National Research Ethics Service) Committee North East-Tyne & Wear South (Ref: 15/NE/0025) on 20 January 2015.

All women were followed up through linkage via electronic health records for cancers and deaths as previously detailed [5,30] (NHS Digital, England and Wales; Northern Ireland Cancer Registry and NI Health and Social Care Business Services Organisation, NI). Women also completed two follow-up postal questionnaires; 3–5 years after randomisation, and in April 2014. As for the mortality analysis previously undertaken [5], cancer registrations received up to 5 April 2015 (England, Wales), and 9 April 2015 (NI) were used.

For all women with a possible diagnosis of ovarian cancer (one of 19 ICD-10 codes) [5], medical notes were requested and reviewed by a member of the independent Outcomes Review Committee (two pathologists and two gynaecological oncologists) who were masked to the randomisation group [5]. The Outcomes Review Committee [5] confirmed the final diagnosis—the primary cancer site (WHO 2014) [24]; the stage and morphology; and where possible, classified invasive tubo-ovarian cancer (WHO 2014 classification) [24] which included epithelial ovarian, fallopian tube and the primary peritoneal cancer as per WHO 2003 classification into Type I (low-grade serous, low-grade endometrioid, mucinous, clear cell) or Type II (high-grade serous, high-grade endometrioid, carcinosarcomas, undifferentiated) cancers or Type uncertain [32].

4.2. Sample Set and CA125, HE4, CA72-4 and Anti-TP53 Autoantibody Assays

The cases were all women in the MMS group diagnosed with invasive tubo-ovarian cancer [24] during follow-up, who had ≥2 serial samples taken within 5 years of diagnosis. Women with borderline epithelial and non-epithelial ovarian cancer were excluded. The controls were randomly chosen from the remaining women who did not have primary malignant neoplasm of the ovary. The cases were matched (1:1) to controls in terms of the number of annual samples available and age (±6 months) at randomisation.

The sample set for the study included all serial samples in the cases and controls where >2 mL serum was available in the cryorepository.

Once assayed for CA125 (Roche Diagnostics, Burgess Hill, UK), the excess serum was stored in liquid nitrogen in an off-site commercial cryorepository until it was retrieved for this study.

CA125 measurements (Roche, Burgess Hill, UK) completed as part of the UKCTOCS screening protocol were used along with anti-TP53 autoantibody values assayed during a previously reported study [19]. HE4 and CA72-4 (Roche Diagnostics, Burgess Hill) were assayed on all samples using the Roche Cobas analyser at the UCL Department of Women's Cancer Proteomics laboratory.

4.3. Method of Mean Trends (MMT) Algorithms Incorporating CA125, HE4, CA72-4 and Anti-TP53 Autoantibody

The MMT that evaluates the dynamics of longitudinal CA125 measurements has been described previously [16].

In brief, the serial pattern of a particular biomarker $Y_{i,j},\ j = 1 \ldots T$ of each woman "i" was mapped into a five-variable space. The new variables included the mean derivative weighted to the most recent measurement, the mean area under the time series (1), the coefficient of variation (2), the "centre of mass" of the time series (3) and the most recent measurement.

$$\left(\sum_{j=1}^{T-1} \frac{\left(Y_{i,j+1} - Y_{i,j}\right)\left(t_{i,j+1} - t_{i,j}\right)}{2} \right) / (T-1) \tag{1}$$

$$\sqrt{\frac{\sum_{j=1}^{T}\left(Y_{i,j} - \overline{Y}_i\right)^2}{T}} / \overline{Y}_i \tag{2}$$

$$\frac{\sum_{j=1}^{T} Y_{i,j} t_{i,j}}{\sum_{j=1}^{T} t_{i,j}} \tag{3}$$

The mean derivative was evaluated as $\sum_{j=1}^{T-1} w_{ij} \frac{Y_{i,j+1} - Y_{i,j}}{t_{i,j+1} - t_{i,j}}$ where weights w_j were computed for each interval between two consecutive measurements as $w_{ij} = \frac{1}{t_{i,T} - \left(t_{i,j+1} + t_{i,j}\right)/2}$. Here, $t_{i,T}$ was the age of the patient at the time of the most recent sample, while $t_{i,j}$ was age of the patient when the j-th sample was taken.

To use this approach to incorporate multiple serial biomarkers, for each of the proteins, the aforementioned five variables were evaluated and combined together into a logistic regression with AIC (Akaike information criterion) used to select the predictors that explain the labels of the patients (control = 0, case = 1) in the most optimal way.

With the MMT approach, we generated four separate models for the prediction of the risk of ovarian cancer using the serial measurements of multiple biomarkers:

- CA125-HE4-MMT1, where variable selection was made only over HE4 indices added to the reported CA125-MMT model [16];
- CA125-HE4-MMT2, where five indices for both CA125 and HE4 were used with further variable selection;
- CA125-HE4-CA72-4-MMT, where five indices for CA125, HE4 and CA72-4 were used with further variable selection;
- CA125-HE4-CA72-4- anti-TP53-MMT, where five indices for CA125, HE4, CA72-4 and anti-TP53 were used with further variable selection.

The performance of these models was evaluated against the original CA125-MMT approach as well as the actual biomarkers levels.

4.4. Statistical Analysis

The cases and controls were randomly split into "training" and "validation" sets in a 1:1 ratio. Longitudinal CA125 MMT described previously [16], and four separate longitudinal multi-marker (CA125-HE4-MMT1, CA125-HE4-MMT2, CA125-HE4-CA72-4-MMT and CA125-HE4-CA72-4-anti-TP53-MMT) algorithms were built using all available serial samples from the cases and controls in the "training" set by OB. OB then applied them to the blinded "validation" set.

Statistical analysis was undertaken by MB to ensure blinding. The performance characteristics of the newly constructed algorithms as a first-line test were evaluated and compared with the CA125-MMT in terms of the following: (1) sensitivity at a fixed specificity of 87.6% similar to ROCA in UKCTOCS [11];

(2) average lead time for all cases detected (the date of detection is the date when risk given by algorithm is abnormal and for all further annual measurements it remains abnormal); (3) the area under the receiver operating characteristic (ROC) curve (AUC). Inference for the ROC curves was based on cluster-robust standard errors that accounted for the serially correlated nature of the samples [33]. At fixed specificity (87.6%), the performance characteristics of CA125 and HE4 cut-offs were compared with those of the newly derived algorithm.

Only annual samples were included in this analysis. The last blood sample was considered as true positive (if within 1 year from diagnosis) and all prior annual samples as true negatives. In the controls, all samples were included as true negatives.

To investigate whether any of the algorithms identified invasive tubo-ovarian cancer cases earlier than CA125-MMT, we performed lead time analysis, where the mean interval from detection to diagnosis was compared for all algorithms. For each algorithm, the average interval was calculated in days for only those cases that were detected as abnormal by the algorithm. Here, we assumed that an algorithm identified a cancer case at a particular measurement if both at this and at all subsequent measurements it classified the risk as abnormal. A further analysis explored how many of the cancers missed by ROCA during the trial (trial-screen negative cases) would have been detected by each of the algorithms.

5. Conclusions

In the context of screening, our study suggests that the additional value of HE4, CA72-4 and p53 autoantibodies to CA125 as a first line test in screening for ovarian cancer of postmenopausal women from the general population is limited. Further work on the value of these markers as a reflex test following elevated risk may show promise and strengthen the confidence in cancer diagnosis and thus shorten the period between the screening test and surgical intervention.

Author Contributions: Conceptualisation, U.M., A.G.-M., O.B., A.Z., A.R., R.C.B.J.; literature search, U.M., A.G.-M.; support and development of CA72-4 and anti-TP53 autoantibody assays, K.L., W.-L.Y. and R.C.B.J.; preparation of the dataset, A.G.-M., A.R.; development of the MMT algorithm, O.B., A.Z.; trial conduct, C.K., R.G., J.K.K., A.D., R.M., M.P., S.J.S., I.J.J.; statistical analysis and preparation of figures and tables, O.B., I.P.M., M.B., J.F.T. All authors have read and agreed to the published version of the manuscript.

Acknowledgments: We are particularly grateful to the women throughout the UK who have participated in the trial. We thank all the staff involved in the trial for their hard work and dedication. We thank the Data Monitoring and Ethics Committee and the independent Trial Steering Committee members. has co-licensed software for the Risk of Ovarian Cancer algorithm to Abcodia. All other authors declare no competing interests.

References

1. CRUK. Ten Most Common Causes of Cancer Death in Females. Available online: https://www.cancerresearchuk.org/health-professional/cancer-statistics/mortality/common-cancers-compared#heading-Two (accessed on 8 January 2019).
2. van Nagell, J.R., Jr.; Miller, R.W.; DeSimone, C.P.; Ueland, F.R.; Podzielinski, I.; Goodrich, S.T.; Elder, J.W.; Huang, B.; Kryscio, R.J.; Pavlik, E.J. Long-term survival of women with epithelial ovarian cancer detected by ultrasonographic screening. *Obs. Gynecol* **2011**, *118*, 1212–1221. [CrossRef] [PubMed]
3. Buys, S.S.; Partridge, E.; Black, A.; Johnson, C.C.; Lamerato, L.; Isaacs, C.; Reding, D.J.; Greenlee, R.T.; Yokochi, L.A.; Kessel, B.; et al. Effect of screening on ovarian cancer mortality: The Prostate, Lung, Colorectal and Ovarian (PLCO) Cancer Screening Randomized Controlled Trial. *JAMA J. Am. Med. Assoc.* **2011**, *305*, 2295–2303. [CrossRef] [PubMed]

4. Kobayashi, H.; Yamada, Y.; Sado, T.; Sakata, M.; Yoshida, S.; Kawaguchi, R.; Kanayama, S.; Shigetomi, H.; Haruta, S.; Tsuji, Y.; et al. A randomized study of screening for ovarian cancer: A multicenter study in Japan. *Int. J. Gynecol. Cancer Off. J. Int. Gynecol. Cancer Soc.* **2008**, *18*, 414–420. [CrossRef]
5. Jacobs, I.J.; Menon, U.; Ryan, A.; Gentry-Maharaj, A.; Burnell, M.; Kalsi, J.K.; Amso, N.N.; Apostolidou, S.; Benjamin, E.; Cruickshank, D.; et al. Ovarian cancer screening and mortality in the UK Collaborative Trial of Ovarian Cancer Screening (UKCTOCS): A randomised controlled trial. *Lancet (Lond. Engl.)* **2016**, *387*, 945–956. [CrossRef]
6. CRUK. Ovarian Cancer Survival by Stage at Diagnosis. Available online: http://www.cancerresearchuk.org/health-professional/cancer-statistics/statistics-by-cancer-type/ovarian-cancer/survival#heading-Three (accessed on 12 December 2018).
7. Lu, K.H.; Skates, S.; Hernandez, M.A.; Bedi, D.; Bevers, T.; Leeds, L.; Moore, R.; Granai, C.; Harris, S.; Newland, W.; et al. A 2-stage ovarian cancer screening strategy using the Risk of Ovarian Cancer Algorithm (ROCA) identifies early-stage incident cancers and demonstrates high positive predictive value. *Cancer* **2013**, *119*, 3454–3461. [CrossRef] [PubMed]
8. Menon, U.; Skates, S.J.; Lewis, S.; Rosenthal, A.N.; Rufford, B.; Sibley, K.; Macdonald, N.; Dawnay, A.; Jeyarajah, A.; Bast, R.C., Jr.; et al. Prospective study using the risk of ovarian cancer algorithm to screen for ovarian cancer. *J. Clin. Oncol. Off. J. Am. Soc. Clin. Oncol.* **2005**, *23*, 7919–7926. [CrossRef] [PubMed]
9. Skates, S.J.; Horick, N.; Yu, Y.; Xu, F.J.; Berchuck, A.; Havrilesky, L.J.; de Bruijn, H.W.; van der Zee, A.G.; Woolas, R.P.; Jacobs, I.J.; et al. Preoperative sensitivity and specificity for early-stage ovarian cancer when combining cancer antigen CA-125II, CA 15-3, CA 72-4, and macrophage colony-stimulating factor using mixtures of multivariate normal distributions. *J. Clin. Oncol. Off. J. Am. Soc. Clin. Oncol.* **2004**, *22*, 4059–4066. [CrossRef]
10. Skates, S.J.; Pauler, D.K.; Jacobs, I.J. Screening Based on the Risk of Cancer Calculation From Bayesian Hierarchical Changepoint and Mixture Models of Longitudinal Markers. *J. Am. Stat. Assoc.* **2001**, *96*, 429–439. [CrossRef]
11. Menon, U.; Ryan, A.; Kalsi, J.; Gentry-Maharaj, A.; Dawnay, A.; Habib, M.; Apostolidou, S.; Singh, N.; Benjamin, E.; Burnell, M.; et al. Risk Algorithm Using Serial Biomarker Measurements Doubles the Number of Screen-Detected Cancers Compared With a Single-Threshold Rule in the United Kingdom Collaborative Trial of Ovarian Cancer Screening. *J. Clin. Oncol. Off. J. Am. Soc. Clin. Oncol.* **2015**, *33*, 2062–2071. [CrossRef]
12. Drescher, C.W.; Shah, C.; Thorpe, J.; O'Briant, K.; Anderson, G.L.; Berg, C.D.; Urban, N.; McIntosh, M.W. Longitudinal screening algorithm that incorporates change over time in CA125 levels identifies ovarian cancer earlier than a single-threshold rule. *J. Clin. Oncol. Off. J. Am. Soc. Clin. Oncol.* **2013**, *31*, 387–392. [CrossRef]
13. McIntosh, M.W.; Urban, N. A parametric empirical Bayes method for cancer screening using longitudinal observations of a biomarker. *Biostatistics* **2003**, *4*, 27–40. [CrossRef]
14. Whitwell, H.J.; Blyuss, O.; Menon, U.; Timms, J.F.; Zaikin, A. Parenclitic networks for predicting ovarian cancer. *Oncotarget* **2018**, *9*, 22717–22726. [CrossRef] [PubMed]
15. Vázquez, M.A.; Mariño, I.P.; Blyuss, O.; Ryan, A.; Gentry-Maharaj, A.; Kalsi, J.; Manchanda, R.; Jacobs, I.; Menon, U.; Zaikin, A. A quantitative performance study of two automatic methods for the diagnosis of ovarian cancer. *Biomed. Signal Process. Control* **2018**, *46*, 86–93. [CrossRef] [PubMed]
16. Blyuss, O.; Burnell, M.; Ryan, A.; Gentry-Maharaj, A.; Marino, I.P.; Kalsi, J.; Manchanda, R.; Timms, J.F.; Parmar, M.; Skates, S.J.; et al. Comparison of Longitudinal CA125 Algorithms as a First-Line Screen for Ovarian Cancer in the General Population. *Clin. Cancer Res. Off. J. Am. Assoc. Cancer Res.* **2018**, *24*, 4726–4733. [CrossRef]
17. Whitwell, H.J.; Worthington, J.; Blyuss, O.; Gentry-Maharaj, A.; Ryan, A.; Gunu, R.; Kalsi, J.; Menon, U.; Jacobs, I.; Zaikin, A.; et al. Improved early detection of ovarian cancer using longitudinal multimarker models. *Br. J. Cancer* **2020**, *122*, 847–856. [CrossRef] [PubMed]
18. Simmons, A.R.; Fourkala, E.O.; Gentry-Maharaj, A.; Ryan, A.; Sutton, M.N.; Baggerly, K.; Zheng, H.; Lu, K.H.; Jacobs, I.; Skates, S.; et al. Complementary Longitudinal Serum Biomarkers to CA125 for Early Detection of Ovarian Cancer. *Cancer Prev. Res.* **2019**, *12*, 391–400. [CrossRef] [PubMed]
19. Yang, W.L.; Gentry-Maharaj, A.; Simmons, A.; Ryan, A.; Fourkala, E.O.; Lu, Z.; Baggerly, K.A.; Zhao, Y.; Lu, K.H.; Bowtell, D.; et al. Elevation of TP53 Autoantibody Before CA125 in Preclinical Invasive Epithelial Ovarian Cancer. *Clin. Cancer Res. Off. J. Am. Assoc. Cancer Res.* **2017**, *23*, 5912–5922. [CrossRef]

20. Cramer, D.W.; Bast, R.C., Jr.; Berg, C.D.; Diamandis, E.P.; Godwin, A.K.; Hartge, P.; Lokshin, A.E.; Lu, K.H.; McIntosh, M.W.; Mor, G.; et al. Ovarian cancer biomarker performance in prostate, lung, colorectal, and ovarian cancer screening trial specimens. *Cancer Prev. Res.* **2011**, *4*, 365–374. [CrossRef]
21. Anderson, G.L.; McIntosh, M.; Wu, L.; Barnett, M.; Goodman, G.; Thorpe, J.D.; Bergan, L.; Thornquist, M.D.; Scholler, N.; Kim, N.; et al. Assessing lead time of selected ovarian cancer biomarkers: A nested case-control study. *J. Natl. Cancer Inst.* **2010**, *102*, 26–38. [CrossRef]
22. Russell, M.R.; Graham, C.; D'Amato, A.; Gentry-Maharaj, A.; Ryan, A.; Kalsi, J.K.; Ainley, C.; Whetton, A.D.; Menon, U.; Jacobs, I.; et al. A combined biomarker panel shows improved sensitivity for the early detection of ovarian cancer allowing the identification of the most aggressive type II tumours. *Br. J. Cancer* **2017**, *117*, 666–674. [CrossRef]
23. Pepe, M.S.; Feng, Z.; Janes, H.; Bossuyt, P.M.; Potter, J.D. Pivotal evaluation of the accuracy of a biomarker used for classification or prediction: Standards for study design. *J. Natl. Cancer Inst.* **2008**, *100*, 1432–1438. [CrossRef]
24. Kurman, R.J.; Carcangiu, M.L.; Herrington, S.; Young, R.H. *WHO Classification of Tumours of Female Reproductive Organs (IARC WHO Classification of Tumours)*, 4th ed.; IARC: Lyon, France, 2014; Volume 6.
25. Simmons, A.; Fourkala, E.O.; Gentry-Maharaj, A.; Ryan, A.; Baggerly, K.A.; Zheng, H.; Lu, K.H.; Jacobs, I.; Skates, S.J.; Menon, U.; et al. Validation of longitudinal performance of a multi-marker panel for the early detection of ovarian cancer. *Cancer Prev. Res.* **2019**, in press.
26. Mariño, I.P.; Blyuss, O.; Ryan, A.; Gentry-Maharaj, A.; Timms, J.F.; Dawnay, A.; Kalsi, J.; Jacobs, I.; Menon, U.; Zaikin, A. Change-point of multiple biomarkers in women with ovarian cancer. *Biomed. Signal Process. Control* **2017**, *33*, 169–177. [CrossRef]
27. Thiha, A.; Ibrahim, F. A Colorimetric Enzyme-Linked Immunosorbent Assay (ELISA) Detection Platform for a Point-of-Care Dengue Detection System on a Lab-on-Compact-Disc. *Sensors* **2015**, *15*, 11431–11441. [CrossRef] [PubMed]
28. Moore, R.G.; Miller, M.C.; Eklund, E.E.; Lu, K.H.; Bast, R.C., Jr.; Lambert-Messerlian, G. Serum levels of the ovarian cancer biomarker HE4 are decreased in pregnancy and increase with age. *Am. J. Obstet. Gynecol.* **2012**, *206*, 349.e1–349.e7. [CrossRef]
29. Menon, U.; Gentry-Maharaj, A.; Hallett, R.; Ryan, A.; Burnell, M.; Sharma, A.; Lewis, S.; Davies, S.; Philpott, S.; Lopes, A.; et al. Sensitivity and specificity of multimodal and ultrasound screening for ovarian cancer, and stage distribution of detected cancers: Results of the prevalence screen of the UK Collaborative Trial of Ovarian Cancer Screening (UKCTOCS). *Lancet Oncol.* **2009**, *10*, 327–340. [CrossRef]
30. Menon, U.; Gentry-Maharaj, A.; Ryan, A.; Sharma, A.; Burnell, M.; Hallett, R.; Lewis, S.; Lopez, A.; Godfrey, K.; Oram, D.; et al. Recruitment to multicentre trials–lessons from UKCTOCS: Descriptive study. *BMJ* **2008**, *337*, a2079. [CrossRef] [PubMed]
31. Blyuss, O.; Gentry-Maharaj, A.; Fourkala, E.-O.; Ryan, A.; Zaikin, A.; Menon, U.; Jacobs, I.; Timms, J.F. Serial Patterns of Ovarian Cancer Biomarkers in a Prediagnosis Longitudinal Dataset. *BioMed Res. Int.* **2015**, *2015*, 681416. [CrossRef] [PubMed]
32. Kurman, R.J.; Shih Ie, M. The origin and pathogenesis of epithelial ovarian cancer: A proposed unifying theory. *Am. J. Surg. Pathol.* **2010**, *34*, 433–443. [CrossRef] [PubMed]
33. Rogers, W. Regression standard errors in clustered samples. *Stata Tech. Bull.* **1993**, *13*, 19–23.

Permissions

All chapters in this book were first published by MDPI; hereby published with permission under the Creative Commons Attribution License or equivalent. Every chapter published in this book has been scrutinized by our experts. Their significance has been extensively debated. The topics covered herein carry significant findings which will fuel the growth of the discipline. They may even be implemented as practical applications or may be referred to as a beginning point for another development.

The contributors of this book come from diverse backgrounds, making this book a truly international effort. This book will bring forth new frontiers with its revolutionizing research information and detailed analysis of the nascent developments around the world.

We would like to thank all the contributing authors for lending their expertise to make the book truly unique. They have played a crucial role in the development of this book. Without their invaluable contributions this book wouldn't have been possible. They have made vital efforts to compile up to date information on the varied aspects of this subject to make this book a valuable addition to the collection of many professionals and students.

This book was conceptualized with the vision of imparting up-to-date information and advanced data in this field. To ensure the same, a matchless editorial board was set up. Every individual on the board went through rigorous rounds of assessment to prove their worth. After which they invested a large part of their time researching and compiling the most relevant data for our readers.

The editorial board has been involved in producing this book since its inception. They have spent rigorous hours researching and exploring the diverse topics which have resulted in the successful publishing of this book. They have passed on their knowledge of decades through this book. To expedite this challenging task, the publisher supported the team at every step. A small team of assistant editors was also appointed to further simplify the editing procedure and attain best results for the readers.

Apart from the editorial board, the designing team has also invested a significant amount of their time in understanding the subject and creating the most relevant covers. They scrutinized every image to scout for the most suitable representation of the subject and create an appropriate cover for the book.

The publishing team has been an ardent support to the editorial, designing and production team. Their endless efforts to recruit the best for this project, has resulted in the accomplishment of this book. They are a veteran in the field of academics and their pool of knowledge is as vast as their experience in printing. Their expertise and guidance has proved useful at every step. Their uncompromising quality standards have made this book an exceptional effort. Their encouragement from time to time has been an inspiration for everyone.

The publisher and the editorial board hope that this book will prove to be a valuable piece of knowledge for researchers, students, practitioners and scholars across the globe.

List of Contributors

Phichayut Phinyo
Department of Family Medicine, Faculty of Medicine, Chiang Mai University, Chiang Mai 50200, Thailand

Jayanton Patumanond
Center for Clinical Epidemiology and Clinical Statistics, Faculty of Medicine, Chiang Mai University, Chiang Mai 50200, Thailand

Panprapha Saenrungmuaeng
Department of Obstetrics and Gynecology, Faculty of Medicine, Mahasarakham University, Maha Sarakham 44150, Thailand

Watcharin Chirdchim
Department of Obstetrics and Gynecology, Phrapokklao Hospital, Chanthaburi 22000, Thailand

Tanyong Pipanmekaporn
Department of Anesthesiology, Faculty of Medicine, Chiang Mai University, Chiang Mai 50200, Thailand

Apichat Tantraworasin
Department of Surgery, Faculty of Medicine, Chiang Mai University, Chiang Mai 50200, Thailand

Theera Tongsong and Charuwan Tantipalakorn
Department of Obstetrics and Gynecology, Faculty of Medicine, Chiang Mai University, Chiang Mai 50200, Thailand

Ludwig Kiesel and Ariane Baumeier
Department of Gynecology and Obstetrics, University of Münster Medical School, Albert-Schweitzer-Campus 1, 48149 Münster, Germany

Christine Eichbaum
Department of Gynecology and Obstetrics, University of Frankfurt Medical School, Theodor-Stern-Kai 7, 60596 Frankfurt, Germany

Michael Eichbaum
Department of Gynecology and Obstetrics, Helios Dr. Horst-Schmidt-Kliniken Wiesbaden, Ludwig-Erhard-Str. 100, 65199 Wiesbaden, Germany

Thilo Dörk and Peter Hillemanns
Department of Gynecology and Obstetrics, Comprehensive Cancer Center, Hannover Medical School, 30625 Hannover, Germany

Clemens Tempfer
Department of Gynaecology, Marien-Hospital, Ruhr University of Bochum, 44625 Herne, Germany

Julius Breu and Markus C. Fleisch
Department of Gynecology and Obstetrics, University of Witten/Herdecke, 42283 Wuppertal, Germany

Anthony Howell, Ashu Gandhi and Sacha Howell
Nightingale Breast Screening Centre & Prevent Breast Cancer Unit Wythenshawe Hospital, Manchester University NHS Foundation Trust, Manchester M23 9LT, UK
Manchester Breast Centre, The Christie Hospital, Manchester M23 9LT, UK
Division of Cancer Sciences, Medicine and Health, University of Manchester, Manchester Academic Health Science Centre, Manchester M23 9LT, UK

Mary Wilson, Michelle Harvie, Lester Barr, Andrea Wilding, Rosemary Greenhalgh, Jenny Affen, Andrew Maurice, Sally Cole and Julia Wiseman
Nightingale Breast Screening Centre & Prevent Breast Cancer Unit Wythenshawe Hospital, Manchester University NHS Foundation Trust, Manchester M23 9LT, UK

Anthony Maxwell and Elaine Harkness
Nightingale Breast Screening Centre & Prevent Breast Cancer Unit Wythenshawe Hospital, Manchester University NHS Foundation Trust, Manchester M23 9LT, UK
Division of Informatics, Imaging & Data Sciences, School of Health Sciences, Faculty of Biology, Medicine and Health, University of Manchester, Manchester M13 9PT, UK

Susan Astley
Nightingale Breast Screening Centre & Prevent Breast Cancer Unit Wythenshawe Hospital, Manchester University NHS Foundation Trust, Manchester M23 9LT, UK
Manchester Breast Centre, The Christie Hospital, Manchester M23 9LT, UK
Division of Informatics, Imaging & Data Sciences, School of Health Sciences, Faculty of Biology, Medicine and Health, University of Manchester, Manchester M13 9PT, UK

Mary Pegington
Nightingale Breast Screening Centre & Prevent Breast Cancer Unit Wythenshawe Hospital, Manchester University NHS Foundation Trust, Manchester M23 9LT, UK
Division of Cancer Sciences, Medicine and Health, University of Manchester, Manchester Academic Health Science Centre, Manchester M23 9LT, UK

Andrew Baildam
Nightingale Breast Screening Centre & Prevent Breast Cancer Unit Wythenshawe Hospital, Manchester University NHS Foundation Trust, Manchester M23 9LT, UK
Department of Surgery, King Edward VII's Hospital, London W1G6AA, UK

Penelope Hopwood
Nightingale Breast Screening Centre & Prevent Breast Cancer Unit Wythenshawe Hospital, Manchester University NHS Foundation Trust, Manchester M23 9LT, UK
Clinical Trials and Statistics Unit, The Institute of Cancer Research, London SM25PT, UK

Julie Wisely
Nightingale Breast Screening Centre & Prevent Breast Cancer Unit Wythenshawe Hospital, Manchester University NHS Foundation Trust, Manchester M23 9LT, UK
Department of Psychology, University Hospital of South Manchester NHS Trust, Wythenshawe, Manchester M23 9LT, UK

Fiona Lalloo
Nightingale Breast Screening Centre & Prevent Breast Cancer Unit Wythenshawe Hospital, Manchester University NHS Foundation Trust, Manchester M23 9LT, UK
Manchester Centre for Genomic Medicine, Manchester University Hospitals NHS Foundation Trust, Manchester M23 9LT, UK

David P. French
Division of Psychology and Mental Health, School of Health Sciences, Manchester Centre of Health Psychology, University of Manchester, Manchester M23 9LT, UK

D. Gareth Evans
Nightingale Breast Screening Centre & Prevent Breast Cancer Unit Wythenshawe Hospital, Manchester University NHS Foundation Trust, Manchester M23 9LT, UK
Manchester Breast Centre, The Christie Hospital, Manchester M23 9LT, UK
Division of Informatics, Imaging & Data Sciences, School of Health Sciences, Faculty of Biology, Medicine and Health, University of Manchester, Manchester M13 9PT, UK
Manchester Centre for Genomic Medicine, Manchester University Hospitals NHS Foundation Trust, Manchester M23 9LT, UK
NW Genomic Laboratory Hub, Manchester Centre for Genomic Medicine, Manchester University Hospitals NHS Foundation Trust, Manchester M13 9WL, UK
Faculty of Biology, Division of Evolution and Genomic Sciences, School of Biological Sciences, Medicine and Health, University of Manchester, Manchester Academic Health Science Centre, Manchester M23 9LT, UK

Ailish Gallagher
Research Department of Behavioural Science and Health, University College London, Gower Street, London WC1E 6BT, UK

Jo Waller
Cancer Prevention Group, School of Cancer & Pharmaceutical Sciences, King's College London, Guy's Hospital, Great Maze Pond, London SE1 9RT, UK

Ian Jacobs
Department of Women's Health, University of New South Wales, Australia, Level 1, Chancellery Building, Sydney 2052, Australia

Saskia Sanderson
Research Department of Behavioural Science and Health, University College London, Gower Street, London WC1E 6BT, UK
Early Disease Detection Research Project UK (EDDRP UK), 2 Redman Place, London E20 1JQ, UK

Anna Trebo, Christina Kuhn, Helene Hildegard Heidegger, Christine Zeder-Goess, Thomas Kolben, Bastian Czogalla, Sven Mahner and Anna Hester
Department of Obstetrics and Gynecology, University Hospital, Ludwig-Maximilians-Universität (LMU) Munich, 81377 Munich, Germany

Nina Ditsch and Udo Jeschke
Department of Obstetrics and Gynecology, University Hospital, Ludwig-Maximilians-Universität (LMU) Munich, 81377 Munich, Germany
Department of Obstetrics and Gynecology, University Hospital Augsburg, 86156 Augsburg, Germany

Elisa Schmoeckel
Institute of Pathology, LMU Munich, 81377 Munich, Germany

Faiza Gaba and Dhivya Chandrasekaran
Wolfson Institute of Preventative Medicine, Barts CRUK Cancer Centre, Queen Mary University of London, Charterhouse Square, London EC1M 6BQ, UK
Department of Gynaecological Oncology, St Bartholomew's Hospital, Barts Health NHS Trust, London EC1A 7BE, UK

Oleg Blyuss
School of Physics, Astronomy and Mathematics, University of Hertfordshire, College Lane, Hatfield AL10 9AB, UK
Department of Paediatrics and Paediatric Infectious Diseases, Sechenov First Moscow State Medical University, Moscow 119146, Russia
Department of Applied Mathematics, Lobachevsky State University of Nizhny Novgorod, Nizhny Novgorod 603098, Russia

Xinting Liu, Shivam Goyal and Nishant Lahoti
Wolfson Institute of Preventative Medicine, Barts CRUK Cancer Centre, Queen Mary University of London, Charterhouse Square, London EC1M 6BQ, UK

Margarida Kurzer
Department of Gynaecological Oncology, St Bartholomew's Hospital, Barts Health NHS Trust, London EC1A 7BE, UK

Jatinderpal Kalsi and Anne Lanceley
Department of Women's Cancer, Elizabeth Garrett Anderson Institute for Women's Health, University College London, London WC1E 6AU, UK

Munaza Ahmed
Department Clinical Genetics, North East Thames Regional Genetics Unit, Great Ormond Street Hospital, London WC1N 3JH, UK

Lucy Side
Department of Clinical Genetics, University Hospital Southampton NHS Foundation Trust, Southampton SO16 6YD, UK

Yvonne Wallis
West Midlands Regional Genetics Laboratory, Birmingham Women's NHS Foundation Trust, Birmingham B15 2TG, UK

Andrew Wallace
Manchester Centre for Genomic Medicine, 6th Floor Saint Marys Hospital, Oxford Rd, Manchester M13 9WL, UK

Craig Luccarini, Xin Yang, Joe Dennis, Alison Dunning, Andrew Lee and Antonis C. Antoniou
Centre for Cancer Genetic Epidemiology, Department of Public Health and Primary Care, University of Cambridge, Strangeways Laboratory, Worts Causeway, Cambridge CB1 8RN, UK

Rosa Legood and Zia Sadique
Department of Health Services Research and Policy, London School of Hygiene & Tropical Medicine, London WC1H 9SH, UK

Garth Funston and Victoria Hardy
The Primary Care Unit, Department of Public Health and Primary Care, University of Cambridge, Cambridge CB1 8RN, UK

Gary Abel and Willie Hamilton
University of Exeter Medical School, University of Exeter, Exeter EX1 1TX, UK

Emma J. Crosbie
Gynaecological Oncology Research Group, Division of Cancer Sciences, University of Manchester, Manchester M13 9WL, UK
Department of Obstetrics and Gynaecology, Manchester University NHS Foundation Trust, Manchester Academic Health Sciences Centre, Manchester M13 9WL, UK

Jon Emery and Fiona M. Walter
The Primary Care Unit, Department of Public Health and Primary Care, University of Cambridge, Cambridge CB1 8RN, UK
Centre for Cancer Research and Department of General Practice, University of Melbourne, Melbourne, VIC 3000, Australia

Marina Pavanello, Amir Ariff and Susan J. Ramus
School of Women's and Children's Health, Faculty of Medicine, University of New South Wales, Sydney 2052, Australia
Adult Cancer Program, Lowy Cancer Research Centre, University of New South Wales, Sydney 2052, Australia

Isaac HY Chan
School of Women's and Children's Health, Faculty of Medicine, University of New South Wales, Sydney 2052, Australia

Paul DP Pharoah
Strangeways Research Laboratory, University of Cambridge, Cambridge CB1 8RN, UK

Simon A. Gayther
Center for Cancer Prevention and Translational Genomics, Cedars Sinai Medical Center, Los Angeles, CA 90048, USA
Applied Genomics, Computation and Translational Core, Cedars Sinai Medical Center, Los Angeles, CA 90048, USA

Li Sun
Wolfson Institute for Preventive Medicine, CRUK Barts Cancer Centre, Queen Mary University of London, London EC1M 6BQ, UK
Department of Health Services Research and Policy, London School of Hygiene & Tropical Medicine, London WC1H 9SH, UK

Shreeya Patel
Wolfson Institute for Preventive Medicine, CRUK Barts Cancer Centre, Queen Mary University of London, London EC1M 6BQ, UK

Olivia Evans
Wolfson Institute for Preventive Medicine, CRUK Barts Cancer Centre, Queen Mary University of London, London EC1M 6BQ, UK
Department of Gynaecological Oncology, Barts Health NHS Trust, Royal London Hospital, London E1 1BB, UK

Johannes Berkhof and Janneke Wilschut
Department of Epidemiology and Biostatistics, Amsterdam UMC, Vrije Universiteit Amsterdam, 1081 HV Amsterdam, Netherlands

Ana Carolina De Freitas Lopes and Patricia Coelho De Soarez
Departamento de Medicina Preventiva, Faculdade de Medicina FMUSP, Universidade de Sao Paulo, 01246903 Sao Paulo, Brazil

Adam Brentnall and Stephen Duffy
Centre for Cancer Prevention, Wolfson Institute of Preventive Medicine, Queen Mary University of London, London EC1M 6BQ, UK

Li Yang and Bin Cui
School of Public Health, Peking University, Beijing 100191, China

Zakir Husain
Department of Humanities & Social Sciences, Indian Institute of Technology, Kharagpur, West Bengal 721302, India
Department of Economics, Presidency University, Kolkata 700073, India

John Hopper
Centre for Epidemiology & Biostatistics, Melbourne School of Population & Global Health, Faculty of Medicine, Dentistry & Health Sciences, University of Melbourne, Victoria 3010, Australia

Asima Mukhopadhyay
Tata Medical Centre, Kolkata,West Bengal 700160, India

Northern Institute for Cancer Research, Newcastle University, Newcastle upon Tyne NE2 4HH, UK

Amanda Dibden, Stephen W. Duffy and Rhian Gabe
Centre for Cancer Prevention, Wolfson Institute of Preventive Medicine, Queen Mary University of London, Charterhouse Square, London EC1M 6BQ, UK

Judith Offman
Comprehensive Cancer Centre, School of Cancer & Pharmaceutical Sciences, Faculty of Life Sciences & Medicine, King's College London, Innovation Hub, Guys Cancer Centre, Guys Hospital, Great Maze Pond, London SE1 9RT, UK

Oleg Blyuss
School of Physics, Astronomy and Mathematics, University of Hertfordshire, Hatfield AL10 9AB, UK
Department of Paediatrics and Paediatric Infectious Diseases, Sechenov First Moscow State Medical University, Moscow 119991, Russia

Richard Gunu, Jatinderpal K. Kalsi and John F. Timms
Department of Women's Cancer, Institute for Women's Health, University College London, London WC1E 6BT, UK

Anne Dawnay
Clinical Biochemistry, Barts Health NHS Trust, London E1 8PR, UK

Ines P. Marino
Department of Biology and Geology, Physics and Inorganic Chemistry, Universidad Rey Juan Carlos, 28933 Madrid, Spain

Ranjit Manchanda
Wolfson Institute for Preventive Medicine, CRUK Barts Cancer Centre, Queen Mary University of London, London EC1M 6BQ, UK
Department of Gynaecological Oncology, Barts Health NHS Trust, Royal London Hospital, London E1 1BB, UK
MRC Clinical Trials Unit at UCL, Institute of Clinical Trials & Methodology, Faculty of Population Health Sciences, University College London, London WC1V 6LJ, UK

Karen Lu, Wei-Lei Yang and Robert C. Bast, Jr.
University of Texas M.D. Anderson Cancer Center, Houston, TX 77030, USA

Steven J. Skates
Massachusetts General Hospital and Harvard Medical School, Boston, MA 02114, USA

Ian J. Jacobs
Department of Women's Cancer, Institute for Women's Health, University College London, London WC1E 6BT, UK
University of New South Wales, Sydney 2052, Australia

Alexey Zaikin
Department of Paediatrics and Paediatric Infectious Diseases, Sechenov First Moscow State Medical University, Moscow 119991, Russia
Department of Women's Cancer, Institute for Women's Health, University College London, London WC1E 6BT, UK
Department of Applied Mathematics, Lobachevsky University of Nyzhniy Novgorod, Nizhniy Novgorod 603105, Russia
Department of Mathematics, University College London, London WC1H 0AY, UK

Aleksandra Gentry-Maharaj, Andy Ryan, Matthew Burnell, Chloe Karpinskyj, Mahesh Parmar and Usha Menon
MRC Clinical Trials Unit at UCL, Institute of Clinical Trials & Methodology, London WC1V 6LJ, UK

Index

www.ingramcontent.com/pod-product-compliance
Lightning Source LLC
LaVergne TN
LVHW081012210926
848485LV00004B/847